HEALTH WALK MEDICAL CLINIC

A breakthrough in lowering cholesterol, weight,
and the risk of cardiovascular and Alzheimer disease
through knowledge of your body's genes

The Apo E
Gene Diet

Pamela McDonald, FA, WHCNP, PNP, FNP
Integrative Medicine Fellow

Penscott Medical Corporation
Integrative Medicine Clinic
4165 Blackhawk Plaza Circle, #125
Danville, CA 94506
Penscott Medical Corporation is a division of Penscott Management Corporation.
www.ApoEGeneDiet.com

Library of Congress Cataloging-in-Publication Data

McDonald, Pamela.

The Apo E Gene Diet: A breakthrough in lowering cholesterol, weight, and the risk of cardiovascular and Alzheimer disease through knowledge of your body's genes / Pamela McDonald.—1st ed.

   p. cm.

Includes bibliographical references.

ISBN: 978-1-60070-038-5

1. Genetics. 2. Nutrition—Genetic aspects. 3. Alzheimer disease—Alternative treatment. 4. Cholesterol. I. Title.

QP141.A1M33 2007

576.5—dc22

                           2007017209

Library of Congress Control Number: 2006928892

Before you use any suggestions in this book, please consult with your medical provider. The goal of the book is to provide helpful information, not to replace medical care. Working with a licensed medical or clinical practitioner is strongly recommended while undertaking this program.

For

Granddad,
Richard,
Victoria,
Alison,
and Paige.

Contents

ACKNOWLEDGMENTS

In completing this project I am indebted to numerous family, friends, and colleagues. Expressing my personal gratitude to all who contributed their time, patience, and understanding while I undertook this endeavor cannot be accomplished with a mere "thank you." And so I want to offer a personal tribute to the individuals mentioned below. The completion of the manuscript would not have been possible without each and every one of them.

At the top of my list is Robert Superko, MD. This man had the courage to make it his personal mission to find new ways to prevent heart disease. His drive, passion, and determination inspired me to write this book. Dr. Superko has shared his knowledge with me in many ways. It benefited not only me, but also hundreds of my patients, and particularly my husband, Rick. For that, I will always be grateful. It was my fierce desire and commitment to solving my husband's heart health mystery that led me to Dr. Superko's work. Today, at my Integrative Medicine Clinic in Danville, California, hundreds of patients are being provided answers to many of medicine's mysteries. Dr. Superko made this possible, and I will always be grateful for his knowledge and continued support.

After being blessed with Dr. Superko's knowledge, I was directed to Kona, Hawaii, by a colleague. It was there, at the Integrative Medicine Cardiology Conference, that I first met Andrew Weil, MD. Since then Dr. Weil has given me so much that the words "thank you" cannot express the depth of my gratitude. It is his knowledge, obtained through my fellowship in the Integrative Medicine Program at the University of Arizona that helps me facilitate change in my patients with chronic heart disease and other chronic illnesses.

This fellowship took me on a most amazing journey, one I would encourage any physician or nurse practitioner to explore. It provided me with a unique and personal education for healing-oriented medicine that takes the whole person into account—body, mind, emotions, and spirit, as well as the surrounding environment—and makes use of all appropriate healing therapies, both conventional and alternative.

Besides Drs. Superko and Weil, I would like to thank John Roberts, MD, J. B. Humphrey, MD, Claire Humphrey, MD, Thomas Gregory Quinn, MD, Tieraona Low Dog, MD, Victoria Maizes, MD, Dan Shapiro, PhD, Randy Horwitz, MD, and Howard Silverman, MD. These people have taught me about so much more than medicine; they have taught me, through their depth and integrity, to be a better person.

In addition, cardiologist Nelson Gwinn, MD, has supported me for what seems like a thousand years, and to him I offer a personal thank you. I would also like to thank Bridget Bongaard, MD, Julie LaGuardia, NP, Rich Cazin, PA, Christine Aday, NP, Brenda Garret-Superko, RN, Kim Evans, NP, Kalama Hochreiter, MSW, Catrina Morefield, MPH, RD, MS, and Molly McCormick, MS, exercise physiologist.

I cannot forget my many fantastic co-workers and friends such as Lynne Schurga, Betty Johnson, Mary Silva, Diane Rozakis, Joanne Clark, Adrianna Molina, Susan Copeland, Lacy Richmond, Kristin Bedford, Bella Iranitalab, Mr. R.S. Kushwaha, and Rita Southammavong. I thank them, each and every one. I extend a very special thank you to my dear friend and colleague Barbara Barclay, whom I have known for what seems like multiple lifetimes. Her daily gifts of unconditional support have been invaluable. She is a friend, a sister, a gentle and giving person who has an exceptional understanding of the business of integrative medicine. She balances the needs of operating a viable business with the immediate and personal needs of patients for gentle care. Without her, our clinic and this project would not be what it is today. Thank you.

A special thanks to my sisters Heather, Irene, and Lynne, and to my dear friends Carla Enea, Monique Cary, Cleve Palmer, Kristin Bedford, Hyein Hong, Stacey Moore, Amanda Roberts, and Nancy Vasko, CPA. I give a thank you in loving memory to my dear friend Cindy. She, and her husband, Doug, assisted me during the beginning of my private practice.

It is one of my hopes that, in some small way, my work will be an extension of the exceptional contributions that Amy Roberts, PhD, gave to the field of disease prevention before her death. I dearly miss both Cindy and Amy. A very big thanks to Kirsten Beal, who has supported me and helped so much over the past 10 years that she is a close member of my family and is one of the nicest, kindest people I could ever have in my life.

Lastly, I deeply appreciate my husband, Rick Cassidy, for supporting me unconditionally for over 20 years in all my hopes and dreams, both professionally and personally, and my children—Victoria, 22, Alison, 12, and Paige, 8—for being so patient.

Health care does not progress through the efforts of professionals alone—patients' feedback is a significant and integral part of each new discovery. So to all those patients past, present, and future, I express great gratitude to you. Without you, I could not have made this journey.

Warm regards,
Pam McDonald

WHY I WROTE THIS BOOK

Cure sometimes, heal often, support always.
—Hippocrates

During my 28 years as a medical professional working in Great Britain and the United States, I have witnessed, firsthand, illness and disease at all stages. I have seen everything from simple coughs and colds to the most deadly cancers. Unfortunately for most of us, disease shows up when least expected and can create life-shattering consequences. Disease brings with it many painful problems, yet very few of the associated problems are more devastating than the emotional distress and panic that people experience when diagnosed with a life-threatening illness. Observing firsthand the response people have to these diagnoses has, unfortunately, been the worst side of my job. For each patient who feels panic, I feel and internalize the panic myself. (In fact, I believe almost all patient-oriented practitioners do the same.) My immediate response is to help them deal with their initial pain. However, my long-term goal is to help prevent disease from occurring in the first place, and I consciously undertake this task one patient at a time.

For instance, some of my patients can count themselves among the millions of obese Americans—not only adults but now even children as young as toddlers. All of them face unpleasant health futures, with heart disease, hypertension, and diabetes poised to walk in the door opened by extra weight. I tell my overweight patients that, despite all the general diet and information available, each individual's approach to weight loss must be a personalized endeavor, and I work with them to create individual weight-loss programs based on their own variation of the Apo E gene. Often, I begin by discussing with them the reasons why obesity has reached epidemic proportions in the United States.

I believe the main reason is our move away from whole, natural foods to highly processed food products. We have also left behind healthy home-cooked meals in favor of fast food and restaurant meals, having little control over the contents. The food in many restaurants, fast-food establishments, schools, and even hospitals is highly processed and often preserved in ways harmful to the body. Furthermore, we tend to eat too fast, with little emphasis on mindful eating, which would strengthen our mind-body-spirit connection and enhance our enjoyment of life. Then, as we gain weight, we jump into the latest in-vogue diet, trying to find a quick way out of unhealthy eating patterns we have been following for years. All of this only encourages obesity, chronic inflammation of the body, and the development of chronic illness.

As a culture, we need to recognize and understand that the most favorable diet for the human body requires understanding of the connection between each person's genetic makeup and the nutritional environment, specifically how the body is exposed to the macronutrients (the big-food groups) we consume: carbohydrates, fats, and protein. Among my own patients who want to lose weight, the confusion factor is the number one problem. Many people today don't know what to eat to be healthy, at least partly because the medical community doesn't give clear messages about nutrition. This is, sadly, understandable because doctors themselves receive no meaningful training in nutrition.

Over the past few decades, however, the medical field has been jolted into noticing how powerfully nutrition can affect a person's health. We can thank Dr. Robert Atkins for *Dr. Atkins' Diet Revolution*, Dr. Robert Superko for *Before the Heart Attacks*, Dr. Arthur Agatston for *The South Beach Diet*, and Dr. Dean Ornish for *Stress, Diet and Your Heart*. Without question, these diets produced some interesting information about how different eating patterns can be a powerful tool and affect a person's health in both the short and long term—in both positive and negative ways. These diets gained not only the attention of the lay public but also of the medical community. In particular, the Atkins diet shifted so many people's weight in such a significant way (although perhaps not the best way) that the medical community couldn't help but notice. For the first time, the medical community in general began to consider the notion that maybe diet really does make a difference in a person's health, and we should pay attention to nutrition as a useful tool to battle obesity and disease prevention.

However, all these diets, no matter how good or bad, are recommended for the general population as "one diet fits all" plans. Fortunately, medical science has concluded that diets are an individual matter, with no particular popular diet working well for everyone. We now have enough information to shift from mass diet recommendations to the safer science of nutritional medicine, delivered by trained, licensed medical professionals who have the scientific training, the knowledge of the human body, and the understanding of how the human body functions in tandem with the mind and spirit to efficiently utilize food as medicine. In addition, if this tool of nutrition is clearly implemented, patient safety will be taken to a new level. As a medical health care professional, I am not convinced that the local gym or the commercial diet center provide the safest environment for diet and exercise. In those environments, many patients are receiving misinformation and potentially harming themselves. In my opinion, the medical professionals most qualified to offer the best guidance about diet and exercise are the *properly trained* MDs, nurse practitioners, osteopaths, physician assistants, registered dieticians, and exercise physiologists.

It is time that the medical community come together and recognize nutritional medicine as the field that supports the health of the entire nation. With the epidemic of obesity well underway, we can make monumental changes by focusing on the correct nutrition and disease-prevention strategies for *each individual patient.* In my heart and as a scientist, I know the epidemic of obesity, heart disease, stroke, cancer, and all the other chronic illnesses can be greatly slowed or even stopped. However, as a medical community and as a country we need to act now and begin working together to stop this epidemic. This means not only focusing on educating our physicians, osteopathic doctors, nurse practitioners, and physician assistants about disease prevention but also enlisting the total medical community, the food industry, our educational institutions, and our local and national food businesses in a concerted effort to help prevent a human health disaster—and maybe an economic disaster as well. Such a collaborative effort can create a win-win health outcome for all of us.

Truly, this is a monumental task. But we can start by educating ourselves about appropriate care and therapies to help prevent disease. One of the most cost-effective therapies is teaching people how to make appropriate nutritional choices, since good nutrition can have the most positive effect on a person's health. In fact, it is the number one integrative medicine tool used today.

In addition, we should strongly consider utilizing integrative, healing-oriented medicine as a practical method simply because it takes into account the whole person—body, mind, spirit, and physical environment, including all aspects of a person's lifestyle. This kind of medicine gives meaning to the patient-provider relationship and makes use of the best therapies, both conventional and alternative, for the patient at the particular time of need.

Today we live in a world where the patient and the medical delivery system are not matched and where the patient is dealing with new stresses, such as ubiquitous junk food as well as popular but perhaps unhealthy diets advertised in high-powered media. We need new guidelines to be able to move forward in a beneficial, meaningful way to help both the patient and the system make the transition.

During my integrative medicine training I was taught the following powerful principles that can help guide us during this time of transition:

- Focus on and utilize the principles of patient/provider-focused medicine and health care.
- Ensure that patient and practitioner are partners in the healing process.
- Take into consideration all factors influencing health, wellness, and disease, including body, mind, spirit, and physical environment.
- Facilitate the body's innate healing process by the appropriate use of both conventional and alternative methods.
- Use effective natural and less invasive interventions whenever possible.
- Integrative medicine neither rejects conventional medicine nor accepts alternative therapies uncritically.
- Good medicine is based on good science; it is inquiry-driven and open to new paradigms.
- Alongside the concept of treatment, the broader concepts of health promotion and the prevention of illness are paramount.
- Practitioners of integrative medicine should exemplify its principles and commit themselves to self-exploration and self-development.

Stay Focused on Your Goals

Before you read any further, I would like you to keep in mind one simple but essential idea: *Stay focused on what you want, rather than on what you do not want.* There is a simple reason for this: Our subconscious mind will always lead us to take action on what we focus on. If you wish to have good health, then you must focus on having good health, not on being sick, or even on not being sick. With the latter, your energy is still on what you don't want, not what you want.

If you want to lose weight and become more physically fit, then you need to focus on being healthy and physically fit, not on not being overweight and ill. Being overweight is a *symptom,* not the *problem.*

Clear your mind and focus on what you want. *Write it down.* Refuse to let *anything* get in the way of what you want. This may be as straightforward a task as losing weight, or something more complex, such as improving your whole health to prevent or reverse a chronic illness such as arthritis, stroke, high blood pressure, diabetes, or heart disease, etc. At the same time, expand your focus to include your body, mind, spirit, and your physical environment.

The Role of Nutrition and Integrative Medicine

Curbing the escalating rates of chronic illness—from obesity to heart disease, stroke, and cancer—are possible when we recognize the role of nutrition in health and healing, and focus on what is right for each individual patient. We can start by educating ourselves on how to make appropriate nutritional and lifestyle choices to prevent disease. But we need to act now. Good nutrition has a powerful effect on a person's health, and is the number one integrative medicine tool.

To accomplish this we must begin to educate physicians, nurse practitioners, and physician assistants about the role of nutrition in disease prevention, and also focus on bringing the food industry, educational institutions, and media together to serve the health needs of our nation's population. I believe this is both possible and necessary, if we are to prevent a human health disaster—and quite possibly an economic disaster from the widespread decrease of job productivity and spiraling treatment costs, as these unwell people get sicker. Such a collaborative effort can create a win-win outcome for the health status of human beings and the economy.

A major force in forwarding this change will be the training of more integrative medicine practitioners. We will look at the principles and practice of integrative medicine in more depth in a later chapter. For now, it is helpful to understand a basic distinction between allopathic and integrative medicine. Allopathic medicine, using drugs and surgery, is our current norm for treating disease. It is an excellent model for treating many acute symptoms and diseases, but it has limited value in treating chronic illnesses or bringing about healing.

Integrative medicine has a much wider foundation and has been called the medicine of the future, a future that is already here in a number of areas of the country. Integrative medicine providers have been fully trained in conventional allopathic medicine and then undergone additional training in integrative medicine. Integrative medicine takes into account the whole person—body, mind, emotions, and spirit, as well as the physical environment.

At my clinic in Danville, California, we practice integrative medicine. This means that, as well as utilizing medication and surgery, we incorporate diet, exercise, botanical herbs, mind-body medicine, manual medicine, prayer, meditation and/or guided imagery in treatment plans. These are all very effective therapies that gently shift the body and support its own internal healing processes. We have found that to prevent the major diseases such as obesity, diabetes, cardiovascular disease, autoimmune disease, and cancer, we must look closely at each person's specific individual genetic instructions or recipe. Utilizing this recipe as a guide to helping people shape their environment is proving to be a very powerful tool for prevention. I call this creating a gene-supportive environment or GSE.

Many people think they know what to do to be healthy yet cannot seem to take the requisite actions and accomplish their goals. Why? Have you ever wondered why you have not been able to stay with a low-fat diet along with a typical gym's standard high intensity exercise program ("no pain, no gain")? It could be that your body does not have the genetic makeup to be able to tolerate a very low-fat, or low-carbohydrate, or even high-protein diet. Similarly, the body may not like a high intensity exercise program because it may not be able to tolerate that kind of exercise. Just as individuals have different nutritional needs, they have differing predispositions to being supported by particular style of movement.

As already noted, research (see Appendix B) suggests that when a person follows the nutritional guidelines for their genotype, they have a far greater chance of preserving optimum health and avoiding chronic disease. I am very excited by these discoveries and know that we are only seeing the tip of the iceberg. It is in part my excitement at the prospects these discoveries hold for our health that has prompted me to write this book. I want to see this research more widely available to both lay people and professionals, to seed both more research and greater application of what we already know.

I believe that mature adults must be responsible for, and take care of, their own physical and mental health. Daily disease prevention practices are vital for maintaining the good health of the body, mind, emotions, and spirit. Part of this prevention practice is medical screening. With today's advanced technological tools, medical practitioners can detect many medical problems and treat them before they become life-threatening.

How Can This Book Help You Now?

My immediate intention with this book is to share information that can support you in both achieving optimal levels of health and well-being, and in minimizing the likelihood of your developing the debilitating diseases that are normative within our culture today. More specifically, this book can guide you to better health. It can give you important information about the correct diet, exercise, and other gene-supportive environment issues relevant for your Apo E genotype. While there are general guidelines for all the genotypes, I will address the pros and cons of having your Apo E genes analyzed, so that if you decide to be tested and learn your genotype, you can then create a more gene-supportive environment for yourself. What you will be advised to do may be as straightforward a task as losing weight or something more complex as changing many factors in your life to prevent chronic illness. I know this method can work for you because it has worked for hundreds of others at my clinic.

I was asked by many of my colleagues and friends to include some of my experiences while writing this book. As a trained practitioner in allopathic medicine, alternative medicine, and integrative medicine, I believed that this required me to commit myself to self-exploration and self-development before embarking on the writing of this book. So I am including a small part of my own personal journey. In summary, my hope is that this information will help you in making a happier and healthier life for you.

My promise is to bring the very best information on the Apo E gene and its effects on health to my readers and the patients in my clinics. As we learn more about the specifics of each type's gene-supportive environment, I will update this book via my website www.ApoEGeneDiet.com.

※

Introduction

The Apo E Gene Diet is not a book about diets in the usual sense of the word. I debated using the word "diet" in the title for months. Colleagues encouraged me to use it to reach an audience that might not otherwise pick up the book. But it is most definitely not a "diet book." *I define diet as recommendations for individual nutritional and other environmental factors that lead to disease prevention and a healthy life.*

Now that it's in your hands, please expand your thinking about the word "diet."

How to Use this Book

My hope is that the information in this book will help change your health for the better.

When you begin reading, you may first want to flip through the entire book and read any part that attracts your attention. Then, as you begin to move through the book from the beginning, you will see the full picture about how the Apo E gene and the internal environment you create in your body with food, exercise, and stress contribute to your health and to the prevention or creation of certain illnesses, particularly heart disease and Alzheimer disease.

There is an explanation of the Apo E gene, what it does in the body, and the different genotypes or variations of this gene, which everyone possesses. There is a discussion of how to get gene-tested and the necessary cautions regarding such a test. Since this book is based on the principles of integrative medicine, which is based on mind, body, and spirit, I included information on that, as well as how to find a medical practitioner and other supports to guide you through the process in this book.

You will find nutritional information on the Big Three—the macronutrients, or carbohydrates, proteins, and fats—along with a list of beneficial foods and practical advice on exercise, all related to each Apo E genotype.

I included tools you can use to explore who you are, to understand more about where you have come from, and where you and your health could be headed. Then you will find full information, along with further resources, about how to make positive changes in your life and improve your health based on your Apo E genotype.

Next, there is a lengthy list of nutritional recommendations, based on Apo E genotypes and calorie allowances, followed by some delicious recipes. Finally, several appendices will offer additional information for those who are interested.

Many of my patients have used these same procedures, tools, and nutritional advice, and found them to be helpful and healthy. I wish for you the same results.

Chapter One

BACKPACK OR BEDPAN, HEALTH IS A CHOICE

Just as in nearly all life situations, I believe we often have a choice between health and chronic illness. We can choose to be healthy and be out backpacking, or we can choose to be sick, living out our days in an institution where we need to use a bedpan, our independence lost as a result of chronic illness.

Keep in mind that chronic illness does not just show up one day and cause instant problems. Some diseases can take decades to develop, and many of them develop silently, often with very few symptoms, if any. Understanding this and knowing that you do have a choice of taking action—or not—to safeguard your health is the first step in preventing many chronic diseases from gaining a foothold. It's much better to live your life in a way that will prevent disease, instead of learning later that you have developed an illness after it's too late to reverse the accumulated damage of many years. But to do this, we need to become more focused on disease prevention and look a little deeper than we have in the past, asking questions about what is driving these disease processes in the first place.

Diabetes, insulin resistance, glucose intolerance, and heart disease can be well established without giving any major warning signs. Sometimes the first knowledge of such a disease arrives with a full-blown heart attack or stroke. Being overweight or obese is one of the most obvious signs that one or more of these diseases is establishing itself (although even thin people can be over-fat). Keep in mind: Being overweight is not all about body image. Being overweight is a symptom of a serious underlying problem, not the problem itself. Many people think they know what to do to be healthy, yet many of them cannot seem to accomplish this goal. Why? Have you ever wondered why you have not been able to stay with a low-fat diet along with rigorous exercise? It could be that your body does not have the genetic make-up to be able to tolerate a very low fat, or low carbohydrate, or even high protein diet. It is my hope that I can guide you to better health with the information contained in this book.

Remember, we have choices where our health is concerned, and we need to connect our lifestyle with our direct health outcomes. I am committed to helping you with this process and to doing my best to be a role model for my patients. Personally, when I reach the age of 75, I want to be outside *backpacking, hiking, biking, skiing,* with my children and grandchildren, not spending my days institutionalized and needing help going to the bathroom. Historically, public health recommendations focus on what is right for the general public, not for the individual. Therefore, when you read this information and ask, "Should I consider getting these tests?" you should make your decision with a medical provider or practitioner who can help you make the right decision specifically for you—not based on what is believed to be good for the health of the general population. You do not want your health to be determined on the average scale, because what you will end up with is the average heart attack or chronic illness plan.

As you will learn in this book, consistently creating the wrong body chemistry for any of the six Apo E genotypes through the wrong diet and wrong exercise regimen can yield the wrong genetic expression for that genotype—it can create chronic illness. That's why a general diet recommendation such as "Eat a low-fat diet" is not right for everyone. For some Apo E genotypes, for instance, a low-fat diet can actually create heart disease. So, a logical solution is to learn about the Apo E gene and gain information about the right nutritional fuel for you.

Diet and Gene Interactions

With our new understanding of the human genome and the arrival of DNA sorting, it has become increasingly promising to recognize interactions between what we eat and gene function, and how these interactions contribute to disease prevention or development. Polymorphism, or the different "blueprints" of genes, has been shown to play specific roles in either reducing or increasing risk of disease. One example is the variations of the Apo E genotype, which is the subject of this book. Research shows that diet can change genes and that genes can adapt to their environment.

Today we have begun to develop the technological capability to look at our gene types to determine whether we have the potential to develop a chronic disease or illness. If we know what our genetic recipe is, we can make fundamental decisions useful for preventing the development of a particular chronic illness or disease. While we don't yet understand all the genetic information stored in our bodies, we know enough to begin applying our knowledge of gene traits and how they interact with certain dietary regimens so that we can begin making a positive difference in our health today, rather than waiting decades until a disease announces itself with a health crisis.

Therefore, I am going to highlight some common tests for you to consider, which may help to prevent certain chronic illnesses. By no means a complete list, they are just a few important, common examples that have already been used successfully and have shown practical applications for disease prevention. It is extremely important to remember that our passageways to illness vary from person to person, based on each person's combination of genes and the dietary factors that influence them. We are unique individuals in every way when it comes to our personal daily chemistry requirements—our food. Clearly, every human being requires individual dietary recommendations. Research clearly shows that food can be used as nutritional medicine if consumed in the correct manner for a particular genotype.

Genetic Risk and Family History

The human body gains two copies of each of its genes—with each pair receiving one from Mom and one from Dad. The unique body that is "you" is a combination of genes passed down through many generations. Some combinations continue through the generations, while others do not. Looking back at your family's medical history can offer clues to inherited disease patterns as well as how to prevent them.

In this context, though, "inherited" means much more than just the physical, genetic components of your body. It includes the entire scope of your family's culture—beliefs, customs, practices, social behavior, and attitudes. It is also good to be mindful of how strongly you accept these elements of your family's culture, as well as what other beliefs you picked up on your own. All of your beliefs influence your journey through life and will affect your body, mind, spirit, emotions, and your inside and outside environments.

You probably know at least a little about your family's medical history, and even this can be helpful. Perhaps you know that your maternal grandfather was a hard-working farmer and lived to be 97, even though he ate all the "wrong things," at least according to what we believe today. So you assume he had "good genes."

That could be true, but it also could be true that while he had a genetic predisposition to heart disease, his lifestyle of hard physical labor outdoors for many years kept their negative expression in check. He may even have had the worst possible genetic traits for developing heart disease—positive LDL pattern B trait, Lp(a), and an Apo E 4/3 (which you will learn about later in this book)—but still remained healthy thanks to his lifestyle.

So, have you inherited this predisposition to heart disease? There is no way to know without genetic testing, but consider that the environment you live in today is completely different from just two generations ago, with much less physical activity and far fewer whole, healthy foods freely available. If you share Grandpa's genetic traits relating to heart disease but live today's high-stress, nutritionally manipulated, and chemically-exposed lifestyle, you might not be so lucky.

For now, understand that many people have unrecognized hereditary cholesterol factors that can increase their risk of heart attack, even at an early age. Eighty percent of heart disease is said to be genetic, so genetic testing is crucial to knowing your own health status. Just as important is knowing that a family history of heart disease is the most powerful element you and your medical practitioner can use in determining how to reduce your risk.

Chapter Two

AN INTRODUCTION
TO THE APO E GENE

"You're one fit guy, Rick," Dr. Humphrey told my husband. "You have the cholesterol results of a nineteen-year-old."

After his annual physical exam with all the standard and necessary blood tests, including a screening cholesterol panel, this was welcome news. But Rick, age 47, wondered, "Am I truly free of disease?" He wanted more definitive proof, real peace of mind about his health. He wondered if the screening cholesterol test told him all he needed to know.

Rick had good reason to question the test results. When he was 12, he watched his father be transformed from a healthy, active man to one who was bedridden with a heart condition and diabetes. The heart disease meant he could no longer be physically active, which led to his gaining a great deal of weight around his midsection. This in turn led his body to express Type 2 diabetes, which, in a vicious circle, worsened his heart disease. To make matters much worse, he was also battling colon cancer.

Rick's sadness and grief over his father had never left him. One of his most vivid, and terrifying, childhood memories was witnessing his father have a heart attack, after watching his health degenerate over a matter of months.

It motivated Rick to keep himself as healthy as possible; he didn't want his children to watch him die young or to suffer these same health problems. For years, he had followed a low-fat diet and a strenuous exercise regimen, believing the experts who said this was the best way to keep his heart in good shape.

Still, he had his doubts. So even with excellent results from his cholesterol screening, he asked what other tests he could take. Dr. Humphrey didn't believe any further testing was necessary, but in the face of Rick's determination, he recommended a heart scan. I decide to join him.

A few weeks later, Rick and I went for heart scans near our home in Walnut Creek, California. Mine showed no evidence of heart disease. When Rick's scan was complete, he hopped off the table, eager to see his results. We were stunned. His heart scan revealed coronary plaque, the beginnings of artery disease. Rick was silent on the ride home, and when we arrived, he disappeared. I found him sitting on the edge of our bed and crying, terrified about the condition of his heart. "Am I going to die?" he asked. In reply, I promised I would do everything possible to solve this mystery. It's true that arterial inflammation can be stopped and reversed, but 50 percent of people who have heart attacks also have normal cholesterol levels and no other apparent reason for the heart attack.

When Dr. Humphrey heard Rick's results, he was also surprised. How could someone apparently as fit and healthy as Rick—someone who had religiously followed the recommended guidelines for maintaining a healthy heart—have coronary heart disease?

For three weeks, I scoured the scientific literature to find the answer to that question. What I discovered about the genetic heart disease risk factors and the Apo E genotype not only changed Rick's health for the better but also broadened my work with heart disease and began leading to improved outcomes for many of my patients.

In brief, Rick was eating the wrong foods for his Apo E genotype. His low-fat diet did not provide enough long-term fuel in the form of fats, which, combined with his strenuous exercise routine, meant he was not eating enough of the right foods for his genotype, placing harmful levels of stress on his body's systems. He was eating the wrong kind of protein for his genotype—too much animal protein and not enough from plant sources, which turned on a genetic pattern related to LDL cholesterol production that increased his arterial plaque production by 50 percent. Furthermore, the small amount of fat he was eating came mostly from meat containing saturated fat, which increases arterial inflammation. And finally, in a double whammy, his high intake of carbohydrate foods elevated his insulin level, which also has been shown to encourage arterial plaque.

Rick began eating correctly for his genotype: more non-inflammatory fat in the form of olive oil and nuts, soybeans and avocados; fewer high-glucose carbohydrates; and more plant protein, including beans, soy nuts, and lentils. His LDL cholesterol normalized, his percentage of body fat decreased, and his insulin resistance—a precursor to Type 2 diabetes—resolved. He also cut back on exercise.

Despite following the guidelines touted in recent decades as being the best, and perhaps only, way to prevent heart disease, Rick was actually killing himself by following them. To be fair, genetic testing was not available when the guidelines were developed. However, in light of what we now are learning about the Apo E genotypes, simply evaluating total cholesterol in terms of LDL and HDL is not enough. It is also important to evaluate 13 other kinds of total cholesterol. Finally, to complete the picture, it is necessary to determine a person's Apo E genotype, which will reveal the correct diet and exercise regimen that will truly maintain heart health and also help prevent serious illness such as vascular diseases and Alzheimer disease.

It is becoming common to hear media reports about new research that clearly shows how many of our diseases have genetic components. Since the completion of the Human Genome Project of 1987, scientists have found many genes that are involved in a variety of disease states. Genetic research will doubtless continue to make new discoveries in this area, supporting more disease prevention through practical applications of this newfound information. It is possible that in the near future, the Apo E gene will be linked to a lot more disease states than are currently proven.

What exactly do we mean by genes? When you want to build a house, you have an architect draw blueprints. Your builder then looks at the blueprints to figure out exactly what to build. The same process occurs with the body—only our genes are the blueprints for our body. *And*, unlike a house, the body is being rebuilt every second of every day.

Besides the builder and the blueprint, another major factor in house building is the quality of the materials used. When built with poor quality materials, buildings deteriorate rapidly. When built with high-quality materials, structures, such as St. Paul's Cathedral in London, can stand for hundreds of years. Your body follows the same process—if you use high-quality materials, it will last much longer. *This book is about choosing the right materials to go with your specific blueprint.*

What is the Apo E Gene?

The human body has 23 pairs of chromosomes. Each chromosome is made up of many genes. We will look mainly at a particular gene on chromosome 19—the Apo E gene—that was discovered in the early 1970s. We single out this gene because certain variants of it—the specific pair of Apo E genes you inherited from your mother and father—influence your predisposition to certain illnesses.

There are three Apo E gene variations, or *genotypes,* that occur naturally in humans: Apo E 2, Apo E 3, and Apo E 4.

Since genes come in matching pairs, and we each have two copies of every gene, one from each parent, there are six possible combinations of pairs. If you received an Apo E 2 from each parent, the shorthand description would be E 2/2. The other five combinations are E 2/3, E 3/3, E 4/2, E 4/3, and E 4/4.

As you can see from the table below, the most common gene, Apo E 3/3, is found in approximately 64 percent of the population. It is considered the "neutral" Apo E genotype.

Percentage of Apo E Genotypes in the General Population		
Apo E 2	2/2	1%
	2/3	10%
Apo E 3	3/3	64%
Apo E 4	4/2	2%
	4/3	18%
	4/4	5%

Combinations that include either the Apo E 2 or Apo E 4 are considered "alternative" expressions of the more common Apo E 3 pairing; and they process foods differently from the way in which an Apo E 3's body will.

For optimal health, you need to match your particular genotype with the most gene-supportive environment (GSE) you can create. You do that through what you eat, how you exercise, and how you respond to stress, which is largely determined by how you think.

What Does Apo E Mean?

Our body has evolved a very complex biochemical method of moving fats around inside it. Why all this complexity?

You already know that oil and water don't mix. That's what our body (water-based) is up against when it must absorb and use fats (oil-based). Our blood is a water-based solution for moving nutrients and oxygen around to the cells. Any fats that need to travel in it won't dissolve; they would just clump up and clog the system.

To get around this inconvenience, our body has created a wonderful method of packaging the fats and oils in molecular "suitcases" that keep the fats from coming in contact with the water of our blood.

That's where this strange word "Apo" with an "E" attached to it comes in. Apo is short for *apolipoprotein*.[1] It has the letter "E" because it's one of a whole series of apolipoproteins—A, B, C, D, etc. The Apo E *gene* gets its name from the fact that it's the blueprint in charge of synthesizing apolipoprotein E, an important component of cholesterol metabolism.

In a larger sense, the Apo E gene is involved in the energy system of the body—and energy is key to every system in the body. Apo E can be found in many places: blood, spleen, liver, intestine, brain, kidney, and other peripheral parts.

Making Connections: Genotype, Gene-Supportive Environment, and State of Health

The Apo E gene can either *provide good health* if the body is given the correct foods and other gene-supportive environment (GSE) factors for its Apo E type. On the other hand, the Apo E gene can also *impair good health* if the body is given the wrong foods and other gene-unsupportive environmental (GUE) situations.

---

1   Derivation of apolipoprotein: Apo•lipo•protein. Apo = separated from or derived from; lipo=fat; proteins are made of amino acids and essential to all cellular structures. The apolipoproteins are the protein components of lipoproteins that remain after the lipids to which the proteins are bound have been removed.

The Apo E gene is the key to making the right match. Here's where knowing your Apo E genotype can help determine the environment that will best support you in developing and maintaining a safe, optimal level of cholesterol in your system.

Before we go any further, let me further clarify what I mean by "environment." Everything that surrounds or goes into your body or mind is an element in your environment and subsequently impacts your health. This means your thoughts become as much a part of you as does the food you eat. So while your food intake is an important element in your environment, you are much more than just the food you eat.

Your environment, so defined, largely determines your health. More specifically, it consists of:

- what you eat
- the way you move and exercise your body
- the quality of your mental and emotional experiences (including how you deal with stress and emotional energy)
- the strength and quality of your intention for what you want
- what you think others want from you
- the physical environment that surrounds you—is it pleasing or stressful?
- your spiritual beliefs

With today's affordable technology for analyzing people's genotype, we can easily learn a person's Apo E genetic recipe. While we have a lot to learn about what each of the thousands of genes we have in every cell actually does, we can make excellent use of the ones that we do understand—like the Apo E gene—to make recommendations for the ideal gene-supportive environment for any individual.

Inflammation: A Poor Match Between Environment and Genotype

Chronic diseases such as diabetes, obesity, gouty arthritis, hypertension, cardiovascular disease, multiple sclerosis, chronic kidney disease, Parkinson disease, and cancer all have in common the long-term presence of low-grade cellular inflammation that is largely the result of *a poor match between environment and genetic makeup—the gene-unsupportive environment* (GUE) that I described above. I will describe the mechanisms of inflammation in detail in a later chapter, but for now, it's important to know that when a normal healthy cell is exposed to an inflammatory environment over a long period of time, the cell becomes aplastic (unable to replicate properly). How this *dis-ease state* manifests in your body can range from high cholesterol levels, cardiovascular disease, and vascular dementia, to cancer, Alzheimer disease, Parkinson disease, and more. In most cases these degenerative killer diseases are the result of imbalances of the body's ability to regulate its processes that are usually present for 30 or more years before they are noticed. Some can even begin before birth, in a toxic womb environment.

Put simply, the wrong environment for a particular Apo E genotype can push the body to produce high levels of cellular inflammation as it attempts to fight the affects of its environment. This can result in chronic illnesses, including cancer.

Remember, it's about the gene and the environment the gene is exposed to. The body knows what to do when it has an occasional or brief imbalance. But when it becomes chronically overwhelmed and unbalanced from consistent exposure to an unsuitable environment, it cannot function as it should. Such an imbalance between genotype and environment will likely lead to chronic illness.

This means that while you may, over many years, be eating a "health-conscious" diet like the popular low-fat diets and never develop a disease, another person may follow the very same diet and develop a serious illness. Could this be, in part at least, because the so-called "healthy diet" advocated by the media may not be right for everyone?

*We are unique individuals in every way, even when it comes to our personal daily dietary requirements. Knowing this, food can be used as nutritional medicine if we eat the appropriate foods in the correct amounts. This is why I developed the Apo E Gene Diet. My experience has shown me again and again that **one diet does not fit all.***

The foundation of the Apo E Gene Diet and your optimal gene-supportive environment is a nutritional plan that focuses on eating the optimal percentages of The Big Three—carbohydrates, fats, and proteins, called the macronutrients. There is a unique optimal combination of these which creates the ideal diets for each of the six Apo E genotypes. Creating this optimal balance in your diet is a prerequisite of good health. Why?

The Apo E gene has been shown to be the number one factor affecting how your body uses The Big Three, and this influences the likelihood and severity of your developing some diseases. It is very important to eat the right balance of The Big Three.

We have all heard the saying "You are what you eat." Now, more than ever, research shows this to be true. The food you eat today becomes the cellular makeup of your tissues tomorrow—food that goes into your body becomes your body. Eating the right diet for your Apo E genotype is one of the best investments you can make in your health. A healthy diet can be delicious and health-promoting, supplying the nutrition your body needs, based on your current health and Apo E genotype.

※

Chapter Three

THE CONNECTION BETWEEN DISEASE AND THE APO E GENE

All Apo E genotypes seem to require a specific fat combination, and the Apo E Gene Diet provides the recommended amounts and types of fats for optimal cell health. Your Apo E genotype can guide you in choosing the type and amount of dietary fat to consume so you will have the correct percentages of fuel needed to function properly. The Apo E 4s have the greatest difficulty clearing fats from their bodies, especially the more complex inflammatory fats, and must significantly limit saturated and trans fats. However, everyone, no matter what their Apo E genotype, should minimize inflammatory fats.

You can't change your genes, but you can change how they perform by creating a gene-supportive environment (GSE) for them to function in. But first, let's look at what can happen in a gene-unsupportive environment (GUE), using some of the research that has established a clear connection between the Apo E gene and cardiovascular disease plus other chronic illnesses such as Alzheimer disease. Please keep in mind that *statistics never relate to the individual person because no situation or circumstance is ever quite the same for any two individuals.*

It is important to realize that the presence of Apo E 4 does not cause cardiovascular disease and other diseases like Alzheimer disease. Nor does it necessarily mean that the person will develop such diseases. What is important is matching your diet and lifestyle to the needs of your genes. Since each Apo E genotype has an individual set of dietary recommendations linked to it, knowing your type can prevent diseases that are common to your genotype.

Cardiovascular Disease and the Apo E Gene

Cardiovascular disease accounts for the number one (heart attack) and number three (stroke) causes of death in the United States. Combined, these account for 40 percent of all deaths. Cardiovascular disease is a progressive, deteriorating, inflammatory disease leading first to damage of cells, major organs, and eventually whole body-systems. It is a gradual process that can begin in childhood—as young as 5 years old. Upon reaching a certain age, usually around 40 to 50 but sometimes younger, the risk of heart attack jumps dramatically. Following a heart attack, many people fail to make a full recovery, with approximately 40 percent dying within a year. Within six years, nearly half of those surviving have become disabled.

The work performed by the heart is demanding and never-ending. Your heart is only the size of two fists, but the energy produced by this tireless little machine over a 50-year period could move a battleship. It beats thousands of times a day, pumping hundreds of gallons of blood. Never stopping day or night, your heart works twice as hard as the largest muscles in your body. A damaged heart means almost inevitably a damaged life.

The heart requires a constant supply of blood to provide it with oxygen and the necessary nutrients, via three main coronary arteries. If a blockage occurs in one of these arteries, the heart becomes deprived of oxygen, resulting in the death of some of its cells—a heart attack.

Cardiovascular disease is a disease of inflammation, but the impact of inflammation is not limited to the arteries. Inflammatory disease can occur anywhere in the body, down to the deepest crevices between cells, sparing nothing and generating a complex chain reaction.

When the body gets the wrong fuel for its genetic makeup, it creates the wrong internal environment. This causes a reaction that harms the major fluid delivery systems of the body—the arteries—and leads to the deterioration of entire body systems because these "rivers" of the body have become a toxic waste dump and are spewing toxins and inflammatory chemistry everywhere.

As the body tries to heal itself from the inflammation resulting from overexposure to the wrong nutrients (LDL), it loses the ability to clean itself (from low HDL) quickly enough to reverse the damage. See the illustration on page 20. Specialized immune cells, clotting substances, and proteins, along with seven kinds of "bad" lipoproteins (LDLs) then form a scab in an attempt to protect the inner cells and heal the lining of the arteries. See the section below, Looking Deeper Into the Cholesterol *Pot.* Arterial plaque is similar to the plaque that forms in your mouth if you don't floss, but plaque on your teeth won't kill you. Inside your plumbing, it's a different matter. Everyone "knows" that too much cholesterol is bad for us—but it's not quite that simple. First, we need to learn more about two components of cholesterol that few people understand—low-density lipoproteins (LDL), the "bad" type of cholesterol, and high-density lipoproteins (HDL), the "good" cholesterol.

While the cholesterol inside LDL lipoproteins is called the bad cholesterol, it is not the cholesterol that is *bad*; it is instead *how* and *where* it is being transported, and in what amounts, over time, it is being delivered to the artery wall.

Besides the "bad" cholesterol (LDL) wreaking havoc by inflaming your arteries, the problem is compounded if your genetic makeup doesn't provide you with enough of the "good" cholesterol (HDL), your body's arterial self-cleaning ability will not be adequate for the job. This means there will be more rapid plaque buildup, with arteries clogging even faster. While many other factors are involved in the development of arterial plaques, it is the Apo E gene that determines your levels of HDL and LDL.

Again, we find that knowing your Apo E geneotype is crucial in determining how your body will respond to its environment, and particularly, what food components are helpful and which are toxic for your genotype.

Looking Deeper into the Cholesterol *Pots*: LDL and HDL

To understand the impact of cholesterol on your health, we need to look more closely at the components of cholesterol.

The Specifics

The usual blood tests, called a cholesterol panel, done during routine checkups, are for the main categories of cholesterol and fat. They are:

- total cholesterol
- total LDL (bad cholesterol)
- total HDL (good cholesterol)
- triglycerides (fatty acids)

But testing for just these basic groups reveals only so much. In fact, the testing most commonly done does not even measure the LDL directly but calculates it from a formula based on the other three values. Furthermore, research shows that 80 percent of patients who developed coronary artery disease have the same total cholesterol level as those who did not develop the disease. To learn what's *really* going on in our arteries, we must look more deeply at several of the 12 different subtypes of cholesterol particles contained in the two major cholesterol groups—LDL and HDL. I often refer to these major categories of cholesterol as "pots." To see inside these pots requires more sophisticated testing than the typical cholesterol panel. Fortunately these tests are now available and affordable, so that what we find inside these pots can tell us a lot more about the health of our arteries.

There are actually seven kinds of cholesterol particles in the LDL pot, of which three concern us the most. There are five kinds in the HDL pot, only one of which is important to us here. The composition of the 12 types in these two pots is determined first by what type of Apo E genes you have and more importantly—because you can change it—the gene-supportive environment you create for your arteries by what you eat, what kind of exercise you get, and how you think.

First, the Bad News: LDL Cholesterol, Large and Small

How does an artery become damaged? Understanding how our body's vascular plumbing system—especially the arteries—becomes damaged by imbalances in the cholesterol it creates is critical to understanding what causes chronic heart disease.

LDL's job is to carry cholesterol and fatty acids from the liver, where it is synthesized, to the cells where it is used by your body in a variety of ways. This sounds reasonable, so how does LDL get such a bad rap?

Well, first you need to know that LDL cholesterol comes in seven sizes, called type I, IIa and IIb, IIIa, IIIb, IVa and IVb (the larger the number, the smaller the size). LDL's bad rap comes from three of these. The first is IVb, the smallest of the stew. If you have elevated levels of IVb, you have a much greater risk of developing artery damage. But that's not all—having more than 15–20 percent of the IIIa and IIIb types also puts your arteries at risk.

So why are these three smaller ones bad for you? They are so small that they can easily slip in between the cells that line the insides of your arteries. In fact, they are twice as likely as the larger types of LDL to do this. When they do this slippery thing, they cause the arteries to become inflamed in reaction to the invasion, and that's not good.

One way to think of these culprits is as little metal chips with spikes on them that, once they get inside the artery's lining, make a multitude of cuts that then need to be healed by your immune system. The smaller the chip, the more places it can cause damage. When the inflammation reaches a certain level, your immune system becomes overwhelmed. Plaques of hardened calcium and cholesterol then form in your arteries in a misguided attempt to seal the damage off.

Here's where the Apo E genotypes come in. They determine what happens to the different types of fats, proteins, and carbohydrates that you eat. For example, if you have the Apo E 4 gene—either the 4/4, 4/2 combination or the 4/3—and eat a lot of fat, the likelihood of inflammation in your arteries is higher. To a lesser extent, arterial inflammation occurs with the Apo E 2 gene—either the 2/2 or the 2/3 combination.

Each genotype has both an ideal kind and combination of fats, proteins, and carbohydrates for arterial health—and hence heart health—so knowing the right balance for your particular genotype is crucial.

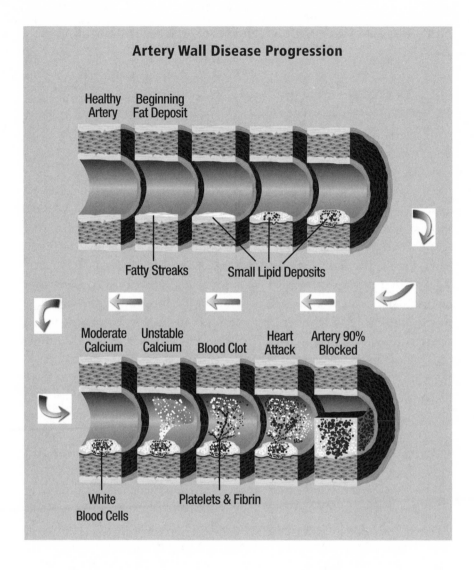

APL (LDL Pattern B): Why is it Dangerous?

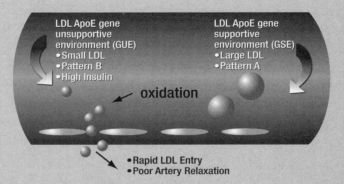

Individuals have different environments for expressing their genotype, meaning how the genetic data appears in their body or tissue structure—think blue eyes, a long nose, or LDL particle size. While eye color and nose length don't change, LDL particle size *can change*, depending on the type of diet and other gene-supportive environmental factors. What matters is how this gene's requirements are being met. An example is LDL Pattern B.

Approximately one in four people have another genetic risk factor—a cholesterol disorder known as "LDL Pattern B" (small dense, bad cholesterol). Even though this disorder is associated with three times the risk of heart attack, the standard cholesterol test will not find this condition, common as it is.

In the case of the LDL Pattern B trait, eating the wrong dietary balance, based on a person's Apo E genotype, "turns on" the Pattern B type gene, giving the body a genetic instruction resulting in the production of smaller LDL particles in the liver. If the gene is not present, it cannot be turned on. Approximately 50 percent of men and 30 percent of pre-menopausal women with heart disease have the Pattern B trait.

What does "turning on" a particular gene mean? The expression "turning a gene on" may conjure up an image of a little man standing by the DNA double helix in a plumber's suit holding a wrench and waiting to be called upon to turn a gene on or off. However, what actually happens is that if the body contains a gene that prefers a certain mix of nutrients in its diet but cannot find it, the body becomes unbalanced. This compromised state then encourages the body to try to find its own balance.

The Good News: HDL2b

While the various components of the LDL pot carry cholesterol out to your cells, HDL carries the surplus back to the liver where it is recycled. In this way, HDL provides our body with a natural artery-cleaning service. You simply cannot have too much of this good type of cholesterol, and later we will see how the Apo E Gene Diet and exercise program can cause even more HDL to be produced.

In my experience, the Apo E 2 and the Apo E 3 genotypes tend to have higher levels of HDL, especially HDL2b.

So how does HDL2b relate to artery disease? If you have too much bad LDL and not enough good HDL, especially HDL2b, your body can't clean its arteries properly, and the cholesterol accumulates and causes them to narrow—and thus begins cardiovascular disease.

HDL2b works for the body's vascular system in at least two ways. It lowers blood "thickness"—a tendency to clot inappropriately—and it is a powerful antioxidant that stops molecular damage to the vascular system.

Having levels of HDL2b greater than 20 percent for men and 30 percent for women contributes to optimum artery health. To achieve these levels I advise patients to first be tested for HDL2b because despite high HDL levels, I often see very low HDL2b levels. Unless your HDL2b levels are normal or above, your ability to clean your arteries is hindered.

It's important to know that not all advanced cholesterol-testing methods are the same—some can be off by as much as 40 percent—leading to the wrong treatment plan.[2] Once you know your true levels you can make any necessary dietary and lifestyle changes.

---

2   Comparison of traditional and alternative laboratory methods. Determination of lipid measurement Lp (a) and LDL phenotype. Presented by H. Robert Superko MD at American Heart Association 42nd annual Cardiovascular Disease Epidemiology and Prevention. Honolulu, HI April 23-26 2002

Optimal Cholesterol Panel Results		
	Situation	**Optimal Level**
Total cholesterol	You do not have heart disease	less than 200 mg/dl
	You have heart disease	less than 150 mg/dl
Total LDL	You do not have heart disease	less than 100 mg/dl
	You have heart disease	less than 70 mg/dl
Total HDL	Men	greater than 50 mg/dl
	Women	greater than 60 mg/dl
Total triglycerides	All situations	less than 150 mg/dl
HDL2b	Men	greater than 20 mg/dl
	Women	greater than 30 mg/dl
LDL small particle size		
IIIa + b	All situations	less than 15 mg/dl
IVb	All situations	less than 5 mg/dl
Lp(a)	All situations	less than 30 mg/dl
Blood glucose	Normal range	65 to 99 mg/dl
		Note: 100 to 125 means you are glucose-impaired. Greater than 125 mg/dl means you are diabetic.

Your Cholesterol Level and the Apo E Gene

Maintaining a healthy level of cholesterol is essential to your cardiovascular system. Although researchers are not completely certain about the exact level of cholesterol for optimum health, it appears to be below 70 mg/dl (that's milligrams per deciliter—there are almost 30,000 milligrams in an ounce, and a deciliter is 1/10 of a liter, or about 3.3 fluid ounces—not very much!).

Of the three kinds of Apo E genes, the 4s (especially that 5 percent of the population who have two of the Apo E 4 genes) are the most sensitive to high-fat diets and need more carbohydrates than the other types, or their cholesterol will be higher.

The Apo E 2s are the reverse, having the best ability to handle fats but an inability to process elevated levels of carbohydrate without increasing their cholesterol levels. This genotype is able to process the complex and low glycemic load carbohydrates (grains, legumes, fruits, and vegetables—see chapter 11, page 118) but not refined processed carbohydrates.

If you have cholesterol problems, it's important to know which Apo E genes you have. You can then adopt the dietary recommendations that can prevent this disease from being expressed.

The Interconnections Between Environmental Factors

Your arterial health depends not only on your genotype but on many environmental factors—from your body composition, diet, and exercise program, to the psychological factors of the way you think, how you manage stress, how you view the world, and how you think the world views you. These factors are not independent of each other but *highly interconnected.* For example, the way you think influences the chemistry in your brain, which, in turn, changes your body's food needs. This is an aspect of that ever-present, but often ignored, mind-body connection I will describe in more detail below.

The Apo E Diet takes into account not only your diet and exercise program, but also how your stress levels are influencing your LDL and HDL levels because excessive stress affects how your body performs. If you are in a constant state of stress, your body is constantly in the fight-flight-or freeze response, producing ever more cholesterol in anticipation of this pattern continuing. Knowing what genes you have gives you the power to intelligently create a gene-supportive environment through what you eat, how you exercise, and how you think.

Alzheimer Disease and the Apo E Gene

Cognitive decline in old age has been described throughout history. However, it was not until the early part of the 20th century that a collection of brain cell abnormalities was specifically identified by a German physician, Alois Alzheimer, for whom the dread disease was named.

Nearly a century later, a high risk for Alzheimer disease was associated with the Apo E 4 gene. Immediately following this discovery, ethical dilemmas associated with genetic testing led to the conclusion that medical records should be kept private in order to protect the rights of patients. Guidelines for genetic testing for Alzheimer disease determined that individuals should not be tested without their primary medical providers' support and guidance. In 1997, President Clinton proposed a law that would help make it a crime for employers or insurance companies to discriminate on the grounds of genetic testing data they obtained. While his proposal did not become law, half the states in the United States have adopted this policy.

Not all people with Apo E 4 develop Alzheimer disease, especially those who have created a gene-supportive environment. But without that, 90 percent of the 4/4 combination and 49 percent of the 4/3 and 4/2 variants develop the disease. This is a relatively exclusive Apo E club since it is estimated that only 5 percent of the population has the Apo E 4/4. The percentage of the population with the Apo E 4/3 and 4/2 genotype totals 20 percent.

Conversely, not all people with Alzheimer disease have the Apo E 4 genotype. What I do know from my clinical practice is that Apo E 4s who eat a high-fat diet have a very high cholesterol level. My patients with two copies (Apo E 4/4) consistently have total cholesterol levels in the 300s and 400s with LDL in the 200s and 300s. Extremely high levels of LDL (bad) cholesterol cause high levels of inflammation in the blood vessels, including those in the brain. Therefore, a connection between Alzheimer disease and one's diet is not surprising.

As with all chronic diseases, Alzheimer disease results from the interaction of genetic, environmental, and lifestyle factors over many years, causing changes in brain structure and function. While it is a complex disease with no single, clear-cut cause, for those with a 4/4 genotype, careful matching of your nutritional environment will likely postpone or prevent the development of Alzheimer disease.

In summary, of the many theories about this disease—from toxic factors like aluminum or zinc to smoking being the causative agent—having an Apo E 4 gene (or two) seems to have the strongest connection with Alzheimer disease and provides a connection between elevated cholesterol and fats, with a resulting cellular inflammatory process in the brain.

In my clinical practice I am often able to discern trends in diseases. From these examples, I hope that you can see that the Apo E gene is a powerful component of our total genetic blueprint—a major factor in our overall state of health. For this reason, I believe this gene will be the focus of much future research in the areas where it interacts with our specific environment—our diet, exercise, thought patterns, and any medications we're taking, as well as its connection with heart disease, cancer, and many other chronic diseases, especially those involving the immune system.

In my opinion not enough attention is being paid to the nutritional connection of these diseases with the Apo E gene. With more attention paid to that connection and with the right nutritional adjustments, reducing the risk of chronic disease is possible, and the risk of cardiovascular disease and Alzheimer disease in particular can be lowered.

Furthermore, I think the risk for Apo E 4 genotypes extends beyond just Alzheimer disease and heart disease. Given that my clinical experience has shown that patients with certain genotypes have certain disease clusters or associated illnesses, the development of many chronic illnesses may turn out to stem from imbalances within each Apo E genotype and how the person's environment supports (or doesn't) their specific genotype.

Genetic Risk and Family History

Looking back at your family's history can provide ideas of what diseases have occurred in your family. That gives you an idea of what you might have inherited and what might be needed to prevent a reoccurrence of untimely deaths. Remember that not only do you inherit the physical components of your body but also the entire scope of your family's culture, which you inherited through exposure to their beliefs, attitudes, customs, practices, and social behavior.

In addition to what has been imprinted by your family, the culture you live in also creates much of your belief structure. It's important to understand this, since it is your beliefs that shape your mind, body, emotions, spirit, and soul and show up in the environment you create around you. All of these factors will influence your journey through life.

Even a casual examination of your family's medical history can be helpful, but uncovering it can be difficult because with families scattered all over the world, as many are today, their health information is scattered with them. My patients often give a description like, "Grandpa lived until he was 97 years old. He was a farmer, and he lived in all that fresh air. But he ate all the wrong things. He must have had good genes to live that long." Perhaps he did indeed have good genes, but the question that begs to be asked is: Was his environment gene-supportive? He could have had so-called "bad genes" but perhaps his genes had not "turned on" or been expressed negatively to adversely affect his health.

A farm diet, despite being high in animal fats, was usually replete with pure, whole foods—produce from the garden, eggs from free-range chickens, regular eating patterns without skipped meals, and a higher quality of life with a positive attitude of creating and producing—a sound foundation and mission. All that plus a high amount of physical exercise could have promoted perfect health for Grandpa. The question then becomes: What have his descendents inherited? Is there a risk of genetic heart disease or not?

Many people have unrecognized hereditary cholesterol factors that can increase their risk of disease. Therefore, an accurate family history—or at least as accurate as you can gather—can help you decide whether or not to consider a more advanced cholesterol test. Selective testing can then assist your medical provider in evaluating the true risk of vascular disease.

The social milieu and working environment our family of origin likely experienced is not the same as the more sedentary lifestyles most of us live today. Even if Grandpa had a positive LDL Pattern B trait, Lp(a), and even an abnormal Apo E 4/3, eating whole foods and staying extremely active for his entire life might have kept these traits from "turning on," so that he lived a long and healthy life. Today, however, with today's high-stress, nutritionally manipulated, chemically exposed, less active lifestyle, he might not have been so lucky.

Remember, we know that a large percentage heart disease is genetic, so getting genetically tested is important. A family history of *any* chronic disease, however, is the most powerful message you can get for the importance of a risk reduction program targeting that disease.

A Patient's Story: Sam

Having been in the medical field for more than 26 years, I can safely say I've seen my share of interesting situations. One I've encountered frequently is patients with the "doc in a box" mentality, where they demand a test right away just because they want it right then, without even understanding what the test is all about or what the results might mean to their lives.

Many people have come to our office, insurance card in hand, demanding to have "this new Apo E test." They say a friend who's had the test referred them, and then they hold out their arm to have blood drawn, and "Oh, by the way, you can just call me with the results." But we don't operate this way.

One day, a man named Sam walked into our office, handed his insurance card to Barbara, our office manager, and said he was ready for his blood test.

Barbara looked at the schedule and didn't see his name listed. Neither did she recognize him.

"I don't seem to have you on the schedule," she said. "Are you sure you're in the right place?"

"Isn't this Pam McDonald's office?"

"Yes."

"Then I'm here for that Alzheimer disease test."

Barbara asked if he meant the Apo E gene test. He agreed that was the one.

"Have you seen Pam before?" she asked. "Are you her patient?"

"No. I've never met her," Sam said. "I was just looking at getting that test today. I understand you don't have to fast for it. I have good insurance, and they'll pay for it. And if they don't, you can bill me."

Barbara knew that Sam had no idea what the Apo E test was all about and asked why he was interested.

"I've got Alzheimer disease in my family," Sam replied, "and I want to get tested to know if I'm going to get it."

When Barbara recommended that he make an appointment for a consultation to learn more about Apo E gene testing, he became agitated. "I want this test done today," he insisted as he pulled out his credit card and placed it on the counter. "I have a lot of money. I can pay for the test."

I came around the corner at that moment and saw the distress on Barbara's face. She asked Sam to take a seat and filled me in on the situation.

I invited him into my office and asked him to sit down so I could tell him more about the gene test and the Apo E gene. Still upset, he wasn't inclined to listen, but I asked him to give me about 20 minutes of his time to provide some critical information, and then I would answer all his questions. Ten minutes later, he returned his credit card to his wallet in very slow motion. He began to relax and sat back in his chair. When I had finished talking, his face showed surprise at what he had learned.

"Wow," he said. "Thank you. I had no idea this test was so powerful and important. Thank you."

Sam did return later for Apo E gene testing, along with other tests so that we could see the larger picture of his health. He chose not to know his Apo E gene type, saying as long as I knew it and could prescribe the right nutrition, exercise, and stress reduction plan for him, that was just fine. He knew that if he ever changed his mind and wanted to know the test result, all he had to do was ask.

Sam began following the appropriate plan for his Apo E genotype and now says his health has never been better.

How Different Genotypes Use Fuel Differently

The digestive system basically consists of various organs that function to break down food into components the body can use. The goal is to transform healthy, whole food into small nutritionally loaded fuel packages that can be placed in the cells. Now we must ask how fuel use relates to the Apo E gene.

Each Apo E genotype has a preference for different types of fuel from the foods eaten. These are summarized in the following table.

Food-type Preferences of Apo E Genotypes	
Apo E 2/2	Prefers more long-term fuel
Apo E 2/3	Prefers more long-term fuel
Apo E 3/3	Prefers a balance of long and short-term fuel
Apo E 4/2	Prefers a balance of long and short-term fuel
Apo E 4/3	Prefers more short-term fuel
Apo E 4/4	Prefers more short-term fuel

The Apo E 4 combinations cannot effectively use fat in high amounts. Apo E 4 genotypes need to rely on moderate glycemic load, complex carbohydrates.

The Apo E 3 genotypes have neutral or normal ability to use cholesterol, fat, and glucose as fuel. A balanced combination of moderate fat and carbohydrate intake is required for this genotype, avoiding all high glycemic load, simple carbohydrates. In my clinic, I often see trends related to genotypes, such as more insulin resistance and Type 2 diabetes with the Apo E 3/3 genotype than any other. I am not sure what the reason is, but one interesting consideration is that Apo E 3/3 people cannot tolerate a low-fat diet or imbalance in the Big Three—they require 25 percent of their calories to come from healthy fats.

The Apo E 2 genotype tends to utilize fat as the preferred source of fuel, rather than carbohydrates. This genotype should avoid all high glycemic load, simple carbohydrates in preference to moderate glycemic load, complex carbohydrates.

You need to take into consideration the quality, quantity, and usability of any fat, protein, or carbohydrate based on your genotype. This next diagram shows blood glucose levels with both incorrect feeding and correct feeding habits.

Table 3.1: Incorrect Fuel Delivery

Incorrect Morning Fuel Eaten	Incorrect Lunch Fuel Eaten	Incorrect Dinner Fuel Eaten
Blood sugar increases quickly, blood glucose decreases rapidly in response to insulin production.	Blood sugar increases quickly, blood glucose decreases rapidly in response to insulin production.	Blood sugar increases quickly, blood glucose decreases rapidly in response to insulin production.
If additional blood glucose is not available, gluconeogenesis occurs.	If additional blood glucose is not available, gluconeogenesis occurs.	If additional blood glucose is not available, gluconeogenesis occurs.

Breakfast	Breakfast Snack	Lunch	Lunch Snack	Dinner	Dinner Snack

GREY GRAPH SHOWS NORMAL RISING AND FALLING GLUCOSE LEVELS

Gluconeogenesis is the making of new glucose. Glucose is the only fuel used by the brain, red blood cells and kidneys and other systems.

Table 3.2: Correct Fuel Delivery

Correct Morning Fuel Eaten	Correct Afternoon Fuel Eaten	Correct Evening Fuel Eaten
Breakfast and Morning snack. Normal blood glucose level maintained with balanced short and long term fuel. No Gluconeogenesis. Body fuel remains stable.	Lunch and Afternoon snack. Normal blood glucose level maintained with balanced short and long term fuel. No Gluconeogenesis. Body fuel remains stable.	Dinner and Supper snack. Normal blood glucose level maintained with balanced short and long term fuel. No Gluconeogenesis. Body fuel remains stable.

Breakfast	Breakfast Snack	Lunch	Lunch Snack	Dinner	Dinner Snack

GREY GRAPH SHOWS NORMAL RISING AND FALLING GLUCOSE LEVELS

Caloric Requirements and Your Optimum Health

In today's complex and fast-paced technological world, many people are willing to open a bottle of pills or try almost any kind of treatment that promises fast weight loss, including extreme diets with no science behind them. More and more people are becoming overweight and adopting a sedentary lifestyle. But we don't *have* to give up good health in today's world. We can live a healthier life if we become mindful of creating a gene-supportive environment and choose with care our food and our physical activities, as well as use some time-tested preventive and treatment methods based on an integrative medical approach.

The first thing to determine is how much fuel your body actually needs to maintain optimal daily functioning. In order to accomplish this, we must understand what a calorie is and how this may effect our fuel requirements.

Your body needs energy every second of every day. Every single bodily function, from thinking a thought to the complex operation of growing a body, requires fuel to energize it. Fuel is measured in calories, with one calorie being the amount of energy required to increase the temperature of one gram of water by one degree Celsius. This fuel comes from carbohydrates, protein, and fat— macronutrients, or what I like to call The Big Three—and is delivered via the intestines throughout the day. For some people, a fourth fuel is alcohol, but at the expense of getting no other nutrients, just empty calories. Caloric needs are individual, and everyone has a set calorie requirement per day to function well. Here are the fuel ratings for The Big Three, plus alcohol:

- 1 gram of carbohydrate provides 4 calories
- 1 gram of protein provides 4 calories
- 1 gram of fat provides 9 calories
- 1 gram of alcohol provides 7 calories

In addition to the proper amount of calories, it is important to divide calories among foods that are effective and beneficial to your body. It is very easy to overfeed your body by eating more than is necessary. For maximum benefit, your caloric intake should be spread throughout the day in smaller meals. Most of us are in the habit of three meals a day, at set times, but there is no conclusive evidence to support any benefits from this pattern. In fact, many of my patients don't even eat breakfast, so starting with lunch, they have a concentrated feeding schedule over about six to eight hours, leaving the other 16 to 18 hours with no food fueling the body.

We can learn a lot about how our bodies *should* be fed by seeing how long it takes to digest a normal portion of carbohydrates, proteins, and fats. In terms of quantity, we need to look at the size of the stomach. Should we be eating smaller meals, more frequently? The answer is yes. Frequent meals with smaller amounts are better suited to fulfill our fuel needs.

So how to split 2000 calories over a 15-hour period? With properly sized meals, the ideal spacing between them is about three hours. This means six meals, which will maximize the body's balance of blood glucose and other nutrients. Here is a sample meal schedule, but be aware that individual caloric requirements will vary.

Sample Meal Schedule

7 a.m.	Breakfast	400 calories
10 a.m.	Morning snack	200 calories
1 p.m.	Lunch	500 calories
4 p.m.	Afternoon snack	200 calories
7 p.m.	Dinner	500 calories
10 p.m.	Evening snack	200 calories

This is an ideal eating schedule, and the only difference in its applicability between one person and the next is the caloric amount and when they sleep. For example, a very physically-active person will have a higher caloric need than someone sitting behind a desk all day. The following represents a way to determine your own required daily intake of calories.

The first step is to calculate your daily caloric requirement. (We will look in detail at just how you can do that, in Chapter 17)

The second step is to start to learn the caloric content of your typical meals. Read the labels on food products so you know their caloric content. Serving size is important. Learn to recognize what a healthy serving—for you—of different foods looks like. Many people will be surprised to learn that a nutritionally balanced serving of carbohydrate, fat, and protein is far different than what we are used to eating. Serving sizes are included in the individual diet section (see page 258-325).

In the beginning, using a timer can remind you to eat a meal or snack at appropriate times of the day (many cell phones have countdown timers). Many people find that their stomach works like clockwork after a very short time. I usually eat breakfast at 6:00–6:30 a.m. and by 9:30 or 10 a.m. I am ready for my snack. I can tell the time by my stomach—I am not one to miss a meal.

The next important step is to eat the correct foods so your calorie intake is just right for you—not for your friend, your husband, or your wife—*you*. While making dietary changes, you must regularly double-check your diet with your body composition to be sure that you are neither gaining nor losing an excessive amount of lean or fat mass too quickly. Once you reach the ideal weight, your body composition should be checked at least twice a year. Make food enjoyable by trying new recipes with new spices and whole food ingredients.

Multi-Level Stress

Stress can be caused by mental, emotional, or physical strain. Stress comes in many different forms, some of which are related to emotional negativity, others to major life events such as getting married, a death, or job change. Stress can sometimes be tolerated, and sometimes not. What is stressful for one person may not be stressful to another. For example, some people consider a wedding to be a calm, beautiful, positive event. For most of the people involved, however, a wedding is a high-stress event. No matter what causes the stress, it requires and produces a host of chemicals and hormones within the body, the emotions, and the mind. Our physical body and nervous system, when stressed, require a large and continuous flow of fuel (glucose) in our bloodstream. When we do not eat correctly and keep our bodies fit and healthy, we are less able to tolerate stressful events.

Feeling stressed all day long is hard enough on a body, but skipping meals only causes it more stress. Not taking time to eat and rest properly causes the body to attempt to feed itself internally, causing stress on the cells. Typically, a busy person who does not eat may feel fatigued and take a caffeine drink to correct this feeling. But the caffeine stimulates the nervous system, which in turn requires more fuel or blood glucose, so it becomes a Catch-22, creating ever-more stress. Fundamentally, this is the internal cell stress we do not see. But if it goes on for an extended period of time, we begin to see chronic illness creeping into the body. The body shows very few signs that chronic illness, silent at first, is developing.

Let's look in more detail at a day in the life of a highly stressed person:

6 a.m. Wakes up. Skips breakfast. The body now has to make its own fuel because, during prolonged fasting like this, the body needs energy and will break down muscle to get it. Gluconeogenesis, or the breaking down of body tissue to feed itself, is set in motion. The by-products of gluconeogenesis are urea and ammonia, which create inflammation in the body—so an inflammatory process is now activated.

7 a.m. Drives to work. With a stressful drive, cortisol production increases. More fuel is required. More fuel required means gluconeogenesis continues, with still no food intake.

8 a.m. Gets to work. Drinks a cup—or two—of coffee. Coffee is a stimulant. Still no food, work stresses are beginning to build, cortisol is produced in still higher amounts. Gluconeogenesis continues—further inflammation.

11 a.m. or noon. The body begins to feel highly compromised. Keep in mind that the last time this person ate was probably dinner time, around 7 p.m. the night before. It is now 11 a.m. We are looking at 16 hours without eating. The body can become very fatigued very quickly.

This person's day is an abnormal, self-imposed, multilevel, internal stress event. But this type of eating behavior is common among my patients. Why? Because people believe that if they don't eat, they will not gain weight. This cycle can be changed, but first it must be identified as an unhealthy behavior.

The symptoms of stress can vary from butterflies in the stomach to life-threatening, pure panic events. These, in turn, can elevate blood pressure and create heartbeat irregularity. Many people spend their lives with their nervous systems turned on high, and when coupled with poor fuel intake, this translates into more stress chemistry. This high-stress setting requires a lot of fuel in the way of glucose. It is as if the body has the gas pedal pushed to the floor and the engine is revving at top speed, but the wheels are not moving. When the nervous system goes into overload due to stress, we can begin to manifest physical symptoms, and extended stress with no relief can lead to chronic illness and depression.

The body doesn't have any way to counteract or use this level of stress—physically a fight-or-flight reaction—unless it runs or fights. The natural physical preparation of a fight-or-flight reaction is to increase fuel in the blood, increase oxygen and blood to the brain and large muscles, decrease fuel to the gut, and improve lung function to take in more oxygen. These are all basic reactions to be able to either fight or run.

If you are sitting in a meeting and are given some stressful information, and stress in the past has trained your body to prepare for either fight or flight, then your body becomes over-stressed with no outlet. This can harm you on many levels, physical and psychological. However this harm manifests is unique to each person.

You can control or change your reaction to a stressor. It just takes practice and patience. What does your body need at this point? It needs to shift out of this fight-or flight reaction state into a calmer, restful state, so that you can logically think about the situation you are experiencing. An excellent way to calm the autonomic nervous system is by breathing deeply and slowly. Using the breath to help lower an elevated stress reaction is very effective (see page 210). Our breath is a connector between our conscious mind and our sympathetic and parasympathetic nervous systems, those automatic unconscious systems that function without our having to think about them.

As important as many other heart disease risk factors are, knowing your family history, your genotype, and how to intervene in multilevel stress events is of utmost importance in ensuring you'll end up with a backpack rather than a bedpan.

Let's now look in more detail at what I believe to be our best path to developing and sustaining a healthy body, mind, emotions, and spirit—the Apo E Gene Diet.

A Patient's Story: Dr. Amanda

Amanda, 49, is a cardiology specialist who came to me both for personal and for professional reasons. She wanted to learn more not only about her own health but also gain some knowledge so she could help her patients.

She had some real concerns about her own health. Her cholesterol levels had been high in the past, she had recently been diagnosed with elevated glucose levels—a warning sign for future diabetes— and her family had a history of cardiovascular disease and stroke. And, she added with a laugh as I took her medical history, "Can you do something about these terrible hot flashes and night sweats?" Then, in a more serious tone, "I'm sick and tired of feeling so terrible because of them."

As a cardiology specialist, Amanda was a busy professional, and she also had a family—two children and a husband—who depended on her at home. She struggled with balancing all aspects of her life, including her own health. Typically, she got up at 7 a.m. to get herself ready for work and the kids for school, feeding them a quick breakfast of toast or cereal and then simply grabbing a glass of juice and a cup of coffee for herself before rushing out the door to drop the kids at school then get to her office or the hospital. She usually didn't eat before 10 or 11 a.m., unless she grabbed a snack bar from the box she kept in her desk.

Her blood tests revealed that her total cholesterol was 243, her LDL was 164, and her blood glucose was 108—all high. She also had an elevated Lp(a), which is an element of cholesterol not tested in the standard cholesterol panel. Lp(a) at high levels has a tendency to increase the risk of heart attack and stroke, and Amanda's was twice the safe level. Her Apo E genotype was 3/3 (not able to tolerate a low fat diet or long periods of fasting), and her body composition was 34 percent body fat. She also kept a diet log for a week, which showed her diet was low in fat—something she believed necessary to keep her weight down—and that she frequently skipped meals.

These results motivated Amanda to make some changes in her life. First of all, she underwent a full cardiovascular screening to see if she had developed any disease so far. Fortunately, her results were negative. We worked together to set some goals. For the first week, she focused on her daily schedule so she would have time to eat right and exercise. Since this would take the cooperation of her family, she called a meeting to explain what she needed to do and why she wanted to do it. Her family easily agreed to help out.

With her new, healthier schedule, Amanda got up earlier so she could have time to eat a healthy breakfast based on her Apo E 3/3 requirements and walk for exercise every day. Throughout the day, she began to eat her meals and snacks on a regular basis. She also changed her schedule at work so she could have a break in the morning and afternoon to relax and eat a nutritious snack and have a soothing cup of green tea. Amanda treated herself to fresh flowers on her desk and bought a beautiful new teacup so she could enjoy her breaks even more.

Six weeks after beginning her new way of living, Amanda's total cholesterol had dropped to 187, her LDL was 84, her Lp(a) had dropped by a third, and her fasting blood glucose was a normal 89. While she still had night sweats, her daytime hot flashes had decreased. She had lost three pounds and 3 percent of her body fat while increasing her lean muscle mass.

Amanda saw very clearly how her old eating habits and stressful schedule were harming her health—and how the changes she made were reversing that trend. Not only was she sold on the Apo E Gene Diet plan for herself, she began using the new information in her own cardiology practice.

＊

Chapter Four

SETTING THE STAGE
FOR THE APO E GENE DIET

As an integrative medicine nurse practitioner, I am dedicated to the cause of disease prevention. I have developed the Apo E Gene Diet disease prevention program by drawing on the knowledge and experience I have gained through my formal medical education, my clinical practice, and my integrative medicine fellowship, as well as my life experience. I began using this program with patients in 2002 and as of this writing have seen several hundred patients (The Heart Health Watchers program, Danville, California).

As noted earlier, the Apo E Gene Diet is not a diet in the usual sense of the word. I use the word "diet" to mean *a series of specific recommendations for individual nutritional and other environmental factors that lead to disease prevention and a healthy life,* based on your individual Apo E genotype. A personalized plan for your genotype—your gene-supportive environment—will guide you in choosing the optimal:

- fat content, with the correct types of fats
- carbohydrate content, with the correct types of carbohydrates
- protein content, with the correct types of proteins

- caloric content, for your needs
- amount and kind of exercise
- balance of stress and relaxation in your life
- quality of mental and emotional environment
- type of energy and intentions you allow into your life (the spiritual component)
- physical environment (esthetics and other factors in the physical space around you)

Besides these general recommendations, the elements of this program draw strongly on the principles of integrative medicine. According to the University of Arizona's Program in Integrative Medicine, which is internationally recognized as the leader in Integrative Medical Education, integrative medicine is a healing-oriented medicine that takes account of the whole person (body, mind, and spirit), including all aspects of lifestyle. It emphasizes the therapeutic relationship and makes use of all appropriate therapies, both conventional and alternative. The Principles of Integrative Medicine[3] are as follows:

- Patient and practitioner are partners in the healing process.
- All factors that influence health, wellness, and disease are taken into consideration, including mind, spirit, and community, as well as the body.
- Appropriate use of both conventional and alternative methods facilitates the body's innate healing response.
- Effective interventions that are natural and less invasive should be used whenever possible.
- Integrative medicine neither rejects conventional medicine nor accepts alternative therapies uncritically.
- Good medicine is based in good science. It is inquiry-driven and open to new paradigms.
- Alongside the concept of treatment, the broader concepts of health promotion and the prevention of illness are paramount.
- Practitioners of integrative medicine should exemplify its principle and commit themselves to self-exploration and self-development.

---

3   Based on the program in Integrative Medicine, University of Arizona, School of Medicine.

My experience in supporting patients in implementing the changes required by the Apo E Gene Diet has led me to develop a number of general recommendations that apply to all, regardless of their particular genotype.

General Recommendations for Implementing The Apo E Gene Diet

In order to make changes in a current lifestyle, the following general recommendations will help you be successful in those changes.

- Use the principles of integrative medicine that:
  - take into account the whole person—body, mind, emotions, spirit, environment, and lifestyle
  - emphasize a supportive, caring, therapeutic relationship
  - make use of all appropriate therapies, both conventional and alternative, and
  - use culturally appropriate, natural, effective, minimally invasive interventions whenever possible

- Find a practitioner who is:
  - trained in integrative medicine, since nutrition and exercise are two very powerful tools of integrative medicine
  - committed to a healthy lifestyle, self-exploration, and self-development

- You will then be guided and supported in:
  - stimulating your body's innate healing with foods that match its genetic instructions
  - utilizing all three food categories (fats, proteins, carbohydrates) in an optimal balance for your genotype (unless a medical condition prevents this)
  - focusing on foods that do not cause inflammation and are easily assimilated, metabolized, and cleared by your body
  - counting *all* calories (if weight is an issue)
  - choosing natural, whole (that is, unprocessed) foods whenever possible
  - utilizing routine blood chemistries and physical evaluations to make adjustments as treatment progresses
  - implementing the exercise program that is best for your individual Apo E genotype

♦ managing life stressors (includes use of proven gentle therapies, such as stress reduction, breathing techniques, prayer, or meditation)

♦ choosing and using appropriate natural supplements

While an understanding of the whole picture, starting with the Apo E genotype, is necessary to make appropriate recommendations for an *individual*, the more general recommendations below apply to all types.

General Recommendations for Optimal Health

Improving Your Nutritional Intake

It has been my experience that the right diet is one of the most important factors for good health. The physiological environment you create as a result of the foods you eat, combined with your Apo E genotype, are crucial factors in preventing dis-ease and maintaining your cellular balance. These elements are all part of creating the right internal environment:

• Choose organic, whole foods.
• Eat plenty of fruits and vegetables.
• Eat balanced amounts and types of protein, carbohydrate, and fats.
• Eat slowly.
• Choose appropriate food portions.
• Cut back on excessive caffeine and alcohol.
• Avoid eating gmo, chemically treated, and processed food.
• Stop eating on the run.
• Eat foods that taste delicious and feel good to your soul as well as your body.

Regular Physical Activity

Regular physical activity is as important as good eating habits. The following routines are a few examples of beneficial activities that contribute to optimal health. Whether it's one of these, a combination, or other activities, you'll get the greatest benefit if you do them regularly.

• aerobic (cardiovascular) exercise
• anaerobic (strengthening) exercises
• flexibility exercises
• daily walks

Greater Self-Awareness

As you make your lifestyle changes, you can enhance the process by documenting it as you go along. Self-expression activities are a great vehicle for keeping in touch with how you feel about personal changes. Be sure to choose an activity that you feel comfortable with and can do regularly. These are a few examples.

- painting, sculpting, or other art practice
- music
- journaling or writing

Relaxation or Stress-Reduction Practices

These examples are just a few techniques my patients have used successfully. Try one that appeals to you:

- meditation or contemplation
- mindfulness practice
- balancing your time between work and play

Spiritual Practices

While the following examples may be unfamiliar, you can find out if they can help in your life by trying them on for size. This is no different than trying new foods. If you don't like the flavor of the activity, then find something else.

- inward disciplines (meditation, prayer, study)
- outward disciplines (simplicity, solitude, submission, service)
- incorporate disciplines (confession, guidance, worship, celebration)
- remember the things that matter to you

Other Recommendations

The following suggestions are general recommendations for overall health and well being.

- Improve your sleep patterns.
- Start a new class (for instance, educational or development class, yoga, tai chi).
- Practice preventive oral hygiene (flossing, regular dental checkups).
- Stay connected with friends and family.
- Be optimistic.
- Be caring and kind.

Unhealthy Practices or Behaviors to Eliminate
Practicing the positive behaviors above will likely make it easier to eliminate unhealthy behaviors. Take some quiet time to think about particular behaviors that might be in your best interest to change. The following are examples of typical behaviors to eliminate:

- poor food intake
- poor exercise and movement habits
- drug/alcohol usage
- driving too fast
- tobacco use
- negative thinking

Chapter Five

APO E GENE TESTING

Besides the genetic testing, it's useful to counsel with your practitioner to determine if you want to do the advanced cholesterol testing to learn your cholesterol sub-fractions—those components in "pots" discussed previously.

While our medical system has not yet fully embraced genomic information, nor applied it effectively to clinical medicine, we have some high-quality testing programs that can give effective assessment and treatment options. One example is the subject of this book: advanced cholesterol testing coupled with Apo E testing. It is now possible to use genetic testing to help prevent some of the serious chronic illnesses that are appearing in near-epidemic proportions.

Just because you do not currently exhibit any signs of disease, this does not mean you will not develop them. Now is the best time for prevention. A high blood cholesterol level, as well as other risk factors, can lead to serious problems in the future, so finding out your total cholesterol, HDL, LDL, and triglyceride levels—the basic cholesterol panel—is an important first step in determining your risk for heart disease and Alzheimer disease.

In addition to these routine blood tests, two advanced kinds of testing can be valuable, and these are the subject of this chapter. One test is for the Apo E gene, while the other is an advanced cholesterol test. The Apo E gene is the number one gene affecting cholesterol. So if you are considering getting an Apo E test, you should also consider the advanced cholesterol testing panel.

However, there are important issues to be considered before deciding to have these tests. And they must be done with the support of a health care provider, who may not even be familiar with them. In this chapter, my intention is to help you decide if either test is appropriate for you.

If you decide to do either or both tests, you can send for a kit (see information in the back of the book) that will make it easy for your provider to order the tests for you, since they can only be ordered by a licensed professional. They are simple blood tests that can be drawn at a local lab and then sent off to a special lab for analysis. About a week later your provider should have the results. In the meantime you can study chapter 6, page 53, which will help prepare you for possible changes that the tests may indicate are advisable in creating your optimal gene-supportive environment.

Apo E Gene Testing and You

A large percentage of heart disease is known to be genetic. So, as experience with patients has also shown me, even more important than looking beyond total cholesterol levels is testing for the number one gene that affects cholesterol and heart disease—Apo E.

Most people are still not sure how they feel about genetic testing or what to do with genetic testing results if they have been tested. Because it is such a new technology, most people have never discussed a genetic test with a medical provider, let alone had one performed. Yet if you have had a baby born into your family in the past few years, chances are the baby has had a genetic test for phenylketonuria (PKU). The routine genetic testing of newborns can identify genetic disorders that must be treated early in life and is the most widespread use of genetic testing. All 50 states have passed laws requiring that newborns be tested for PKU because if it is not identified and treated very early with dietary restrictions, it causes mental retardation.

While the medical industry is in its infancy with respect to genetic testing and handling the results of that testing, we know enough to say that proper genetic testing can provide you with some important information that can help you determine how to best protect or improve your health. This does not mean that everyone should be gene tested. Gene testing has some involved, complicated medical and ethical issues associated with it. I won't get into the debate about genetic testing from a philosophical standpoint, but rather, share with you certain conditions under which you may—or may not—want to consider genetic testing. Your decision about whether or not to take the Apo E genotype test should be made with the help of a practitioner, ideally the one who will then order the test for you if you decide in favor. I will offer guidelines below to help you and your practitioner in making the right decision for you.

Drawbacks of Testing

The decision to get tested for the Apo E gene is not easy, and one of the main reasons is because your health insurance company and your employer could find out that you have an above average risk of developing Alzheimer disease or cardiovascular disease. Besides their knowing, you might rather not know that unless you make major changes to how you live your life, you have a 90 percent chance of developing Alzheimer disease. If you are considering the test because your family has a history of Alzheimer disease, or you have very high cholesterol, you should talk with a medical provider who has experience performing these tests and can help keep your test results confidential.

The Apo E test, along with an advanced cholesterol test, can give you clear nutritional direction and guidance. The question then becomes whether *you* need an Apo E test, or just advanced cholesterol testing. Personally, I think it depends on what you want, need, and are willing to do. I do not recommend that testing be done just to find your risk of contracting Alzheimer disease. Rather, the decision to be tested should be based on your desire to obtain the information necessary for proper nutritional guidance and assistance in preventing chronic illness.

Reasons for Doing Genetic Testing

Indications and warning signs that may be a reason for genetic testing are a personal history of:

- severe cardiovascular disease
- Alzheimer disease
- Parkinson disease
- severe neurological disease
- gout
- alcoholism
- high triglycerides and/or ldl
- insulin resistance or diabetes
- substance abuse
- morbid obesity
- depression/anxiety disorder or other mood disorders
- confirmation of a high cholesterol disorder potentially being affected by the Apo E gene

- confirmation of a diagnosis of late onset Alzheimer disease in a symptomatic adult or to reduce risk with dietary prescription
- assistance with treatment of multiple sclerosis by dietary prescription
- assistance with treatment of Parkinson disease by dietary prescription

At the same time, if you have one of the following chronic illnesses or conditions and you are not getting better with your current care plan, you may want to consider getting an Apo E test to help improve your dietary patterns.

Here are just a few conditions that I have seen find exceptional success with dietary change related to an Apo E genotype:

- acne
- gout
- depression
- chronic pain
- high cholesterol
- hypertension
- multiple sclerosis
- anxiety
- fibromyalgia
- insomnia
- glucose intolerance
- arthritis
- diabetes
- alcoholism
- ADD and ADHD
- cardiovascular disease
- Parkinson disease
- severe peri-menopausal symptoms
- chronic obesity
- insulin resistance
- menopausal symptoms

I strongly recommend that you find a medical provider who has been trained in the advancing field of genetic heart disease and in integrative nutritional medicine to support you. More information on medical providers can be found at www.ApoEGeneDiet.com.

Advanced Cholesterol Testing

You may also want to consider getting advanced cholesterol testing if you:

- eat an inflammatory diet
- are an Apo E 4 who eats an inflammatory diet
- have high levels of LDL (bad) cholesterol (not resolving)
- have low levels of HDL (good) cholesterol (not resolving)
- are unable to tolerate cholesterol medications
- experience high levels of stress

If the majority of the situations above apply to you, you *might* be at high risk of developing chronic illness, heart disease, or Alzheimer disease.

By contrast, you will have a low risk of developing a chronic illness if you:

- are an Apo E 4 with a normal LDL (bad) cholesterol
- are an Apo E 4 with a high HDL (good) cholesterol
- have a balanced lifestyle
- eat a diet low in inflammatory foods
- pursue a well-established aerobic exercise program
- have healthy relationships
- are happy and involved in life with little or no stress
- are creating and living a life you love

Answering yes to the majority of these indicates you probably wouldn't gain from advanced cholesterol testing.

If you don't know your Apo E genotype and you switch to a low-fat diet and your small, dense LDL level worsens, is it because you are still getting the wrong diet? Genetic testing might show that you are an Apo E 3/3 that can't tolerate a low-fat diet. Or that you are an Apo E 2/3 or 2/2 that needs to eat a much higher-fat diet.

Dietary Options Without Testing

In the absence of knowledge of your specific Apo E genotype, dietary improvements can be accomplished by *trial and error,* seeing what different diets do to your cholesterol levels. This requires monitoring your diet and body composition extremely carefully. I have tried this trial and error approach many times with patients and can tell you, it is not easy—it requires accurate detailed diet documentation, a strict exercise log, multiple testings, and office visits. It is time-consuming, and patients get fed up with the rigid process quickly. The frustration rate is very high, but if you are willing to monitor your diet, perform the exercise, commit to the testing, stick with the logging journal for your diet and body composition, and are patient, it will work. Rarely in this trial-and-error plan do you or your health provider ever find your Apo E genotype. You follow a general "what's good for one, is good for all" nutritional plan, and a "general" exercise plan, and watch to see what your cholesterol does.

A Patient's Story: Dora

For 16 years, Dora had been working with her primary care doctor to solve her cholesterol mystery. Despite trying many different medications, reading all the books about lowering cholesterol and following their advice, and even trying some of the popular diets, Dora was never able to bring her cholesterol level below about 400—*double* the recommended maximum level for good heart health. When this lovely 75 year old woman came to see me, she was not following any particular cholesterol-lowering program because she was stymied, as was her primary care doctor, about what approach to try next. Nevertheless, she was still determined to reduce her cholesterol levels.

She had good reason. As she told me while relating her medical history, nearly every immediate family member suffered from severe heart disease, and many had already died. Clearly, she faced multiple risk factors for heart disease, and perhaps even Alzheimer disease, since certain Apo E genotypes carry a higher risk for both. People with the Apo E 4/4, in particular, are more prone to Alzheimer disease, although Dora said none of her family members had exhibited symptoms. I saw no hint of cognitive impairment in Dora, whose delightful sense of humor never failed to cheer me. Very no-nonsense and polite, she was also bright, aware, alert, and happy. She is also one of the most determined people I know: While her children were young, she worked nights as a telephone switchboard operator to support them, coming home in time to get them off to school and then sleeping during the day while they were gone. It was this same brand of perseverance that motivated her to solve the perplexing mystery of her cholesterol levels.

Once I explained that advanced cholesterol testing and an Apo E test could give her very detailed information, Dora eagerly agreed to have the tests done. The results showed extremely high total cholesterol and high LDL—not unexpected—as well as Apo E 4/4, passed to her from both of her parents.

Her test results of January 4, 2005, blew the top off the charts with a total cholesterol level of 489 and an LDL level of 381—both extremely high. Her HDL was 67, in the high range.

Now we had a very specific genetic road map, which we could use to structure her particular diet and exercise program. Since Dora had never been able to physically tolerate either drugs or botanical supplements typically used to lower cholesterol, we decided on a non-medicine approach using only diet and exercise in line with her Apo E 4/4. These top two integrative medicine tools would be a true test of the right program for her genotype.

I recommended a diet for Dora that would reduce all her cholesterol levels. She was to make the changes slowly so her body could adjust. First of all, it was important for her to avoid skipping meals, with breakfast, lunch, dinner, and three healthy snacks spaced three hours apart. She was to eat 1600 to 1800 calories a day, divided this way: 25 percent protein from plant sources and fish (very little red meat, limited to only once every 24 to 48 hours), 55 percent carbohydrates from low-glycemic foods such as whole grains, and 20 percent fat in monounsaturated and polyunsaturated forms. In addition, Dora was to begin walking on a treadmill every day, beginning with 10-minute sessions and slowly increasing the time.

A month later, Dora's total cholesterol was 243, her total LDL was 160, and her HDL was 57. At the time of her third test, on March 11, 2005, her results had improved even further: total cholesterol of 214, total LDL of 142, and total HDL of 65. The final result: One very happy patient with exceptional results. A summary of her progress is as follows:

January 4

Total cholesterol:	489 mg/dL *(Optimal: below 200. High: over 240)*
LDL cholesterol:	381 mg/dL *(Optimal: below 100. Very high: over 190)*
HDL cholesterol:	67 mg/dL *(Low: 40. High: 60)*

After a month of Apo E 4/4 genotype diet and exercise protocol with no medications:
February 8

Total cholesterol:	243 mg/dL
LDL cholesterol:	160 mg/dL
HDL cholesterol:	57 mg/dL

March 11

Total cholesterol:	214 mg/dL
LDL cholesterol:	142 mg/dL
HDL cholesterol:	65 mg/dL

Two years later, Dora still comes to see me occasionally, and she's holding her own.

Protecting Your Medical Records

As I mentioned earlier, in 1997 President Clinton proposed a law making it a crime for employers or insurance companies to discriminate on the grounds of any genetic testing data they obtained, but only half of the states in the United States adopted this policy. In any case, it's essential to protect patients' medical records to prevent discrimination as a result of such testing data.

With our current public policy, genetic testing can be a double-edged sword, helping to save lives and improve the quality of life for some, but causing financial loss for others, such as when a person's job, medical coverage, or both are lost based on genetic testing. Therefore, until we get our genetic medical record protection policies in place, I recommend that patients pay for the Apo E gene test privately to keep the results confidential.

Another option is to use an identification number rather than your name. I have set up a foundation, described in Appendix C, for anonymous Apo E gene and advanced cholesterol testing that will help protect patients and their medical records.

How To Get Tested

If you have decided to have advanced testing, see Appendix C for information on ordering a kit that you can take to a practitioner to order for you.

Chapter Six

NOW THAT YOU KNOW
YOUR APO E GENOTYPE

After getting your Apo E gene test results, you may have to devise a clear plan with respect to your current health and what you want to accomplish for your future health. Therefore you must carefully consider your options.

Option 1
You might have been curious to find out your Apo E genotype, but you do not want to change your current behavior. Now that you know your genotype, you may choose to do nothing and simply continue living your life in the same way, allowing your behaviors and environment to determine your health outcome. For example, you now know you are an Apo E 4/4, but you choose to just wait and see if any health complications arise, taking your chances in the nutritionally manipulated environment of conventional foods. With this option, you now have a better understanding of the risk involved, but I do not recommend taking it.

Option 2

Having been tested, you may now know that you have a higher-risk type of Apo E gene but believe that certain medications will help reduce your risk of chronic illness even though you are not able or willing to make big lifestyle changes. When choosing this option, make sure you find a good medical provider who is up-to-date on the latest treatment options and supports your request to reduce your risk of chronic illness over your lifetime, not just in the short term.

Medication is a powerful tool, but not the only answer. You need the *right* medications. This means that finding a provider trained in the advanced field of lipid science and metabolic disease is very important when choosing to take the medical treatment route.

Option 3

If the test showed that you have a higher risk genotype and you're willing to follow a lifelong prevention program that includes all possible options, you can draw on allopathic medicine and alternative methods to reduce your risk of chronic illness—the path of integrative medicine. The full disease prevention program you will develop with your medical provider will probably engage you in the most comprehensive process you have ever undertaken, yet it could yield some of the best possible long-term positive health benefits.

Now that you have decided to take the path of integrative medicine and optimize your health and well-being, you need to be sure that you have a medical provider who will support you in your endeavors to enhance your health.

My Story: Pam

As an integrative medicine practitioner, I never want to recommend a treatment or perform any procedure on a patient unless I have either first thoroughly researched it or experienced it myself. So, soon after I began testing and working with the Apo E gene materials, I had myself tested for two reasons: One, so I could better understand what my patients would go through; and two, when a family member's results came back and we discovered she had an abnormal Apo E genotype, I wanted to see if I also had an abnormal variant.

While I was curious to know my own Apo E genotype, did I want to know if I had an abnormal variant, especially 4/4? Given that I knew the possible outcomes of having such a variant—none of them good without intervention—I wasn't sure if I could face that knowledge. But then, I figured, not knowing and not intervening with the correct diet, if necessary, was worse.

I went to see my physician, who is also a friend and colleague, and explained what and why I wanted to have this gene test. He agreed with me and signed the order to have my blood drawn. I took it to my dear friend Betty, a medical assistant and phlebotomist, so she could take the necessary sample. I put my arm down so she could reach the vein at the crook of my elbow, but just as she moved the needle toward my arm, I jerked it back.

"Not so fast," I said. "Betty, do I really want to do this?"

Understanding my reason for hesitating, she asked, "Do you want to talk to the doctor again?"

"No." But I didn't put my arm back down on the table, either.

Betty sat down and looked me in the eyes. "Think about why you're doing this. You just told me that you want to have yourself tested so you can experience what your patients will experience, yes?"

I had to agree with her. "You're right. I need to know how this feels. Go ahead."

I surrendered my arm, and Betty drew the vial of blood.

A few weeks later, I walked into the building where my doctor has his office. He was walking down the hall toward me.

"Hi, Pam. Did you see your results? You're Apo E 4," he called down the hall and continued into his office.

I stopped in my tracks, feeling as if all the blood in my body had suddenly gushed from my body. Shaking and speechless, I just stood there. I couldn't believe the results—and I couldn't believe my doctor would deliver them in such a public, insensitive way. Finally, I walked into his office and sat down in the chair across from him.

"Are you all right?" he asked.

"Wow. Do I have one 4 or two?" I knew that an Apo E 4/4 is the worst variant; a 4/3 would at least be a little better.

"You're a 4/3. What does that mean?" No wonder he had been so breezy about delivering the results. Not familiar with the Apo E gene, he didn't know what they meant.

So I explained my own gene test results to my doctor. While the "3" is a good transporter of fats and cholesterol, I told him, the "4" is the one that doesn't work so well and can cause serious health problems with the wrong nutrition.

Seeing that I was still upset, he comforted me with the truth.

"Think about it, Pam. You are a healthy person," he said. "You have extremely low cholesterol, your subfraction cholesterol is completely normal, you have a negative heart scan. Plus, you exercise regularly, and your diet is the right diet for you. You've created the right environment for your genotype without even knowing it. And with these results, we know you're living the life journey you created, and your purpose is much bigger than you knew."

He was right. I was healthy, and now knew how to stay that way. I was actually very lucky, since I was one of the people who could actually tolerate a low fat, higher carbohydrate diet because of my specific Apo E gene combination. I decided to remember his words and continue living my life as I had been.

This was an important lesson for me. I had received Apo E test results in the worst possible way. However, I believe that this happened exactly the way I was supposed to experience it: I now knew how not to deliver painful or frightening results to my patients if they chose to have the Apo E gene test. I became even more protective about all my patients and careful about how I explain the test and the results. Yes, my experience was perfect.

How to Choose a Medical Provider

You must use care when choosing a medical provider so that the outcome provides the most fulfilling of relationships. Selecting the best possible medical provider can be a daunting process even under the best of circumstances, since the health care provider-patient relationship involves something we all value most—our health.

The best time to choose a health care provider is when you do not need one. When you begin looking for a doctor, it's best if you have not waited until you or a loved one is faced with an illness or emergency. However, if you do not already have a medical care provider, know that not all medical providers are created equal, or have the appropriate training. You will usually make the best choices after some research. Write down your requirements for a health care provider and order each according to its importance to you. Then proceed to research the possibilities using the information sources available.

At this point it is helpful to remember the distinction between allopathic and integrative medicine. Allopathic medicine is the model our current medical system uses for treating disease. It derives its name from "allele," which means "opposite," and seeks to find drugs or procedures that will reverse the symptoms. It tends then, to ignore, or at least not directly address, the underlying problem the symptoms are pointing to.

Integrative medicine has been called the future of medicine. It is relatively new on the scene, and there are not very many practitioners as yet. However, I suggest you locate a physician or nurse practitioner trained in integrative medicine if at all possible.

While some medical providers have a philosophy that fits your belief system, others may not. It is vitally important that you inquire about a practitioner's training and background. Many medical providers say they can care for your total health; however, when you question the extent of their specific training, you may see some important deficiencies in their ability to appropriately evaluate and treat your whole health picture.

For example, the therapy provided by a professional chiropractor can be valuable when used with a primary care provider—such as an MD, DO (doctor of osteopathy), NP (nurse practitioner), or PA (physician's assistant)—but not in place of them. I work with some exceptional chiropractors who provide excellent care within the boundaries of their training. However, some patients are under the impression that chiropractors are medical doctors because of the word "doctor" in their degree—DC (doctor of chiropractic), but chiropractors are alternative medicine providers, providing manual medicine to mainly reduce pain by adjusting and manipulating a patient's spine.

The world of alternative medicine is wide and varied. Some practices of alternative medicine are safe, some are very questionable, and some are outright dangerous. Most people do not have the background to discriminate between safe and unsafe practices of alternative medicine practitioners. It is wise to get guidance from a primary care provider trained in integrative medicine before attempting to utilize any nontraditional therapy or practice. Integrative medicine practitioners have been educated in many fields of medicine, not just traditional allopathic medicine. They can help you identify the differences between safe and some of the potentially harmful medical treatments that are sometimes used despite concerns about their efficacy and safety.

Selecting a Medical Practitioner

The following guidelines will help you select a medical practitioner that is appropriate for you.

- Consider your personal likes and dislikes of any potential providers.
- Consider their education, training, and competence.
- Consider choosing an MD, NP, DO, or PA for your main adviser.
- Consider a provider known for caring about his or her patients.
- Consider a provider who takes the time to listen to you and your concerns.
- Choose a medical provider who is able to explain information clearly and at your level of understanding.
- Choose a medical provider who will anticipate potential long-term health problems.
- Choose a provider who practices not only disease management but also disease prevention.
- Choose a medical provider who personally practices what he or she teaches.

Additional factors that might affect your choice of a medical provider include:

- your health insurance plan
- the location of the medical provider's office
- the location of the hospital where the provider treats patients
- the age and gender of the medical provider—some women prefer women and some men choose to see only male providers

- cultural considerations, such as language and belief systems— someone with the same faith or religious beliefs, such as someone who offers prayer and spiritual guidance as an option

Integrative Medicine Resources

The following websites are examples of good programs; they can also direct you to trained integrative medicine practitioners:

Duke Center for Integrative Medicine:
www.dukehealth.org/Services/IntegrativeMedicine

Andrew Weil, MD:
www.DrWeil.com

Scripps Center for Integrative Medicine:
www.scrippshealth.org

University of San Francisco, Osher Center for Integrative Medicine:
www.osher.ucsf.edu

University of Arizona Program in Integrative Medicine:
www.integrativemedicine.arizona.edu

Your main medical provider is a key player with respect to providing you with important information, guidance, and support. Knowing who you are and what you want is also key. Once you have found a medical provider, the following section will help guide you with regard to your next steps.

Learning Who You Are—Self-Exploration

As we mature, we develop a sense of who we are, what we want, and why we want it. Some of us may be more aware of this than others. Regardless of where you are in this process, the following questionnaire will help you think more deeply about who you are, where you have been, how the world influences you, and what you want out of your life.

Integrative medicine puts a lot of emphasis on the value of the patient-provider relationship. As well as deepening your understanding of who you are at this point in your life, this questionnaire will allow your medical provider to learn more about you. This will be helpful when, together, you develop your care plan.

A Patient's Story: Rebecca

Rebecca was 26 when she first came to see me. She was chronically ill, with severe, chronic pain in her feet and ankles. This wasn't surprising since she weighed 254 pounds, with a little more than half her weight, or 51.5 percent, being body fat. For many years, Rebecca had tried most of the popular diet plans—Atkins, Jenny Craig, Weight Watchers— and she had even worked with two local weight-loss providers in her struggle to lose weight and keep it off. None of them had worked. In fact, she had continued to gain weight, even though she had followed each plan religiously. Finally, she came to see me, determined once and for all to lose weight, lose her pain, and be healthy.

As always with new patients, I took a detailed medical history. Rebecca's family had a strong history of heart disease, and she suffered severe headaches, chronic pain, terrible acne, kidney stones, and chronic constipation. Her gallbladder had been removed as a result of gallbladder disease. Not surprisingly, she also suffered with deep depression. Her modest job created high levels of stress for her.

I also gave Rebecca The Integrative Medicine Questionnaire, which contains questions that help both me and my patient understand their past, their beliefs, and what they really want out of life (see page 61 for this questionnaire). I also gave her a physical exam, and she had an Apo E gene test. She was an Apo E 4/3. Now it all made sense why she had never been able to lose weight—and even gained pounds—on the popular alternative low carb, low calorie, and high protein diets that seemed to produce such good results for other people. Relieved and happy to know the reason, she was more than ready to test the nutritional plan that was best for her genotype. More than once, she asked me why no one had ever told her about this process before.

She studied the Big Three food groups—carbohydrates, protein, and fat—and how they applied to her Apo E 4/3. Very slowly, Rebecca began making dietary changes according to her genotype. At her next visit, her weight had increased by two pounds, but that did not deter her. The next time, she weighed 246 pounds—she had lost 10—and by six months, her weight was 223 and her body fat was 46 percent. In addition, her cholesterol improved, her acne had completely disappeared, as had her constipation and chronic pain.

Six months after that, or one year after her first visit, she had slimmed down to 197 pounds and 41 percent body fat. She had lost 59 pounds, of which 42 pounds were fat.

Today, Rebecca continues following her prescribed Apo E Gene Diet and exercise and stress reduction plan. She is happier and healthier than any time in her life, feeling like a beautiful woman who has gained control of her health.

"I've changed my life for good," she says, "and I won't ever look back."

Integrative Medicine Questionnaire

Review this section in a quiet, comfortable, relaxing place. Do not rush through the questions—think carefully, and be open and honest with yourself. You may want to use a separate pad of paper or a journal book on which to write your answers.

Growing Up

- Where were you born?
- Close your eyes and relax for a few minutes and think back to some of your first memories.
- Describe who you were as a child (happy, sad, joyful, carefree, afraid).
- Describe who you were as a teenager (happy, anxious, nervous, carefree, relaxed, isolated, connected).
- Can you identify any major experiences or life lessons from when you lived there?
- Other than being born in a certain place because your parents lived there, can you find or imagine any "higher purpose" or spiritual reason why you were born into that physical place?
- Describe who you are now.
- How would you describe yourself to another person?

- How would someone who knows you very well describe you?
- How would someone who knows you casually describe you?
- Write down some key experiences from your life and how they have shaped you and made you the person you are today; include:
  - any and all significant relationships;
  - any significant events connected to an educational experience or career;
  - how these affect the way you are viewed in, or you view, the world

Who and What is Most Important to You Today?

Rate the areas below on a scale of 1 to 5 (where 5 is best possible) and jot down any thoughts the questions bring up:

_____Health (mind, emotions, body, spirit, environment)

_____Partner (husband, wife)

_____Family (children, grandchildren)

_____Family-of-origin (mother, father, brother, sister, children, aunts, uncles)

_____Self-developed family

_____Career (self-creative mission or supportive mission, and the part you are playing in the world with your work)

_____Friends (lifelong, deep friends to casual acquaintances)

Having identified who and what is most important to you, write your response to the following questions:

- What does family represent to you?
- What do friendships represent to you?
- What do work associates represent to you?
- Are there any other key people in your life?
- Who you can trust and go to in times of stress?
- Are these trusted ones—family, friends, life teachers, helpers, counselors, advisors, tutors?
- Do you communicate openly with these people?
- Do you convey your wishes and desires from your true heart?
- Is open communication an easy or difficult task for you to accomplish?

♦ Does your current creative work create who you are?

♦ Are you satisfied with the work you are currently doing?

♦ Is this current work something that you feel in your heart is the best work for you and your personality?

♦ Have you ever asked yourself what is your purpose on this earth, and does your current work fit with your purpose or heart's desire? The following questions can guide you in determining this:

♦ Do you feel as if your work flows from your heart?

♦ Or do you feel the energy is of a restrictive, unsafe, controlled, limited, constrained nature?

♦ At the end of the day, has the time and effort you have spent with people at work left you with positive or negative feelings?

♦ What kind of relationships do you want to have with others?

♦ What kind of relationship do you want to have with yourself?

♦ How do you want to think (negatively or positively)?

♦ How will having your heart's desires change your current life?

Overall Health

Keep in mind that not everyone functions in an optimal way when a low-stress lifestyle is followed. Some individuals actually function better under higher stress situation than lower stress situations.

• Are you aware of how you best function?

• When stress is excessive, do you focus on excuses or finding blame in others?

• Do you see life situations as opportunities or problems?

• Most of the time do you consider yourself to be healthy or sick?

• Do you think a lot about your health? If so, what aspects do you think are the most important?

• If you think a lot about illness, what are the specifics of the illness? Is it a chronic illness or brief occasional illness?

• Is your health care provider a licensed primary care provider trained in allopathic medicine?

• Is your provider one who fits your needs and can evaluate your entire health, not just a small, specialized piece of it?

• How do you describe your relationship with your current health care practitioner?

- Do you feel restricted in your communication (perhaps due to fear of being rejected if you make a request)?
- Do you feel like you have enough energy every day, or are you fatigued much of the time?
- Do you sleep well?
- Do you get enough sleep?
- Do you have a pre-set bedtime?
- Do you have a sleep routine that works for you?
- Do you take any supplements or medicines to help you fall asleep?
- Do you use any other sleep aids such as alcohol or drugs?
- If you do, is this a chronic habit or done infrequently?
- Do these supplements or medication fit with your belief system?
- Do you wake up within a few hours of going to sleep?
- Do you wake up most nights to go to the bathroom, or for another reason?
- Do you wake up on your own when it is time for you to get up, or use another method such as an alarm?
- How do you feel when you wake up: happy, sad, depressed, fresh, energized?
- Do you include other supplements and vitamins in your daily life?
- Does your primary care provider recommend these supplements?
- What do you know about these supplements?
- Have they been prescribed 100 percent for your benefit, or were they prescribed for a provider's financial gain?
- Is your supplement 100 percent pure (at least according to the label)?
- Are your supplements self-prescribed?
- Do you know if your vitamins or supplements are manufactured under the highest quality conditions?
- Do you know if your supplements interfere with any medication?
- Do you feel 100 percent comfortable with your intake of vitamins and supplements. Are you sure they are the correct ones for you?
- Are you sure that what is on the label of your supplement or vitamin is what is in the bottle or container (vitamins are not FDA regulated)?

Eating
- Are you aware of the type and quality of food going into your body?
- Have you ever explored the different types of food, such as whole foods versus processed?
- Are you mindful or mindless of the foods you are consuming?
- Do you have control of the food you consume? Or is someone else responsible of the food you are eating? Family member, caretaker, restaurant, others?

Exercise
- Do you move regularly during your day, or are you primarily sedentary?
- What are the levels—low, moderate, high—of your daily activities?
- Do you know what physical activity levels and exercise routines are?
- Do you have a daily exercise routine?
- Do you have a weekly routine?
- Are you limited by sickness or injury?
- Do you like exercise, or are you completely turned off by it?
- Has your experience included friends or family who have exercised or who do not exercise?
- Would you like to learn how to exercise and learn to like exercise?

Relaxation
- Do you know how to relax?
- Do you feel you have any time to relax?
- Do you make time each day to relax?
- Can you define what relaxation is for you?
- When you do relax, do you feel guilty?
- Have you ever been given a message that relaxation is a waste of time?
- If you do feel guilty, can you identify reasons why?

Spirituality and Love
- What is spirituality for you?
- Do you feel connected to a higher purpose/spirit?
- Can you describe what brings meaning into your life?
- When you are in a time of stress, do you look to an external source of higher spirit/God for guidance?

- How do you define joy for yourself?
- How do you define happiness for yourself?
- How do you define love for yourself?
- How do you define peace for yourself?
- How often do you acknowledge and express these feelings and emotions?
- Were you encouraged to ignore or suppress them?
- Can you describe and express love, joy, peace, and happiness?
- Do you actively seek to bring these things into your life, or were you taught and have you been focused on expressing anger, fear, hurt, or unkindness?
- Do you love yourself?
- Do you love others?
- Have you been loved in the past?
- Can you express love?
- Do you feel you are loved?
- How is love demonstrated to you and around you?

As you come to the conclusion of this exercise, take some time to think carefully about the information you have explored here. You can use it to help make the changes to improve your health and life. Over the next few days and weeks I recommend that you begin to write down any thoughts that come out of this exercise that surprise you, as well as strong feelings that come up, be they negative or positive. If you need assistance with what you discovered, talk with your primary care provider. He or she can help guide you.

Wherever you stumble, there you will find your greatest treasure.
—Unknown

Chapter Seven

MAKING THE CHANGES YOU WANT TO MAKE

Have you ever tried to make a major change in your daily routine and found that it is not as easy as you thought?

For example, have you ever tried to change your eating habits? What about eliminating sweets, candy, or desserts from your diet? If you have tried to do this, you may have failed because this is not an easy change to make. So here's an important question to ask: Do you *need* to remove these foods from your diet, or can you make them count? Can you make desserts and sweets become part of the important foods you eat?

First, look at your current sweet intake. Is it primarily sodas, candy, and other refined carbohydrates? Then look at the whole foods available to you, and ask yourself if you can make changes where dessert and sweets are concerned, so that you are using whole foods instead of processed foods. The answer is yes, you can. A positive behavioral change process like this will enhance not only the quality of your body but also of your mind, emotions, spirit or soul, and environment.

Changing old habits for new ones poses a significant challenge for most people. However, if you use the right combination of carbohydrates, fats, and proteins from pure, whole foods at each meal, these foods become fun foods and no longer pose a behavioral challenge. For example, if you have a cookie made with poor quality, highly processed ingredients, the cookie will have a negative effect on your body's cells. However if you make a cookie with high-quality, whole food ingredients, it will have a positive effect. The cookie has now become a positive food for the body. Once we start eating whole foods on a regular basis, our taste adapts. We no longer crave the unhealthy foods we once ate. In the recipe section (Chapter 20), I have included some fun foods that contain important calories in the form of whole foods.

Viewing food as a critical ingredient in good health is the first step to making changes in your eating behavior. However, while most people do not connect what they eat with health or disease, making this connection is important. In order to begin changing your behavior, you must first recognize that a change is needed, and then you need to identify how this change will benefit you. Finally, you will have to want to make the change.

Let's look at a method that can support you in this process. It is known as *The Six Stages of Change*, and since developed by James Prochaska, PhD, and Carlo DiClemente, PhD, in the late 1970s, it has become one of the most important approaches to behavioral change. Here is an outline of each stage, ending with actions you can take to move you toward the next level.

The Six Stages of Change[4]

Stage 1: Pre-contemplation
Characterized by the thought, "I don't think I have a problem."

At this level, you are in denial. You see no problem and, therefore, no need to contemplate change. You might say, "There is no problem" or "I don't have to fix what's not broken."

There are no actions you can take at this point since you see no problem or need for change. You may or may not later get a wake-up call and move to the next stage.

Stage 2: Contemplation
Characterized by the thought, "Is change really beneficial?"
You may be saying, "Prove to me that a change is needed."

At this level, you have some knowledge of your disease-promoting behaviors and may be considering making some beneficial changes. You have not yet made a pledge because you are still considering the advantages and disadvantages of a major behavior change.

4   See *Changing for Good*, by James O. Prochaska, John Norcross, Carlo DiClemente, Collins, 2006

Actions you can take: Consider making a plan for initiating change. Keep it simple. For example, you may love to eat at McDonald's three times a week. You should already know that this kind of food, in excess, is not good for achieving and maintaining optimum health. Slowly it may dawn on you that you can't keep this up and expect to remain healthy.

Stage 3: Preparation

Characterized by the thought, "I am going to do this! I'm ready to go for it!"

At this stage, you are ready to get started. You're ready to make a change. You are now developing a concrete plan.

Actions you can take: Develop some clear objectives and precise procedures. Plan short-term and long-term goals that are sensible and achievable, along with a clear idea of how to accomplish them, and in what time frame.

Stage 4: Action

Characterized by the thought, "I'm doing it!"

At this level, you have allocated your time and energy to reaching your goal. Even this is a tremendous step forward. In addition, you may develop a strong belief and have the confidence that what you're doing is good and worthwhile. These feelings will drive you to achieve success—enjoy them.

Actions you can take: Continue to follow up with those assisting you with this change. Their support can be pivotal in linking you to any additional information and resources you may need to maintain and strengthen your convictions that you can make the desired changes. In-person support is best, but you can get good support by phone or Internet if necessary. For example, you might want to eat fast food only twice a week, then drop down to once a week, and also decide that if you eat fast food, you won't "super size" it. Ask your support person to help you stick with these decisions.

Stage 5: Ongoing Maintenance

Characterized by the thought, "It's difficult to think of how I was before."

It may be difficult for you to remember what your behaviors were like before you became dedicated to your good health. When you have sustained the new behaviors for six months to a year, you can consider that you have graduated to ongoing maintenance. When you reach this level, you know the benefits of the behavior change because you can feel and experience it firsthand. At this level, there is only one goal left to focus on: prevention of a setback.

Actions you can take: consider defining some long-term behavior maintenance approaches to prevent reverting to old behaviors. For example, develop a support system, review past journals and logs, keep up with body composition tests, be proud of your improved health, and focus on how you feel and look now versus how you previously felt and looked.

Stage 6: Relapse or Termination
Characterized by the thoughts "How can I get back on track?" or "Am I done with this now?"

Relapse is common, and being prepared to start over again is important. If you have relapsed, see if you learned something new about yourself and about the process of changing behavior. For instance, ask yourself, "I did it for six days, so what made that work?" Shift your focus from failure to whatever promotes problem solving. Get the support you need to re-engage in the change process. Set realistic goals to prevent becoming discouraged and take positive steps toward that behavior change.

Alternatively, you have conquered the problem and no longer feel the temptation to return to your old, poor behavior. Congratulations! Typically, confidence in success peaks after a year, but temptation may linger for another year or two. Once you no longer feel any temptation at all, you know you reached your goal and can enjoy your success.

Identifying Your Current Stage
I hope you now have a clearer idea of what it takes to make real and sustainable changes in your life. If you are not ready to make the changes you sense you would need to become a happier and healthier person, then simply do your best to study and follow the information that tells you how to move toward a level where you will be ready to make the next step. It can be very helpful to find a person who will support you in this, and we will look more closely at this in the following pages. Also, ask your medical practitioner for assistance whenever possible. Read health newsletters of reputable institutions like Harvard, Berkeley, Duke, Johns Hopkins, and Tufts, and Stanford. You can find some very reliable information on the Internet, too.

Connecting With a Support Person

Many times, changing our behavior for good requires a strong support system. It is human nature to want to feel connected to others—and to be understood by them. Sometimes, when we are unable to accomplish something by ourselves, we need to involve another person who can help us shift ourselves out of a negative behavior pattern into a positive one. I suggest you identify a support person and schedule a time, daily or weekly, to discuss your progress and the challenges you are facing.

In your session with your support person, the checklist below may help you focus your thoughts and give you both a deeper understanding of where you are and where you want to be.

Support Person "Check in" Questionnaire

Current Date:_____

Support Person's Name:_____

Medical Provider's Name:_____

Which stage of behavior change are you in?:

____ Stage 1: Pre-contemplation

____ Stage 2: Contemplation

____ Stage 3: Preparation

____ Stage 4: Action

____ Stage 5: Ongoing Maintenance

____ Stage 6: Relapse or Termination

The six steps in each of the following sections correspond to the Six Stages of Change.

My Mind: Thoughts and Feelings

Step 1: Ask yourself, "Am I or have I been focusing my thoughts and feelings on what I want to accomplish, or what I want out of life?" Answer: Yes or No.

Step 2: Given your response to the question above, circle a number on the scale below that represents how you are feeling, right now. 1 represents feeling something really bad, 10 really great.

Negative   Positive
1   2   3   4   5   6   7   8   9   10

Step 3: Discuss your score and the associated feelings with your support person.

Step 4: After you have shared your feelings with your support person, gently acknowledge or simply notice, without judgment, the presence of any negative thoughts. Then, withdraw your attention from these and focus on the positive thoughts and feelings associated with what you want to accomplish.

Step 5: Rate your feelings once again by circling the number on the scale below, as it relates to how you are feeling *now*.

Negative   Positive
1   2   3   4   5   6   7   8   9   10

Step 6: At this time could you benefit from the information or expertise of an additional support person, such as a counselor or medical provider?

If "Yes," I suggest that you do not continue with the following sections until you find an additional support person. If you do not need additional support, continue to the next section.

My Body

Step 1: Ask yourself, "Am I or have I been focused on what I want, with respect to how I care for my body?"

_____ Yes   _____ No

Step 2: Given your response to Step 1, rate how you are feeling in the present moment by circling a number on the scale below.

Negative   Positive
1   2   3   4   5   6   7   8   9   10

Step 3: Discuss these feelings with your support person. If you know you want to make changes to your weight, body composition (percent body fat and lean mass), body mass index (BMI), body measurements, nutrition, and exercise habits, include how you feel about each of them with your support person.

Step 4: After you have shared your feelings with your support person, gently acknowledge, without judgment, the presence of any negative thoughts. Then, withdraw your attention from these and focus on the positive thoughts and feelings associated with what you want to accomplish.

Step 5: Rate your feelings once again by circling the number as it relates to how you are feeling *now*.

Negative   Positive
1   2   3   4   5   6   7   8   9   10

Step 6: At this time could you benefit from the expertise of an additional support person?

My Spirit/Soul
Sit quietly and take several deep breaths to calm and focus your energy. When you are ready, move forward to consider the following questions.

Step 1: Ask yourself, "Am I or have I been focused on what I want to accomplish or what I want out of life with respect to my spiritual/soul life?"

_____ Yes   _____ No

Step 2: Having asked this question, how do you feel, in this moment. Rate your feelings by circling an actual number on the scale below.

Negative   Positive
1   2   3   4   5   6   7   8   9   10

Step 3: Discuss these feelings with your support person.

Step 4: After you have shared your feelings with your support person, gently acknowledge the presence of any negative thoughts. Then, withdraw your attention from these and focus on the positive thoughts and feelings associated with what you want to accomplish.

Step 5: Rate your feelings once again by circling the number as it relates to how you are feeling *now*.

Negative   Positive
1   2   3   4   5   6   7   8   9   10

Discuss your overall feelings of this session.

Step 6: At this time could you benefit from the information or expertise of an additional support person, such as a counselor or medical provider?

My Physical Environment

Step 1: Ask yourself, "Am I or have I been focused on what I want to create in my physical environment?"

_____ Yes   _____ No

Step 2: Having answered this question, how do you feel, in this moment. Rate your feelings by circling an actual number on the scale below.

Negative   Positive
1   2   3   4   5   6   7   8   9   10

Step 3: Discuss these feelings with your support person.

Step 4: After you have shared your feelings with your support person, simply notice, without judgment, the presence of any negative thoughts. Then withdraw your attention from these and focus on the positive thoughts and feelings associated with what you want to accomplish.

Step 5: Rate your feelings once again by circling the number as it relates to how you are feeling *now*.

Negative   Positive
1   2   3   4   5   6   7   8   9   10

Step 6: At this time could you benefit from the information or expertise of an additional support person, such as a counselor or medical provider?

Congratulations! You now have greater clarity on how you feel and where you are with respect to each of these areas of your life. Now, it is time to write down the goals and tasks to be accomplished in the next few days and/or weeks as they relate to each section. Make your goals both meaningful and achievable.

You may want to enlist the help of your support person in doing this! Remember, you can change these as you go along and learn more about what you want and what you can achieve. You may also want to take a look at the chapter "Tools for Change" (Chapter 16).

Discuss with your support person, how you are feeling now. Set a date for your next support meeting.

Remember, there is no better time than right now to begin creating the life you want.

At a Glance—Principles and Behaviors to Always Consider

You may want to copy this page and keep it with you at all times.

Keys to Your Apo E Gene Diet

- Educate yourself about nutrition with regard to your own personal health and Apo E genotype.

- Stay open-minded about nutrition—it is an evolving science.

- Find two or three trusted resources to support you in your ongoing nutrition education.

- Drink a trusted, clean water source. Don't take the water you drink for granted.

- Eat unprocessed—whole food—carbohydrates.

- Eat mostly two type of fats—monounsaturated and unprocessed polyunsaturated fats (omega-3s)—derived from a whole non-processed food source.

- Eat high-quality proteins that contain only non-processed monounsaturated and polyunsaturated fats.

- Eat a variety of fruits and vegetables, of all colors, from an organic, non-GMO origin.

- Support wholesome local farming and dine at restaurants that offer healthy menus. Educate yourself regarding local farming and restaurant practices.

- Know what you are eating and putting into your body each day—mindfulness is the key.

- Only take vitamin supplements as they apply to your health, not what is recommended for the general population. Choose a high-quality product not focused on generating profit. Know the full details behind your personal vitamin (or botanical) prescription. Store them properly (cool, and sometimes refrigerated).

- Know the personal risks and benefits of alcohol as they apply to your own health. Do not follow the general population's recommendation.

- Prepare and display your food with individual cultural purpose. (Consider china, silver, crystal over plastic, styrofoam, paper.)

- Practice stress reduction and align your intention with your goals and desired changes throughout the day.

- Actively and respectfully, move your body daily, using stretching, strength, and aerobic exercise.

- Be aware of your surroundings and environment. Respect Mother Earth, communicate honestly and with love and kindness.

Chapter Eight

FOOD: THE FOUNDATION

Food is grouped into three main categories: carbohydrates, fats, and proteins—The Big Three. Eating the right balance of these foods for your genotype is a prerequisite for your good health. Understanding what these categories of food are and how our body uses them is the first step in choosing the right combinations that meet our bodies' specific fuel needs.

Carbohydrates

Carbohydrates are the simplest of foods. They provide the body with an immediate source of fuel in the form of sugars and starches that are easily digested and enter the blood stream as glucose. Glucose is the most basic nutrient that our body needs and uses—the preferred fuel of cells. However, this fuel is short-term; it's quickly metabolized. One gram of carbohydrate yields only four calories of energy.

Carbs, Glycemic Index, and Glycemic Load

Historically, nutritional scientists have tried to devise a method of categorizing carbohydrates to guide wise food choices. Despite public health messages promoting high-carbohydrate, low-fat, low-calorie diet regimens to achieve weight loss, and the public's knowledge of the health hazards associated with being overweight and obesity, the prevalence of weight problems in the United States continues to rise. Of particular concern are the increased risks associated with obesity—hypertension, Type 2 diabetes, heart disease, and many other chronic disorders. If not controlled, these diseases can pose a significant economic and emotional burden to those afflicted and society.

As I've shown elsewhere, of particular concern is the lack of scientific evidence on the safety and efficacy of low- or no-carbohydrate diets on overall health. Because low-carbohydrate diets derive the majority of calories from protein and fat, there is the potential negative impact on cardiovascular health. It is important to have a clear understanding what carbohydrates really are, and how they are used in the body because I've recommended that people get a minimum of half their calories from carbohydrates—but not just any old carbohydrate; specific ones having a low glycemic load.

What is This Word "Glycemic"?

Glycemic means "causing glucose in the blood." Before 1981 carbohydrates were seen as two main types, simple and complex, based on the number of simple sugars in their molecular makeup. The simple carbohydrates are monosaccharides and disaccharides because they have only one or two sugar molecules. The complex carbohydrates are called polysaccharides because they have more sugars in their molecular structure and take longer to be digested.

In 1981 this concept was expanded with the introduction of the *glycemic index* (GI)—a number assigned to each carbohydrate food indicating how much it raises your blood sugar when eaten. The idea caught on and people began to avoid foods with high GIs. Then in 2002 a refinement was made on the GI concept by taking into account the average serving size because a high GI food consumed in small quantities has the same effect on blood sugar as larger quantities of a low GI food. This number is called *glycemic load* (GL) and is calculated by multiplying the grams of carbohydrate content in a food times its GI, divided by 100.[5]

What happens when you eat a high GL meal? A quick increase in blood sugar level causes your pancreas to lower the blood sugar level by producing more insulin. The high insulin level then drops the blood glucose level, but at a cost to your body. After a time, the overworked pancreas becomes tired and is unable to produce enough insulin—*insulin resistance.* If your diet continues along the same path, Type 2 diabetes will result. If the pancreas is pushed even further, pancreatic cancer may develop.

So this is how high GL foods have given carbohydrates a bad name. Low GL foods do not increase the blood glucose as quickly, so less insulin is needed to keep your blood sugar stable. These are the foods we evolved to have as a major part of our diet, and for optimal health, we need to return to.

A Patient's Story: Alexis

Nineteen-year-old Alexis had been diagnosed with abdominal migraines, which are a variant of migraine headaches that cause spontaneous abdominal pain with terrible nausea and vomiting. Not surprisingly, she was suffering anxiety attacks, and she would often sleep more than 12 hours at a stretch from exhaustion. Finally, she was exhibiting signs of anorexia because she rarely felt hungry and also was often afraid to eat because of the severe abdominal pain. Her primary care doctor had prescribed medications to control the nausea, vomiting, and anxiety, and Alexis frequently required intravenous fluids because of the dehydration caused by vomiting. When she failed to improve, her primary care doctor recommended that she see me, and her worried parents came with her.

---

5   For example, a 100g slice serving of watermelon with a GI of 72 and a carbohydrate content of 5g (it contains a lot of water) makes the calculation 5*0.72=3.6, so the GL is 3.6. A food with a GI of 100 and a carbohydrate content of 10g has a GL of 10 (10*1=10), while a food with 100g carbohydrate and a GI of just 10 also has a GL of 10 (100*0.1=10).

After taking a detailed medical history, I could see that Alexis was healthy and had few other stressors in her life except for the chronic abdominal migraines. Her eating patterns were abnormal and very unhealthy, mostly fast food when she did eat, partly out of habit but also because of her need to have food quickly and that tasted good. Her parents wondered if eating a healthy, nutritious diet would help—I believed that it might—so Alexis agreed to try it. She began eating healthier foods in a regular pattern and felt better for a few weeks, but then the abdominal migraines returned even more severely. So I suggested that she have an Apo E gene test and then refine her nutrition to meet the needs of her genotype.

When her Apo E genotype was revealed to be 4/3, she began eating correctly for that type, which meant more complex carbohydrates on a regular basis. Her health improved dramatically, and the abdominal migraines diminished. She began to sleep much less and her anxiety attacks improved a great deal. I explained the reason for the improvement to Alexis and her parents. Very simply, with her Apo E genotype, her body became extremely stressed when she ate very little and on an irregular basis. Combined with the dehydration, this pattern severely depleted her glycogen stores, which are necessary for providing continual energy to the body, and sent her metabolism into a tailspin. For Alexis, this meant abnormal cell functioning in her intestines, which brought on the abdominal migraines.

Alexis continued her anti-anxiety and migraine medications at previously prescribed levels for a time, and then slowly reduced them under medical supervision.

Fat

Fat is a more complex source of fuel than carbohydrates and is derived from two principle sources—plants and animals. When the body breaks down fat molecules, the end results are compounds called free fatty acids and glycerol. The liver then processes these fats and glycerol into glucose, which can then be used as a fuel source.

Fat, once digested and absorbed, provides a long-term form of fuel in the body because it is a more complex package than carbohydrates and takes longer to break down and use.

The fats in our diet can be classified into four main types: monounsaturated, polyunsaturated, saturated, and trans fat. The monounsaturated and polyunsaturated fats should be consumed in the right proportions for your genotype, or your body can become greatly imbalanced. Again, depending on your genotype, your body can tolerate no saturated fats, or only a limited amount, and we should all avoid all trans fats. More on that later.

As we'll see, contrary to popular opinion, we *need* fats in our diet. We need the right kind, though, so choose your saturated fats wisely. I consume mine every other Friday via a small amount of high-quality cheese. I derive great joy from my excellent quality cheese and consider myself to be a cheese connoisseur, but I must be smart and avoid eating too much. Keep in mind a single gram of fat yields nine calories of long-term fuel for the body, no matter if it comes from monounsaturated, polyunsaturated, saturated, or trans fat.

Protein

In talking about fats, we need to talk about proteins too, since all natural unprocessed foods containing protein also contain fats. It seems we cannot open a magazine or turn on the TV without finding some protein drink, bar, powder, supplement, or some other fad idea about protein. Selling protein is a multibillion-dollar business and industry. The fashionable Atkins Diet trend gave a tremendous boost to the protein industry, and today billions of dollars are wasted on these processed protein products.

Protein is essential for the development and maintenance of individual cell structure and function, as well as regulating hormonal activity. Coming from both plant and animal sources, it is comprised of long chains of amino acids that are linked together and break down into mostly carbon, hydrogen, oxygen, and nitrogen. This last element—nitrogen—is not present in carbohydrates or fats. When the body has to use protein as fuel, rather than as building blocks for cellular repair and maintenance, it produces nitrogen-containing amino acids that are burned and produce a waste product in the liver, urea, which then has to be cleared by the kidneys.

As I said above, protein foods most often contain fat (unless it is processed out). Animal protein contains mostly inflammatory fats, while plant and fish protein contains anti-inflammatory fats. One gram of protein yields only about four calories of energy, so it's not a very good source of energy.

The interaction between fats and protein is complex. If you do not eat enough carbohydrates, the glucose the body is designed to get from the carbohydrates will have to come instead from breaking down the body's fats and proteins. One of the uses of body fat is to store energy for times of fasting, which allowed our ancestors to weather lean seasons. But when that system is abused by chronic dieting or inappropriate food selections, and your fat stores are mostly used up, you can do a lot of damage to your body. In this situation your internal feeding system can cause rapid protein (muscle) loss and decrease your ability to burn stored fat. You use up your body's muscle mass to generate energy-producing fuel, all because you are not eating the carbohydrates your body needs. In the short term this may not be harmful. However, over a longer term, this can cause excessive irreversible cellular damage and chronic illness.

The bottom line is that too much protein and small amounts of carbohydrates—as advocated in the Atkins Diet—means limited fuel for the brain. A high-protein, restricted carbohydrate diet puts the body into glucose-deficiency mode, causing major strain to the intestine, liver, and kidneys. The body ends up having to make its own glucose from internal sources to feed the brain and body. High-protein, low-carbohydrate diets are particularly dangerous to an Apo E 4 because the inflammatory fats are more difficult for this genotype to clear from the body, leading to an inflammatory process in the coronary arteries and elsewhere in the body.

How Food Becomes Fuel

First, food is placed into the mouth and begins to be broken down by the teeth and our salivary digestive enzymes. Food then passes down the throat though the esophagus into a bag-like holding area called the stomach.

Once in the stomach, food is further broken down with hydrochloric acid, protein-digesting enzymes, and mechanical churning. From the stomach, food is moved into the first part of the small intestine, the duodenum. Here, the liver, gallbladder, and pancreas feed in more chemicals, enzymes, and other substances that play a major role in the breakdown of the stomach contents. Then absorption of the nutrients occurs in the jejunum (middle section of the small intestine) and ileum (last section of the small intestine).

Once most of the nutrients have been absorbed in the small intestine, the remains are passed into the large intestine or colon. Here live trillions of friendly *lactobacilli, acidophilus,* and *E. coli* bacteria that are necessary for producing most of our Vitamin K and for further breakdown of the unabsorbed food. Also the colon recovers most of the water and minerals from the digestive juices that are no longer needed. What remains (fiber and a surplus of those friendly bacteria) is first stored in and then passed out of the last part of the colon, the rectum, via the anus.

Your body is now left with a supply of the nutrients absorbed by the intestines, but the ratio of the Big Three needed by the body may not be optimal because one or more of the them were restricted by dietary choices (such as, a diet too low in fat). If so, cellular health can become unbalanced, leading to disease.

Popular Diets Are Harmful to Your Health

Most diet books focus on greatly increasing or removing one of The Big Three. Some of the most popular recent trends have been removing most fats or carbohydrates, or greatly increasing protein intake, in the diet. However, nutritional research shows that these approaches are not only *not* optimal for disease prevention, but may actually be *harmful* to your health.

Let's now look at several of these popular diets and some of the misinformation and misconceptions commonly associated with them.

Low-Fat Diets

Different Apo E genotypes need varying amounts of fat, and *no one* should remove *all* the fat from their diet. There are good fats and bad fats. The good ones are unprocessed polyunsaturated and monounsaturated fats that have a positive reaction on the cell. They include nuts, seeds, olives, and avocados. Over-exposure to the bad ones—trans fats especially and too many saturated fats—causes cellular inflammation, which in turn leads to disease.

If you remove the wrong amount and kind of fat from your diet, your long-term fuel supply becomes unbalanced. The recent epidemic of Type 2 diabetes may have partly occurred because our country has been encouraged to eat a low-fat diet for many years. Based on the popularity of programs like Dr. Dean Ornish's *Program for Reversing Heart Disease,* some of our major health organizations encourage a low-fat diet for better health. However, now that we know more about the importance of fats, it is clear that not everyone can benefit from a low-fat diet. But changing misconceptions this widespread is difficult. Fat has been given such a bad name that a study conducted by the American Dietetics Association discovered a major misunderstanding that people have about it. They found that many people thought they should delete *all* fat from their diet to have good health, believing that the more fat they removed, the better health they thought they will have.[6] This is extremely dangerous.

If we don't eat healthy fats (particularly the essential fatty acids), we cannot survive because fat is part of every cell membrane in the body. Because the brain has a fat content of about 60 percent, the fat content of a healthy brain cell is important for your brain to work correctly.

However, it is extremely important to know what type of fat you are eating. Avoid inflammatory fats such as trans fats and excessive exposure to saturated fats, as well as highly processed polyunsaturated oils and omega-6 fats. This will be covered in more detail in later chapters. At the same time, you must also have the correct amount of inflammatory-reducing fats from a monounsaturated and polyunsaturated omega-3 source. The correct ratio of fats for all genotypes is very important, as we will see in the pages ahead.

Another critical misconception is not realizing that fat generally comes "packaged" with protein. For instance, beef protein comes with beef fat, and beef has the highest inflammatory fatty acid percentage of any of the animal protein foods. You can't get one without the other, unless it's in an unhealthy, highly processed product.

You need also to be aware of the source of fats in your diet. Most fats don't just come as a simple plain fat source like cooking oils, so you need to know what types of fats come packaged with what proteins:

- Animal proteins (meat and dairy) come packaged with saturated and trans fat
- Plant proteins (nuts, seeds, beans, rice, and soy) come packaged with mono and polyunsaturated fats

Most foods are usually a combination of fats, carbohydrates, and/or proteins, yet people generally see foods as belonging to just one of these main categories rather than being a combination. This means that if you succeed in removing all fats from your diet, you're also removing other important nutrients. You need protein, and it's very difficult to get good protein without getting fats. You need to eat good sources of fat with good protein, such as fish and soybeans, two excellent sources of protein with anti-inflammatory fats.

Not knowing these facts can, in time, cause health problems for anyone on a low-fat, high-protein, low-carbohydrate diet.

6   *ADA's Nutrition and You: Trends 2002 Survey.* Survey results are based on telephone interviews with a nationally representative sample of 700 adults conducted in April 2002 by Wirthlin Worldwide. The survey has a confidence interval of plus-or-minus 5 percent in 95 out of 100 cases.

A Patient's Story: Scott

When Scott was first diagnosed with slightly elevated total cholesterol of 219 and an LDL cholesterol of 128, plus a slightly elevated blood glucose level in the low 100s (which could mean the onset of diabetes), he preferred not to take any medications. Instead, he wanted to use diet and exercise to bring the numbers down and improve his health. His family doctor agreed, encouraging Scott to eat a low-fat diet and exercise.

Scott enthusiastically followed this advice. He joined a gym and worked out diligently. He changed his diet so that he ate very little fat. He was confident this strategy would do the trick—wasn't it the method all the experts recommended?

But within a short time, Scott started to feel worse and returned to his doctor. Tests revealed that his total cholesterol had jumped to 271 and his LDL to 189. His HDL was low at 43. His blood pressure was also elevated, at 138/80, and his blood glucose had also increased. Since Scott still preferred to not take medications, his doctor recommended a switch to a high protein diet, along with continued exercise. That didn't help, either: Scott's total cholesterol remained about the same, while his LDL increased to 197. His triglycerides had risen to an alarming 220 (triglycerides are blood fat and the optimum number is less than 150), and his small LDL cholesterol factor called LDL Pattern B was an unhealthy 44 percent. Even so, his doctor recommended that he continue the high protein plan. After several months with no improvement in his cholesterol and a worsening of his blood glucose to 164, Scott agreed to try medications—eventually he was taking six different drugs, some twice a day. Not only did his cholesterol and blood sugar not improve, he also began having constant stomach and intestinal problems. His family doctor referred Scott to a gastrointestinal specialist, and he underwent tests to check for a stomach or colorectal problem, but nothing was discovered. His inflammatory diet and medication were most likely the problem.

Finally, after three years of misery with multiple medications and a continued low-fat, high protein diet with daily exercise, Scott's total cholesterol dropped to 140 and his LDL to 80. However, his glucose level was 132 and another cholesterol factor called HA1c, a long-term look at blood glucose, was too high at 7.0. And he still didn't feel energetic or healthy. Tired of feeling so poorly and hoping to wean himself from at least some of his medications, Scott came to see me.

After a thorough physical and medical history, I recommended that Scott have more lab testing including an Apo E gene test, and he quickly agreed. He is an Apo E 3/3, the "normal" Apo E genotype that cannot tolerate either a low-fat or a high-protein, low-carb diet. We discussed his diet options for his genotype, and he agreed to eat a diet with moderate healthy-fat content, eager to be healthy and to feel good once again. He began making slow dietary changes so that his body could easily make the adjustment, eating anti-inflammatory fats rather than inflammatory ones, whole grains rather than highly refined carbohydrates, and plant and fish proteins. He continued to take his medications.

Scott started to feel better within a few weeks. A new cholesterol test revealed that his total cholesterol was 151, LDL was 83. Four months later, his total cholesterol was 135, LDL was 69, and HDL was 53— all excellent numbers. His triglycerides had improved and his Pattern B had dropped from 44 percent to 16 percent, becoming a healthy pattern A. Best of all, Scott was feeling healthy and vigorous again.

We reduced his cholesterol medication at first by half, and he was eventually able to quit taking it. Since his blood pressure was normalizing, continuing that medication was causing his blood pressure to drop too low and making him dizzy, so we slowly reduced that medication as well until he finally did not need it any longer. Scott is still slowly weaning himself from his diabetes drugs.

Scott's overall health has improved dramatically since he began following the correct Apo E Gene Diet and exercise plan for his Apo E 3/3. All his numbers have improved: body fat 15 percent, total cholesterol 177, LDL 99, HDL 63, and blood sugar in the high 80s to low 90s. He has lots of energy and says his golf game has improved.

"It doesn't get better than this," he told me during one of our visits.

I had to agree with him.

Low-Carbohydrate Diets

Another dangerous fad is the low-carbohydrate diet. While certainly successful for weight loss, the problem here is that most of the weight loss is water and lean mass. Carbohydrate is a short-term fuel. Since the brain, intestines, and other organs function only on glucose, which usually comes from carbohydrates, if you are not eating carbohydrates at every meal your body has to ask the liver to take on the extra job of making some glucose. This is a process with the long name of gluconeogenesis. Essentially, it makes the blood glucose that your body is designed to draw from carbohydrates in your diet, but it comes at a high cost—it steals proteins from your tissues by breaking down those tissues to gain a source of energy. This process can put added stress on your kidneys and liver because the nitrogen from the amino acids must be processed by the liver and excreted by the kidneys. The result is rapid weight loss, but in addition to burning the fat you want to lose, you also lose some of the body's engine (muscle mass). This means that your ability to burn fat in the future is reduced because your muscle mass, your body's fat-burner, is also reduced. It's like killing the goose that lays the golden eggs.

The Atkins Diet is the most popular low-carbohydrate diet. One of its primary shortcomings is a failure to distinguish between "good" fats (olive oil and other mono-unsaturates) and "bad" fats (corn, safflower, sesame and other processed polyunsaturates and saturates). Another shortcoming is that since few fruits and vegetables are included, you get very little of the all-important fiber, vitamins, minerals, and health-protective phytochemicals these foods contain. And, even though a few carbohydrates are allowed, this diet makes no distinction between the healthy low-glycemic load carbs (see chapter 8, page 88) and the less healthy high-glycemic load carbohydrates.

While some studies have shown that short-term use of Atkins-type diets may be safe and effective for weight loss (but you have to ask, what is being lost?), many physicians are concerned about its long-term health risks. And I hope you will be, too! With any diet we need to consider results—are you losing fat, or losing weight in the form of fluids and muscle?

Popular Diet Review

Before we look more closely at a healthy diet, I want to share my view on a few popular diets that I encourage you to review carefully before deciding to follow one.

Dr. Atkins Diet Revolution

Theory: Metabolic imbalance, not calories, causes people to be overweight. Carbohydrates are responsible for some of our most modern diseases. A high-protein, low-carbohydrate, and low-calorie diet can cause rapid weight loss.

Truth: There is an initial rapid weight loss; however, it comes mainly from water loss. The diet is very dangerous to your health because it is very high in artery-clogging fats.

Dr. Dean Ornish's Program for Reversing Heart Disease

Theory: An extremely low fat (fewer than 10 percent of total calories come from fat, or long-term fuel) diet is said to reverse heart disease.

Truth: This diet is extremely difficult to stick to, specifically because it is very low in fat, which provides taste and helps you feel full and satisfied longer. I find that most people don't continue with this type of diet for very long.

South Beach Diet

Theory: Fewer carbohydrates, with good fat, not bad fat, are best for everyone.

Truth: This diet, like the Atkins Diet, showed the public a different side of the diet world. It is much better than most. However, it still focuses on the "one-size-fits-all" dietary approach.

The Zone

Theory: High-carbohydrate diets are largely responsible for the rise in obesity in Americans. This diet claims that 75 percent of Americans have a genetic defect that leads to high insulin levels when a high carbohydrate diet is eaten. The "Zone" targets a ratio of 40 percent carbohydrates, 30 percent proteins, and 30 percent fats at every meal.

Truth: No studies or references exist, just testimonials from satisfied dieters.

Sugar Busters!

Theory: Sugar is toxic. While it is suggested that calories do not count, it offers 1200-calorie plans and asks you to limit portions. It suggests three meals a day, minimal snacking, no eating after 8:00 p.m., reasonable quantities that fit nicely on a plate. No seconds.

Truth: This is a low-calorie, low-fat, low-carbohydrate, high-protein plan that is high in cholesterol, low in calcium, iron, Vitamin A, and folate, yet supplements are not recommended. Conclusions such as "sugar causes resistance to insulin and then obesity" are not supported by scientific evidence. Most researchers believe insulin resistance is a *result* of obesity, not the other way around. Other unsupported statements include "inactivity may not be significantly harmful" and "dietary sugar is recognized as an independent risk factor in heart disease."

You only need to stand at the checkout line of any major grocery store and read the headlines of a tabloid to know that there are hundreds of diets out there all claiming to help you lose weight fast. While the proponents of these diets claim "one size fits all"—that their diet will work for anyone and everyone—recent research is beginning to put a damper on these claims. Keep in mind, research indicates that these "one-size-fits-all" diets may actually be harmful to your health.

The number one principle of any diet should be "do no harm" to the body. I never recommend short-term, quick-fix, weight-loss diets because of their costs to your health in the form of chronic diseases. By eating the correct diet and engaging in the right levels of physical activity for your genotype, you can maintain a healthy body weight and reduce your risk of developing diet-related chronic illnesses, from heart disease to cancer.

Today we know that how our body processes fats, proteins, and carbohydrates is genetically guided. Given this knowledge, the Apo E Gene Diet is about recommending and implementing a comprehensive plan based on your individual Apo E genotype. It is specifically tailored to work in harmony with your own body chemistry. This plan recognizes that while food is a critical element in your health, other environmental factors—such as exercise and relaxation practices—are also of real significance and must also be tailored to suit your individual genotype.

While this program includes recommendations for optimizing the health of your entire environment—mind, body, emotions, and spirit—it is specifically your food environment that I will emphasize in this book. This is the area that I have found to be the most confusing and complex for people to grasp, largely because there is so much misinformation and so many misconceptions surrounding what is a "good" food and what is a "bad" food.

Even for those not following a faddish, one-size-fits-all diet, danger lurks for the uneducated consumer in the thousands of processed foods that contain artificial fats and other substances that our body cannot easily assimilate. Everyone should avoid highly processed and preserved foods. The farther away from its source a food has been processed, the more likely it is harmful to the body. Let's look at why.

Chapter Nine

GOOD FOOD, BAD FOOD

Eating the right diet for your Apo E genotype is one of the best investments you can make in your health; therefore, it is worth paying some serious attention to.

We have all heard the saying, "You are what you eat." Now more than ever, research shows how it could represent more truth than we ever thought. The food we eat today becomes the cellular makeup of our human tissue tomorrow—our food goes from our plates to our cells.

Consider this statement: "There are no naturally bad foods." I first heard this from a doctor during my Integrative Medicine fellowship. My first reaction was one of denial—there must be bad foods! Our system is loaded with them! Walk into any supermarket and you are bedazzled with all types of substances we call food but that are so highly processed only a trace of any "whole" or "natural" food remains in them. Some people call this the SAD—Standard American Diet.

However, as I reflected on this and began to learn more, I finally decided the doctor was right. There are no naturally bad foods. It's what's done to them that makes them bad. In addition to across-the-board bad—highly processed—foods, different Apo E genotypes require differing amounts of fat, carbohydrate, and protein. I believe our genes have been selected by the lifestyles and environments of our past, largely as a survival mechanism.

Highly processed foods are a relatively recent addition to the human diet. Prior to their introduction, we ate whole grains, nuts, and fruits, and we occasionally consumed meat from wild or free-roaming animal sources that fed on native vegetation and provided more omega-3 fats than the omega-6 fats in our foods today. The local environment delivered these foods according to the season, and we ate the fruits and vegetables that grew in our villages and the wild animals that were indigenous to the area.

In today's mega-technological and rearranged world, it is important to ask: Has the integrity of my food intake diminished from that of my ancestors? Is my daily food intake good or bad for me? Do I even know what's good or bad for me?

Whole food is usually good food. Take wheat, for example. Whole grain wheat is an exceptionally good food, containing bran and the germ, which are the parts richest in nutrients, including B vitamins, folic acid, calcium, phosphorous, zinc, copper, and iron. However, what happens to wheat if it is highly processed or genetically modified? After it has been processed, washed, bleached, had man-made fats and preservatives added to it, then been raised and baked, this wheat ends up looking like fluffy white sponges. After all this processing we wrap the fluffy white sponges in plastic bags, add eye-catching colors, write compelling marketing messages on the wrappers, and place it on a shelf in the supermarket. We call this *bread*. This bread is not a whole food by any definition.

Have you ever wondered if there could be a possible connection between the present epidemic of food allergies and chronic illnesses and the practice of converting whole food into processed food? The fact is, we now *know* that processing food causes chronic illness and we must stop pretending otherwise.

Bread manufacturing is only one example of intensive food processing. The food industry is out of control, wantonly adding more and more harmful additives to an ever-growing range of foods. Where did this processing mania originate? I think it is largely the profit motive of megabusiness and its ability to apply technology to our food without considering the ramifications to our health. And as long as we buy the foods, the corporations get the message that we want them and continue to expand their repertoire of processed foods.

The U.S. food supply has largely been taken over by a special interest group of a few huge corporations, focused entirely on maximizing their profits. One of their means of maximizing profits is to "refine" natural foods by taking out their most nutritious components (because they spoil more quickly) and adding back some of what was removed artificially, calling the product "enriched," plus adding preservatives and other chemicals. The end result is good looking, "tasty," but nutritionally deficient pseudo-food that will have a long shelf life and sell well.

Some of the common methods of food preservation—drying, pickling, and curing—are almost as old as humanity. Before the advent of commercial operations, canning and preserving foods was done at home in America and other parts of the world. As the commercial canning and preserving industry grew in the 1950s, and processed foods got cheaper, a family tradition lost its appeal.

We began to make changes in how we stored our food years ago. With the advent of technology, we became much more efficient at preserving and processing through the use of various chemicals and radiation. Most recently on the scene is genetic manipulation via the technology of genetically modified organisms (GMO). This means that the genes of plants are being genetically engineered to delay ripening and make them last longer, among other things.

Even before GMO technology, plant breeders were creating hybrids that are resistant to the usual bruising of shipping and handling, such as the now-ubiquitous "taste-free" tomato that can be stacked 12 deep in a shipping crate without damaging the ones on the bottom. Most consumers' willingness to buy into this lower-cost system has made it increasingly difficult to get access to natural whole foods because they are grown by relatively more expensive labor-intensive methods.

Our natural food sources have given way to a world of highly processed, adulterated foods with multiple man-made substance and chemicals added to them. We do not know the full impact of many of these materials on the human body, but what we do know is not good.

Toxins and Processed Foods

Besides the food itself being toxic and the huge number of chemicals added to it as it is processed, most commercially grown foods come to us with residues of pesticides.

Consider the food chain where animals, including humans, are eating other animals. We are familiar with how mercury concentrates in fish as it moves from those lower on the food chain up to the fish we eat. The same is true with farmed animals, whose food source has been highly manipulated through changed farming practices at all levels. Whenever we consume conventional meats and fish, our bodies are being exposed to the toxic substances in that animal flesh. For many people, this may be as often as two or three times a day. The risk of chronic disease through the ingestion of toxic animal flesh can be greatly decreased both by switching from a diet high in animal protein to one of organic plant-based foods with some organically produced meats if desired.

Say No to These Substances!

Our planet's environment has been severely manipulated and is completely different from that of just two generations ago. Of course, the same is true of the food we eat. These altered foods have been implicated as factors helping to cause a host of illnesses, from the escalating rates of obesity to heart disease. Identifying toxic ingredients in our food is a big job and can be a very confusing process—even for medical professionals, scientists, and nutritionists. The first line of defense: When reading a food label, if you don't know or recognize the ingredients, don't eat the food! Another helpful tip is to not purchase anything in a box or container that lists unpronounceable ingredients or has more than four chemical additives. The second consideration is to eat unprocessed foods as often as possible. Third, consider the source of *everything* you eat and drink, not only foods, but also your fluids, including water.

Our foods contain a lot of harmful chemicals that can seriously damage our health if consumed frequently over long periods of time. The body can handle an occasional exposure, but with more than this it becomes very tired while trying to clear these chemicals. Some of us have the ability to clear these abnormal toxins more easily than others, but they still add up and take a toll.

One could generate an extremely long list of toxic chemical substances that should be avoided. The following partial list provides you with a good starting point of substances to consider avoiding.

- man-made fats, especially hydrogenated vegetable oil
- any food containing heavy metals such as fish with high mercury content
- agricultural pesticides
- hormones
- herbicides
- fungicides
- insecticides
- any artificial foods

- artificial colorings (especially Blue #1 and 2, Green #3, Red #2, 3 and 40, Yellow #5 and 6)
- potassium bromate
- processed vegetable oil
- artificial flavorings
- MSG (monosodium glutamate)
- all artificial sweeteners, including aspartame, saccharin, sucralose (Splenda), cyclamate
- hydrolysate invert sugar
- lactitol
- maltitol
- sorbitol
- brominated vegetable oil
- butylated hydroxyanisole (BHA)
- butylated hydroxytoluene (BHT)
- highly refined corn syrup and corn oil
- dextrose (corn sugar, glucose)
- high-fructose corn syrup
- hydrogenated starches
- mannitol polydextrose

So What Can We Do?

Now that we have apparently created a huge range of health problems for ourselves by learning to process, preserve, and genetically alter food at high levels, how do we get back to finding and eating healthy, whole food?

Should we be processing our food as much as we do, even altering the genetic makeup of the food itself? While some of us are debating whether or not changing food at the genetic level is a good idea, most people are not even *aware* that they are buying and eating genetically altered food.

I encourage you to educate yourself, your friends, and your family with regards to processed and GMO foods. Moving beyond the processing and preserving of food into changing the genetic makeup of the food itself is a big, scary step for humankind. I believe that invading the genes of plants to alter an entire food source is putting the health of the world at risk, since there is no definitive research on what these genetic modifications do to the person consuming them.

Alternatives to these chemicals are natural herbs and spices, and food colorings from plants, flowers, fruits, and vegetables. In addition, staying with organic unprocessed whole foods can help eliminate the ingestion of the above harmful chemicals.

Whole food should stay whole, unrefined, unprocessed, and unaltered genetically until we know for sure that it is not bad for us. The lack of evidence of harm does not equal evidence of no harm.

While it is true that whole food, in its raw state, can taste bland compared to highly seasoned and augmented processed food, this is because the bland has become familiar. Once your taste buds have become accustomed to processed food, you must adapt back to the taste of natural whole foods to maximize your health. This will take some time, on average three to four weeks, or maybe a few months— and then you will wonder how you ever ate all that highly processed stuff!

Here are some websites where you can learn more about the impact of, and options in, food preserving and processing:

www.centerforfoodsafety.org

www.thecampaign.org

www.seedalliance.org

www.ecoliteracy.org/programs/rsl.html

www.saynotogmos.org

www.thefutureoffood.com

www.cropchoice.com

www.ucsusa.org

www.organicconsumers.org

www.rethinkingschoollunch.org

www.calgefree.org

Your health is everything! Although the intention behind modifying, processing, and preserving foods may initially have been a good one, the food industry has taken these practices to the extreme. Why? Because they can, and because they want the profits, which gives them more money to develop the technology and machines to take it to ever more extreme levels. As long as megabusiness knows we will buy their "foods," they will be produced and the standard American diet will persist. We each have a responsibility to vote "No!" to these foods with our every food purchase.

Always keep in mind that there are no naturally bad foods. It is what commercial entities are doing to natural foods and how we expose those foods to our body that makes them bad or good. Food processing and modifying may now be costing us more in disease treatment than the time and money it was supposed to save.

A "Normal" Day's Diet

At this point I want to highlight commonly eaten foods that we don't normally associate with disease. Let's assume for a moment that you are a typical person who eats breakfast, lunch, and dinner. Most of the foods you eat are from your local supermarket, and you buy the "regular" food, nothing fancy. Here then, is a typical food and supplement log of one of my own patients.

Breakfast   cereal, with banana and milk
              toast and coffee
              one vitamin
              one over-the-counter, slow-release niacin tablet

The cereal is likely to be low fiber and processed, containing some form of preservatives. The regular milk contains antibiotics and hormones, and its saturated fat content can often be higher than people realize—2% milk is not 2 percent fat, it is 38 percent fat by volume, and whole milk is much higher in fat. The banana (unless it's organic) probably contains some form of chemical sprayed on it as a pesticide. The toast (usually highly processed white bread) contains preservatives, and the coffee (unless grown organically) could contain added harmful chemicals, and there is some evidence that decaffeinated coffee can raise cholesterol levels. The over-the-counter slow-release niacin tablet to help with high cholesterol was found to contain trans fat to slow the absorption of the niacin. We'll talk more about trans fats, but for now, believe me, this trans fat causes far more harm than the niacin does good.

Decaf Coffee May Increase Disease Risk

Drinking a few cups of decaf every day may increase the risk for metabolic syndrome, a group of several conditions that occur together and may increase risk of heart disease, stroke, and diabetes. Metabolic syndrome is the combination of increased blood pressure, elevated insulin levels, and excess body fat around the waist, all of which can lead to abnormally high cholesterol levels. Having just one of these conditions increases risk of heart disease, and having more than one makes that risk even greater.

A 2005 study funded by the National Institutes of Health and conducted by Robert Superko, MD, showed that decaf coffee drinkers had higher levels of the laboratory marker for metabolic syndrome called Apo B and for nonesterified fatty acids (NEFA), which have been identified as playing a role in heart attacks.

The three-month "Coffee and Lipoprotein Metabolism Study" showed that only drinkers of decaffeinated coffee, and not those who abstained from coffee or those who drank only the caffeinated type, had an 8 percent increase in Apo B levels and an 18 percent increase in NEFA. In short, the cholesterol levels of the decaf drinkers rose.

Superko said the difference could be related to the beans used for decaf and regular coffee. Harsher beans are used for decaf so that they can retain enough flavor in the process used to remove the caffeine. The harsher beans contain more of a substance called deptines, which may cause the rise in NEFA, which then results in more Apo B.

Snack   candy bar
        soda

Candy bars typically contain large amounts of trans and saturated fats as well as sugar and high fructose corn syrup, artificial food colorings and preservatives. The soda contains artificial flavorings and coloring, plus either loads of sugar or artificial sweeteners, and the coffee contains caffeine and any chemicals used to process it, plus any sweeteners and fat from cream or creamer.

Lunch   chicken sandwich and chips
                soda

The chicken likely was fed genetically modified food, and probably hormones to make it fatter. Other chemicals, drugs, and pesticides were likely added to its diet as well. Potato chips are processed potatoes fried in a wide variety of fats, many of which go rancid quickly, which makes normally healthy fats toxic to the body, and loaded with salt and preservatives. Soda usually contains corn sweeteners or artificial sweeteners, artificial flavorings, and coloring.

Dinner   hamburger, fries, and a salad
                soda
                ice cream

Much of this meal's nutritional content depends on whether it was home cooked or from a fast food outlet. The beef can contain saturated and trans fat, the fries are usually fried in trans fat, and the soda contains the same toxic brew mentioned above. While the salad can be healthy if organic vegetables and a healthy dressing are used, it's likely that this isn't the case, particularly if the salad comes from a fast-food restaurant. The ice cream usually contains saturated fat from full-fat cow's milk or cream, sugar, plus artificial flavorings and colors.

The above diet can be extremely toxic to the your body, yet it's very common with many people. Just seeing the type and amount of fat alone in this one-day food log is cause for concern. It reveals a very high exposure to inflammatory fats, which cause inflammation in the body's cells.

As already noted, if you are an Apo E 4, clearing this type of toxic fat is very difficult. While it may take many years of chronic exposure to these toxins to develop disease, an individual who takes in a moderate to high level of these unnatural foods will likely develop disease much sooner than someone who doesn't. On the other hand, *with a diet of completely natural foods, the risk of disease is greatly reduced, or even eliminated in many cases.* Knowing this, we, as a society, must ask ourselves some crucial questions:

- What does defective food do to the minds, emotions, bodies, and spirits of our growing children?
- How do these toxins affect us, the adults?
- Are the long-term effects now showing up in the older members of the population?

While we don't have complete answers to these questions, we do know that the body can handle occasional exposure to these toxic chemistries. It is when we expose our bodies to them over and over again that we put ourselves in distress, which leads to disease. If the intake of toxic food continues for a long time, the body can accumulate so much damage that it may have a difficult time recovering.

The human body can be very forgiving and can also change from dis-ease to ease, if given the right fuel. Many patients recover from chronic illness by giving their body what it needs (natural, whole food), and leaving the rest to the body's 100,000 year old internal healing system.

Toxins, Genotype, and Toxin-Clearing Abilities

One man's meat is another mans poison.
—Anonymous

First, let's define what I mean by a toxin. A toxin is a chemical or substance that brings imbalance to the body's cells, creating an adverse environment. Toxins are a poison, but not the same as arsenic or strychnine. Rather, they can be ordinary foods that act as poison to a particular genotype over a long period of time, simply because the foods are wrong for that type. There are many different kinds of food and food sources that can cause harm to the body, if your body is so predisposed.

The standard American diet delivers high amounts of inflammatory fat, usually more frequently than once in every 24- to 48-hour period. These fats, when eaten in excessive amounts, cause long-term inflammation that block the normal functioning of cells by limiting the delivery of nutrition into the cell membrane. The resulting cellular imbalances can bring about many major chronic illnesses.

Each Apo E genotype combination differs in its ability to clear toxic substances from the body. Educating ourselves to the capabilities of the different genotypes enables us to be more aware of our vulnerabilities to various food toxins. We can then use this information to better protect our bodies.

As we saw earlier, we each have one of the six possible combinations, or genotypes, of the Apo E genes we inherited from our parents. Our genotype determines our body's specific ability to handle toxins from our food: the Apo E 2 genotype provides the most ability to clear them; the Apo E 3 has a more limited ability; and Apo E 4 has a very limited, to no ability at all, to clear toxic substances absorbed from our diet.

The Apo E 4 gene prevents the body's systems from processing certain fats in the diet in a regular and consistent manner. If there are two copies of the Apo E 4 gene present, then you should follow the rules for the 4/4 gene, which includes not exposing your body's cells to any inflammatory fat and proteins that cannot be cleared. As we have seen, bad fat, such as trans fat and saturated fat, causes an accelerated inflammatory response in the body, especially with an Apo E 4.

Many patients with Apo E 4/4 have cholesterol levels in the high 300s to high 400s, with some reaching the 500s. Adhering to the correct diet, and allowing time for the body to recover between exposures, lowers those high cholesterol levels.

The Apo E 3/3 is considered the "normal" Apo E genotype, whose ability to clear and use most fats and proteins is not hindered, but even the Apo E 3/3, with excessive exposure to saturated and trans fats, will have difficulty clearing them. Too much exposure to saturated and trans fats in a 24-hour period may pose problems for the body, and as we will see in Chapter 9, it definitely increases bad cholesterol (LDL) and lowers good cholesterol (HDL). However, apply the correct diet for this genotype, allowing ample time between meals containing inflammatory fats and proteins for them to be processed by the body, and a person's LDL and HDL will become normal.

It has been proven repeatedly that individuals with any of the Apo E 4 combinations will respond better to dietary changes than the other genotypes will. Also, people with the Apo E 2/2 or 2/3 combination are more likely to respond better to moderately higher fat diets, while Apo E 4/4 and 4/3 respond better to low-fat diets. The right balance needs to be provided for each genotype. Keep in mind that:

- The toxicity of our body can be influenced by the individual Apo E. This means bodies differ in their ability to clear toxic chemicals and substances.
- The Apo E 4/4 has limited to almost no ability to eliminate processed foods and toxic chemicals.

Enhancing the Body's Toxin-Clearing Abilities

The following list contains recommendations for behaviors that will enhance your body's ability to clear toxins.

- Avoid foods contaminated with chemicals.
- Avoid refined and processed vegetable oils.
- Avoid processed grains in snack foods.
- Avoid margarine, vegetable shortening, and products made with partially hydrogenated oils.
- Avoid any toxic chemicals and substances that can cause cell inflammation and increase toxic tissue levels.
- Avoid a contaminated water source (including chlorine, heavy metals, and pesticides).
- Identify your body's ability to clear toxic foods and chemicals by knowing your Apo E genotype.
- Help your body clear toxins by getting regular exercise and not consuming excessive calories.
- Always ask questions about the food that is going into your mouth—and body.
- Avoid excessively large portions.
- Choose organic foods and organic farming processes.
- Support the whole-foods industry.
- Support school system education regarding healthy foods.
- Support accurate nutritional education for doctors, pharmacists, teachers, and the representatives of the food industry.
- Believe that whole, healthy food can be a way of life again—safe, delicious, convenient, and affordable—and a win-win for all.

Chapter Ten

FAT CITY

There are many types of fats in our food—ranging from the essential to the disease-promoting. The fats we choose to consume are a primary factor in determining our state of health, and yet we are very confused about fats. So, here is a full chapter looking at this element of our diet. It also includes information on how bad fats cause inflammation and how to prevent it.

Sources of fats in our diet include:

- nuts and seeds
- fruits and vegetables
- fish
- dairy products
- animal proteins

As we just saw in The Big Three, fat is an excellent source of long-term fuel because of its biochemical complexity. Fat is involved in cell protection and communication and is also a major component of cell membranes, which serve as storage tanks for our fatty acids. These storage tanks are important in the production of our hormone messengers that direct the body's immune system responses. They may contain either inflammatory or anti-inflammatory fats, and if we do not eat healthy fats that can be stored, we may die of disease.

Essential fatty acids are vital to health. They cannot be made in the body, so they have to be eaten regularly. If you attempt to remove all fat from your diet, you will become very sick in a relatively short period of time. If you consume too much fat, your body is more than likely to become overfueled and overfed, and much of it will probably cause chronic low-grade inflammation.

When the body is fed a fat it doesn't recognize, or that it has to work very hard to break down—processed, saturated, and trans fats—it produces biochemical waste and inflammatory proteins. It must then deal with this waste because it is toxic to the cells. Forced into a state of toxic stress overload, the body is also deficient in the essential fatty acids it needs to operate properly—not a healthy situation.

The common types of fats found in our diet (grouped by inflammatory level with apologies to Clint Eastwood) are:

The Good

- monounsaturated fats
- polyunsaturated fats

The Bad

- excessive saturated fats
- excessive cholesterol

The Ugly

- trans fat

Fats, Inflammation, and the Immune System

For optimal cellular health and functioning of our immune system, we need to consume mainly fats that don't trigger an immune system response of inflammation—what I call the anti-inflammatory fat sources, such as unprocessed monounsaturated and polyunsaturated. Consuming fats from a source the body can recognize and use promotes a proper immune response to:

- physical trauma
- viral, bacterial, and fungal infection
- allergies
- toxic chemical exposure

How well our immune system works depends partly on the type of long-term and short-term fuel sources it has presently and what was stored in prior times. Inflammation is a natural part of the body's internal healing system, but when it becomes chronic the body has a difficult time clearing the inflammatory substances and, as a result, produces a chronic reactive immune response such as:

- increased fever
- increased pain response
- increased tissue fluid retention
- narrowing of the blood vessels
- decreased circulation
- increased blood clot formation

A standard American diet of pro-inflammatory fats, carbohydrates, and proteins can easily be translated into coronary artery disease, vascular disease, psychological diseases such as mood disorders and depression, autoimmune disease, and even cancer. All Apo E genotypes are prone to disease states from pro-inflammatory fat intake, but Apo E 4s show a greater risk. On the other hand, a diet of anti-inflammatory nutrients, such as those of the Apo E Gene Diet, encourages normal cell function, normal immune system function, decreased inflammatory response, and total well-being.

With a better diet we see improved body functions such as breathing and lung function, relaxed blood vessel walls and better circulation, reduced clot formation, improved joint function, normal stomach and intestinal functions, and better muscular movement with reduced musculoskeletal pain.

APO E GENE DIET
Dietary Environment with Immune System Response

Human cells are made up of fat, and fat is essential for healthy cell function and life. Fat plays a role in cell protection, communication, nutrition intake, and waste removal. In addition, the brain is approximately 60% fat. Humans receive fat from their diet.

The Apo E gene can either provide:

CELL "DIS – EASE": Gene unsupportive environmental (GUE) (A commonly consumed American Diet)

Fats from omega 6's, saturated fat, and trans fat impair good health by providing a cell with the wrong long-term fuel source. This creates a gene-unsupportive environmental (GUE).

Immune System Environment Stimulus

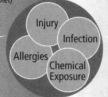

Injury

Infection

Allergies

Chemical Exposure

CELL "EASE: Gene supportive environment (GSE)

Fats from omega 3's, GLA, EPA, DHA, and monounsaturated fat support good health by providing a cell with a source of long-term fuel it can recognize and use. This creates a gene-supportive environment (GSE).

When the immune system is activated by brief or chronic inflammation, allergic reaction, cellular injury, infection, or chemical exposure, fatty acids are released and changed into an immune system messenger or cytokine called eicosanoids. If the correct fatty acids are not available or the body doesn't recognize the type of fat, the body produces inflammatory eicosanoids. If essential fatty acids are released, the body produces anti-inflammatory chemistry that helps optimal immune function.

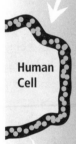

Human Cell

Inflammatory producing fats

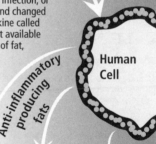

Human Cell

Anti-inflammatory producing fats

Lox Enzyme	Cox Enzyme	Cox Enzyme	Lox Enzyme	Cox Enzyme	Cox Enzyme
LTB-4	**TXA-2**	**PGE-2**	**LTB-5**	**PGE-3**	**PGE-1**
Increases amount and length of inflammation, especially in the lungs and airways	Narrows blood vessels Decreases circulation, increased blood clot formation	Increases ,tissue fluid retention, pain response Narrows airways , decreases circulation increased blood clot formation	Provides optimal blood vessel function, circulation, airway relaxation, providing proper anti-inflammatory response.	Provides optimal blood vessel function circulation, reduced pain response, leading to proper anti-inflammatory response.	Provides optimal muscle function, reduced blood clot formation. Optimal gastro-intestinal function, and improved circulation.

PRODUCES INFLAMMATORY CELLULAR CHEMISTRY

PRODUCES ANTI-INFLAMMATORY CELLULAR CHEMISTRY

The Good: Fats that Decrease Inflammation in the Body

Certain fats, namely unprocessed monounsaturated and polyunsaturated fats, have been shown to decrease inflammation in the body. The body easily recognizes and uses these fats.

Monounsaturated Fats

Monounsaturated fats are the simplest of fats. They are anti-inflammatory if they have not been processed.

Sources of monounsaturated fats include:

- olives and olive oil
- avocados
- canola oil
- palm fruit
- peanut oil

Polyunsaturated Fats

Polyunsaturated fats are also anti-inflammatory, as long as they have not been processed. The essential polyunsaturated fat groups are primarily the omega-3s and 6s.

What Are Omega-3 Fatty Acids?

Omega-3 fatty acids are polyunsaturated fats the body cannot do without. They are a good source of long-term fuel and need to be included in the daily diet.

When you move from a diet of saturated and trans fat to a diet of unprocessed polyunsaturated and monounsaturated fats, the body becomes much more efficient at using fat and produces a lower cholesterol level.

When you change to a diet of unprocessed monounsaturated and polyunsaturated fats, you need to consider eating good fat at most meals. Why? Since your body is now able to recognize and use these essential fats, they get used more quickly, hence the need to eat the correct fat percentages for your Apo E genotype with most meals.

Omega-3 fats come mainly from fish and meats. Additional food sources include:

- canola
- walnuts
- soybeans

- flaxseed

- ocean-borne algae

- whole grains

- very dark green leafy vegetables

If you take it in supplement form—capsule or liquid—know the quality and source. Consider only a fish oil source from wild fish and avoid highly processed supplements. Always follow a medical provider's dosage recommendations for omega-3 fatty acid. I currently recommend omega-3 supplements in dosages ranging from 0.133 grams per day to just over 2 grams per day, but prefer that people get their omega-3s directly from fresh food. Further, I recommend a customized combination of EPA and DHA. Your customized dosing should be discussed with your medical provider.

What Are Omega-6 Fatty Acids?

Just like omega-3s, the omega-6 fatty acids are vital to health. They are usually found in our diet in large amounts and are really not difficult to obtain from common food sources.

Sources of omega-6 fatty acids include:

- nuts

- seeds

- corn

- soy

- safflower

- palm fruit

- canola

- cottonseed

- meats

What Are Omega-9 Fatty Acids?

Omega-9 (oleic acid) is another form of important fatty acids also vital to health. Omega-9 is a monounsaturated fat and can be found in safflower, pumpkin, flaxseeds, and black currants.

The optimal balance between omega-3 and omega-6 fatty acids appears to be a ratio of 1:1 to 1:3–4. Practically speaking, it can be difficult to translate those ratios into our daily food consumption. However, if you stay with non-processed foods, you'll get a more balanced ratio of omega-3 to 6s since higher amounts of omega-6s come from processed foods and cooking oils.

The Bad: Saturated Fats

Primarily found in animal proteins and some vegetable sources, saturated fats can be a powerfully damaging food, more so from some sources than others. However, given the fact that human breast milk contains saturated fat, I do not think that all saturated fat sources have negative effects on the body. Saturated fat is a very concentrated source of fuel, and different types of saturated fat, coming from animal sources especially, have been linked definitively to very high levels of inflammation and disease, especially when we overexpose our bodies more than once in a 24-hour period.

High amounts of saturated fat can cause a rapid increase in the inflammatory process soon after it's eaten. Beginning in the mouth and moving all the way through the digestive tract, this inflammation can end up in the smallest systems of the human cell.

Sources of highly-concentrated saturated fat include:

- cream and all milk except skimmed
- cheese
- lard
- butter, regular ice cream (made from cow milk fat)
- meats (beef, chicken, turkey, pork, lamb)
- processed meats
- coconut oil
- cottonseed oil
- palm seed oil (not the palm fruit)
- chicken fat
- ghee (used in Indian food)

Cholesterol

A related type of lipid, or fat, in our diet is cholesterol, which is found in many foods that also contain fats. We need cholesterol but should avoid excessive amounts of it. Cholesterol occurs naturally in the body and is also absorbed from food. An average body produces around 800–1000 mg of cholesterol and takes in an additional 200–300 mg from food. We need this cholesterol to create and maintain cell membranes, break down fats, and absorb vitamins (especially Vitamin D).

Cholesterol also plays a role in the production of bile and of hormones such as cortisol, aldosterone, progesterone, estrogen, and testosterone. In the brain, cholesterol assists in the maintenance of nerve synapses. Cholesterol also plays an important role in our immune system.

Sources of highly-concentrated cholesterol include:

• eggs

• dairy products

• animal meats, both lean and fat

• organ meats

• lard

The Ugly: Trans Fats

The trans fats in the standard American diet are especially damaging. These mostly man-made fats actually begin as an unsaturated fat, usually a vegetable oil, which is mixed with hydrogen gas and platinum catalysts, then heated to temperatures in excess of 500° F to make it more solid and to give it a longer shelf life. This recipe results in changing the molecular makeup of healthy fatty acids into disfigured, twisted molecules—trans fat—often listed on food labels as hydrogenated fats or oils. Serve them hot or cold, and your body will deliver this toxic, inflammatory mixture to every cell in your body, including your brain cells. Chronic exposure to man-made trans fat found in thousands of processed foods from salad dressings to snacks, margarines to cake mixes can be very toxic to everyone, but extremely toxic to Apo E 4s. It is very difficult for the body to get rid of these types of molecules once they are incorporated in its cellular structure, and this can cause severe chronic disease states.

One of the reasons we have so much trans fat in our diet is due to a very powerful consumer interest group that campaigned to remove saturated fat and palm seed oil from our food. The drive in the early 1980s to remove saturated fats led to the food processors using something even worse—trans fat, but in the early 1990s we began to realize the damage it causes. In January 2006 we saw even more subversive uses of trans fat via legislation with a labeling loophole allowing foods less than 0.5 mg per serving of fat to be labeled *nonfat*. This means that you can still get a dose of trans fat in your "0" trans fat-labeled food. Best read the label and the ingredients!

While trans fat has been produced and used in food for more than 100 years, we still have much to learn about its effects on the development of cell membranes, brain cells, arterial inflammatory plaque development, and growing fetal brain tissue. We do know that our body manufactures cell membranes from the fats we eat, so if our diet is high in inflammatory fats, we are creating defective cell membranes, hormones, and brain cells.

Could this be why we have so much brain pathology, with severe neurological diseases such as Alzheimer disease and Parkinson disease? We do not yet have conclusive evidence, but logic tells us this could be a cause. Once again, we need to take precautions by removing these fats from our diet. Remember that no evidence of harm is not equal to evidence of no harm.

The food processing industry is very powerful. As long as using trans fat saves money, increases food shelf life, and provides more flavor, they will continue to use the hydrogen process, unless forced to stop.

As a medical practitioner on the front lines, I say let logic prevail! We all need to learn more about food so we can make better food choices. Education is our best weapon. Toward the end of your life, it will be your long-term food choices that determine whether you will be playing with backpacks or bedpans. As a consumer, you can change the way the food industry produces the foods you purchase. The choice is simple—don't buy foods with inflammatory trans fats in them. As Marion Nestle, PhD, MPH, author of *Food Politics: How the Food Industry Influences Nutrition and Health* and *What to Eat*, says, "Vote with Your Fork." I agree with Marion, because behind your fork is green power—money!

Important sources of trans fat to avoid include:

- stick margarine
- deep-fried fast food
- commercial cookies
- crackers
- commercial dessert pastries such as pies and cakes
- sports drinks (a popular brand added a "Z factor," which turned out to be trans fat)

How to Avoid Trans Fat

Knowing that trans fat can be hidden, read the ingredient list, not just the percentage of fat on the front. Choose foods that do not contain "vegetable shortening," "partially hydrogenated," or hydrogenated fats and oils. Avoid deep-fried foods from restaurants, fast-food chains, and school kitchens.

Students may want to do a small research project of asking the cooks in their school cafeteria what kind of oil they use in the deep fryers and how often they change it. Is it healthy oil, like canola, or not, like shortening? Do the cooks change it once a day, once a week, once a month, or once a semester? Any cooking oil will oxidize and become rancid (toxic to the body) when exposed to light and heated, but the more unsaturated it is, the more quickly this happens. Therefore, while the cafeteria should be using healthy oils, these oils also need to be changed frequently. You may find that the oil your lunch is cooked in is being changed a lot less often than you think—possibly once a month or even once a semester. Shocking, isn't it! Request that the oil is changed daily.

Consciously purchase lower-fat baked chips and trans fat-free crackers, cookies, pastries, and other processed foods. Use olive or canola oil instead of butter, margarine, or shortening. Foods that are marketed as "cholesterol free," "low cholesterol," "low in saturated fat," or "made with vegetable oil" are not necessarily low in trans, hydrogenated, or partially hydrogenated fats. Once again, read the label and be informed.

In 2004, one of my patients showed me a very popular sports drink bottle and said, "Pam, does this drink have trans fat in it?" My response was "no," but I had never read the label. The bottle he handed me, with "0" fat grams in the nutritional facts, listed partially hydrogenated vegetable oil plus many types of preservatives and artificial dyes. The brand is now being marketed under a new name with flavors such as lemon-lime and strawberry. Their market is our children, and the ads imply "drink enough of this drink and you will look like a professional sports player."

This patient, a world-class triathlete, had made a trip to my office to bring me this information and was understandably very upset. His concern was that this company, involved in every sport as a major drink supplier for better sports performance, is now using trans fat in its products and marketing it to athletes and to parents who give it to their children.

The moral of the story is: *read the label,* for both the nutritional facts and the ingredients. If you find inflammatory ingredients on the label, don't buy them!

Garbage In = Garbage Out (GIGO)

When any digested food enters the intestines, the body is smart enough to recognize the quality of the nutrients and decide if those nutrients should be used, stored, or excreted. A little known fact about fats is what happens after they are stored and then later removed from the body's internal storage tanks to be metabolized as fuel.

Often a person will wise up to the bad fats they've been eating, clean up their diet, and begin to lose weight. What will happen, often unexpectedly, is that all the stored toxic fats with their inflammatory components are released into the body and metabolized, causing the same negative effects as when they first entered the body. It can take many months before all these stored inflammatory fats are removed, so be patient with any symptoms that persist after you have removed the bad fats from your diet. Remember, the garbage you ate and stored will still be garbage on its way out of your body. Keep in mind, though, that it is a finite amount and will be gone when you've emptied those storage tanks. The reverse is true if the stored fats are anti-inflammatory (mono- and polyunsaturated); they will be released and help reduce any inflammation present.

The American Heart Association (AHA) recommends that saturated and trans fat intake not exceed 10 percent of total calories each day for healthy people and 7 percent for those with cardiovascular disease, diabetes, or high cholesterol.

How Much Protein Do We Need?

We can thank Dr. Atkins for his contribution to nutritional medicine, but think twice about his popular diet, especially if you carry an Apo E 4 genotype. Even if you are an Apo E 3 or Apo E 2, I recommend avoiding a high-protein, low-carbohydrate diet because this diet is pro-inflammatory. Keep in mind that animal protein comes packaged with inflammatory fats. You can avoid producing inflammation in your body if you stay away from a diet that consists of excess inflammatory protein and the "bad" fats.

As an integrative health care practitioner, I recommend that people who have liver or kidney disease consume a low-protein diet. In addition, the type of protein should come from milder vegetable sources (see below).

A normal person involved in a routine exercise program needs only 1.2–1.6 grams of protein per kilogram (2.2 pounds) of body weight. That translates into just 3–4 ounces of protein for a 160-pound person. Very few athletes need more. The reality of most protein sources is they include fat—either inflammatory or anti-inflammatory, as follows:

• Beans have protein and mostly *anti*-inflammatory fat.
• Nuts and seeds have protein and mainly *anti*-inflammatory fat.
• Fish has protein and mainly *anti*-inflammatory fat.
• Meat has protein and mainly inflammatory fat.
• Dairy contains protein and inflammatory fat.

The first three are ideal proteins with good, anti-inflammatory fat, which the body can use and eliminate easily.

The body does much better when its protein comes from vegetable sources that provide monounsaturated and polyunsaturated fat. Vegetable protein is better than animal sources because plant protein is a "weaker" form of protein that the body can handle more easily. Does this mean you shouldn't ever eat protein with saturated fat? No, but you need to be very careful how much and how often you do consume these complex sources. Depending on what Apo E genotype you are, this general rule can be defined even more closely:

Apo E 4s will do much better with plant protein and monounsaturated fats, than with animal protein and saturated and trans fats. This is doubly important because you need more time to clear (eliminate) fats, no matter what type of fat it is.

Even the most intense athletes require only a small amount of protein compared to what some fad diets recommend.

Milk Protein

What about milk? Milk is a food that contains protein, yet in its natural form, it's loaded with saturated fat, despite those low sounding 1%, 2%, and 4% fat numbers. Let's look at the real fat content, while not forgetting that milk contains animal saturated fat that is difficult for the body to clear, and that this type of animal fat has been found to cause inflammation in the human body.

Nonfat milk is not non-fat. The dairy industry has dubious standards for what can be called skim or nonfat milk. Many people think it has "no" fat. This is not true, as it is very difficult to remove all the fat from a product. Even skim milk is not totally void of fat, but because it is below the level requiring labeling (0.5 gram/serving) it is reported as fat-free. This is terribly misleading!

Whole milk is advertised as 4 percent fat by volume, but since most of the volume is water, this means that with all the fluid removed, what remains is 48 percent animal fat! What is called "2% milk" is actually 37.5 percent animal fat.

※

Chapter Eleven

INDIVIDUAL MEDICAL AND NUTRITIONAL RECOMMENDATIONS BASED ON APO E GENOTYPE

Now, let's look at some specific information on the benefits of a diet related to your Apo E genotype. Not all foods are created equal. Certain foods create a disease faster in some people than in others. Knowing how to feed your body based on your specific genotype is crucial to your good health. Remember, the Apo E gene directs your body's use of cholesterol and blood fat, so I strongly recommend you have your cholesterol and triglycerides evaluated at the same time as you are tested for Apo E genotype. As we saw in Chapter two, you should consider being tested for the seven subtypes of LDL (bad) cholesterol and the five subtypes of HDL (good) cholesterol. A complete advanced panel can be done to see the full picture of your blood chemistries, not just the tip of the iceberg, as we commonly see in routine screening. Let's look at recommendations for the six Apo E genotypes. Along with differing nutritional needs, genotypes vary with respect to recommended exercise programs, which I note in the following guidelines.

Recommendations for the Apo E 2/2 Genotype

Fat 35%   Protein 15%   Carbohydrate 50%

With a poor nutritional intake and unhealthy environment, this genotype can develop very high levels of cholesterol, triglycerides, and very low-density lipoproteins (vldl). A specific cholesterol condition called Type III high cholesterol is seen in this genotype. Typically, unless a person has a triglyceride level above 150 mg/dl this genotype has no problems. A high triglyceride level is likely to develop with 1) abnormal eating behaviors such as meal skipping or 2) a high body fat percentage from excessive calories and saturated/trans fat intake. In addition, overexposure to saturated fats and high exposure to polyunsaturated oils and margarines, coupled with excessive omega-6 sources, contribute to elevated triglyceride levels. When combined with excessive simple carbohydrate calorie intake along with little exercise, poor health will result. Alcohol is also a significant negative factor for this genotype. This genotype requires a very specific exercise program.

Use the following guidelines for your genotype:

- Make dietary changes slowly.
- Work with your medical provider to check your basic and advanced blood cholesterol and triglyceride levels.
- Be aware that a gene-supportive environment can prevent many chronic diseases, especially neurological ones.[7]
- Have a body composition test to evaluate your percentage body fat and lean mass.
- See page 138, Table 1: Exercise Recommendations for Each Apo E Genotype.

Recommendations for the Apo E 2/3 Genotype

Fat 30%   Protein 15%   Carbohydrate 55%

This genotype is considered a variant combination. We tend to see little dietary influence on bad cholesterol (LDL) levels unless the diet is high in calories from processed foods, inflammatory trans and saturated fats, and processed polyunsaturated fats. A highly inflammatory diet and lack of exercise increases the risk of heart disease.

---

7   Keeping in mind that protein and fat usually come packaged together, pay close attention to the recommended serving sizes, and leave an adequate amount of fat clearance time (24–48 hours) in between eating fish or any animal protein with high saturated fat content.

A significant negative risk factor for alcohol can also be seen with this genotype. Use the following guidelines for your genotype:

• Make dietary changes slowly.

• Work with your medical provider to check your basic and advanced blood cholesterol and triglyceride levels.

• Be aware that a gene-supportive environment can prevent many chronic diseases, especially neurological ones.[8]

• Have a body composition test to evaluate your percentage body fat and lean mass (page 227-228).

• See the exercise recommendations for this genotype in Chapter 12.

Recommendations for the Apo E 3/3 Genotype

Fat 25%   Protein 20%   Carbohydrate 55%

This genotype is considered the normal or neutral genotype and cannot tolerate either a low-fat or high-fat diet. Avoid excessive inflammatory fats. Leave 24 to 48 hours between meals of saturated fats for them to be cleared from your body. This genotype needs balance in both short-term (carbohydrate) and long-term (fat) fuels. Remember, all excess calories are stored as fat. Calories should match the body's ability to clear its fuel source. We tend to see metabolic disease when Apo E 3/3 patients fail to keep to a normally balanced diet and exercise.

Use the following guidelines for your genotype:

• Work with your medical provider to check your basic and advanced blood cholesterol and triglyceride levels.

• See the exercise recommendations for this genotype on Chapter 12).

---

8   Keeping in mind that protein and fat usually come packaged together, pay close attention to the recommended serving sizes, and leave an adequate amount of fat clearance time (24–48 hours) in between eating fish or any animal protein with high saturated fat content.

Recommendations for the Apo E 4/2 Genotype

Fat 25%   Protein 20%   Carbohydrate 55%

For Apo E 4s it is critical to limit all inflammatory trans fats and overexposure to saturated fats, polyunsaturated oils and margarines, and excessive omega-6 sources, utilizing instead monounsaturated and omega-3 fats.

Due to the combination of the 2 and the 4 genes, this genotype must balance between the contrasting needs of the two. With the presence of the Apo E 2, carbohydrate intake must be strictly limited to complex carbohydrates with low glycemic load. Fat and protein sources should be mainly monounsaturated and polyunsaturated fats. Plant protein should be considered over animal protein. It is extremely important for people with this genotype to use aerobic exercise to reduce stored body composition, or fat levels. These patients should work closely with a medical practitioner who is trained in advanced lipid disorders as well as exercise science or sports medicine and be regularly evaluated for all types of cholesterol and triglyceride markers. See specific aerobic versus anaerobic exercise recommendations for this genotype.

Use the following guidelines for your genotype:

• Make dietary changes slowly.

• Work with your medical provider to check your basic and advanced blood cholesterol and triglyceride levels.

• Be aware that a gene-supportive environment can prevent many chronic diseases, especially neurological ones.[9]

• Have a body composition test done to evaluate your percentage body fat and lean mass.

• See the exercise recommendations for this genotype in Chapter 12).

---

9   Besides the risk of cardiovascular disease, research shows an increased risk of developing Alzheimer disease with the presence of the Apo E 4 gene, but the gene alone should not be used to predict Alzheimer disease risk. Research has not shown that Apo E definitely causes Alzheimer disease. Many other factors are involved in the development of disease in this type, especially the nutritional environment. It appears to be not the gene that encourages a disease but the environment. Creating a gene-supportive environment is key to lowering risk.

Recommendations for the Apo E 4/3 Genotype

Fat 20%   Protein 25%   Carbohydrate 55%

With a higher caloric level, the percentages change, due to the body's inability to use more protein:

Fat 20%   Protein 20%   Carbohydrate 60%

Clearing fat and cholesterol from the body is hindered, so exposure to excess amounts of dietary fat and cholesterol causes stress that in turn pushes the body to produce too much LDL. Fat should come mainly from anti-inflammatory monounsaturated and polyunsaturated sources—those the body can recognize and use effectively.

It is extremely important for this genotype to use aerobic exercise to reduce stored fat levels. These people should work closely with a medical practitioner who has had additional training in advanced lipid disorders as well as exercise science and sports medicine. These patients should be regularly evaluated for all types of cholesterol and triglyceride markers. See specific aerobic versus anaerobic exercise recommendations for this genotype.

Use the following guidelines for your genotype:

• Make dietary changes slowly.

• Work with your medical provider to check your basic and advanced blood cholesterol and triglyceride levels.

• Be aware that a gene-supportive environment can prevent many chronic diseases, especially neurological ones.[10]

• Have a body composition test done to evaluate your percentage body fat and lean mass.

• See the exercise recommendations for this genotype on Chapter 12).

---

10   Pay close attention to the recommended serving sizes and leave adequate clearance time (24–48 hours) when a saturated fat has been consumed. This genotype combination contains an Apo E 4, so you need to be mindful when making fat and protein choices.

Recommendations for the Apo E 4/4 Genotype

This gene pattern of two 4s is a critical combination.

Fat 20%   Protein 25%   Carbohydrate 55%

As with the Apo E 4/3, with a higher caloric level, percentages change, due to the body's inability to use more protein:

Fat 20%   Protein 20%   Carbohydrate 60%

This genotype contains two variant 4s. Clearing fat and cholesterol from the body is hindered in the extreme, so any exposure to dietary fat and cholesterol causes stress that pushes the body to produce too much LDL. Fat sources should be primarily monounsaturated and non-processed polyunsaturated.

It is extremely important for this genotype to use aerobic exercise to reduce stored fat levels. These people should work closely with a medical practitioner who has had additional training in advanced lipid disorders as well as exercise science and sports medicine. These patients should be regularly evaluated for all types of cholesterol and triglyceride markers. See specific aerobic versus anaerobic exercise recommendations for this genotype.

Use the following guidelines for your genotype:

• Make dietary changes slowly.

• Work with your medical provider to check your basic and advanced blood cholesterol and triglyceride levels.

• Be aware that a gene-supportive environment can prevent many chronic diseases, especially neurological ones.[11]

• Have a body composition test done to evaluate your percentage body fat and lean mass.

• See the exercise recommendations for this genotype on Chapter 12).

Up-to-date information and self-education, coupled with good common sense, are important when considering any nutritional recommendations. As our body of knowledge grows, it is likely that dietary recommendations will change. The best defense against those that would have us believe that we cannot take care of our own health, is a good arsenal of facts. The one thing that will not change is the importance of common sense in any behavior change plan.

---

11   Pay close attention to the recommended serving sizes and leave adequate clearance time (24–48 hours) when a saturated fat has been consumed. This genotype combination contains an Apo E 4, so you need to be mindful when making fat and protein choices.

Diet, Hygiene, and Dental Health

The right Apo E Gene Diet contributes to healthy teeth and gums.

Gingivitis and periodontitis are conditions of tissue inflammation affecting the gums that cause pain and bleeding. These are commonly found with advancing age, but we are beginning to see this in younger people, I think due to the worsening of the standard American diet. The majority of dental disease, specifically gum disease, can actually be prevented by:

- practicing good daily oral hygiene
- obtaining regular professional dental care
- eating the right Apo E Gene Diet for your genotype

Chapter Twelve

MOVEMENT AND EXERCISE

It's time to move our focus from the dining table to moving our bodies! In this chapter I will identify the common elements of a safe and healthy exercise program. As with dietary guidelines, there are general guidelines. However, one plan does not fit all. If you know your Apo E genotype, you should ask for a personalized exercise prescription for your profile. It is important, whenever possible, to have the correct exercise routine prescribed for you based on your Apo E genotype, taking into account your current fitness level.

Sometimes it seems that I can't open a magazine, watch a television program, or do a search on the Internet without hearing of new "guidelines" for exercise and movement. It can get confusing. But researchers do agree that you should exercise most days, if not every day. The latest recommendation by the American Heart Association is to exercise a minimum of 30 to 60 minutes, three to six days a week.

When we look at the makeup of the physical body, we can see that it was built to move. Most of us move, in some way or other, every day. Not all of us move in the same way or at the same level. I will use the word "movement" here as an umbrella term to refer to activities of daily living or physically changing the position of the human body. I define "exercise" as a subset of movement, to mean the vigorous movement required of certain sports, the rare job requiring extensive physical effort, or a formal exercise routine.

We know that if the human body moves on a regular basis, it will be healthier. The health benefits don't just apply to the physical body but also to the emotions, mind, and spirit. I could easily include five full pages on the benefits of movement and exercise, but I think by mentioning just a few of these, you will agree that movement of the physical body is good for you.[12]

A Patient's Story: Lilian

Lilian was referred to me by her primary care doctor. She was 5' 4", weighed 103 pounds, and had high cholesterol and osteopenia (the precursor to osteoporosis). Several years earlier, she had received a diagnosis of fibromyalgia and depression, for which her doctor prescribed an antidepressant. However, Lilian did not like to take medication and so was not following her treatment plan.

After having many tests performed on recommendation of her primary care doctor, Lilian decided she was done with tests. But then she heard about the Apo E gene test and decided she wanted to know her Apo E genotype.

When she came to my office, I did a complete medical history and a physical. I asked her to keep a diet log for a week, and it revealed only minimal food intake, mostly at dinner, with some coffee and water during the day. Lilian told me she didn't like to eat during the day because she felt uncomfortable eating before exercise, which she did from two to five hours a day.

I suggested that her first step should be to try a normal anti-inflammatory diet. But she was adamant—she would make no changes in her diet or her exercise patterns. She just wanted to know her Apo E genotype. I gently tried to educate her further about this test and how it relates to diet and exercise, but she insisted that she would not make any changes to accommodate the results of the test.

Lilian suffered from depression and anxiety, not to mention some deeply rooted, abnormal dietary patterns that were more than likely contributing to her illnesses. She was eating too little in any case,

<hr>

12   An excellent resource for learning more about the benefits of physical activity is the American College of Sports Medicine, www.acsm.org.

which stressed her body, and then her over-exercising only made the situation worse. When the human body is pushed to these extremes, it's very common for extreme disease to develop.

I recommended some psychological counseling to help her discover the reasons for her extreme eating and exercise patterns, but Lilian was not interested. She continued to demand an Apo E test. In good conscience, I could not order it. What if she was an Apo E 4/4 and then was not willing to make any of the appropriate changes? I think such an outcome would have worsened her condition. With her mind-set regarding diet and exercise, she could have begun an even more extreme routine, which would have caused further harm.

Since I knew Lilian would not listen to me, I recommended she return to her primary care doctor for further direction. She clearly needed help with a strongly rooted alternative-eating pattern. I recommended to her doctor that she not be tested for her Apo E genotype but instead that she learn how to begin normal, healthy eating and exercise patterns through a consultation with an exercise physiologist and a registered dietician with special training in alternative eating patterns. I also recommended that Lilian begin working with a psychological counselor and also continue taking her antidepressant.

Perhaps Lilian would become a good candidate for Apo E testing later, but she clearly was not when I saw her.

Health Benefits of Exercise

Exercise keeps the body functioning at its best by aiding the use of fuel and removing excess waste. Movement helps the body function with ease. If we do not engage in enough movement, our body becomes susceptible to "dis-ease" and illnesses such as cardiovascular disease, dementia, Alzheimer disease, hypertension, diabetes, obesity, and the high multi-level inflammation process of arthritis. It has been shown that as little as 10 minutes of walking each day can help with the prevention of disease!

Exercise helps prevent the loss of cognitive abilities by increasing the body's internal brain chemicals such as morphine-like endorphins. The nervous system's performance is also enhanced by the increase of blood and oxygen flow, and by increasing growth factors that assist in the generation of new nerve cells. Many common chronic illnesses can be helped with just a small amount of regular movement and exercise.

Regular exercise can help prevent:

- premature death
- heart disease and stroke
- high blood pressure
- high cholesterol
- cancers such as colon and breast cancer
- diabetes
- non-insulin-dependent diabetes
- depression and anxiety
- sleep problems
- arthritis
- back pain, osteoporosis
- ADD/ADHD

Regular exercise can also:

- reduce or m aintain body weight or percentage of body fat
- build and maintain healthy muscles, bones, and joints by decreasing inflammation
- improve psychological well-being
- enhance work, recreation, and sport performance

As you can see, the benefits of exercise extend far beyond the usual weight loss goal. As a health-conscious nation, we need to understand and appreciate the many benefits of regular physical activity and know that the right movement and exercise program can help reduce our risk for chronic illness, which will in turn yield an overall improved quality of life.

Now we've seen the benefits of exercise, I hope you're ready to get involved! So let's look at the elements of a safe and healthy exercise program.

Elements of a Safe and Healthy Exercise Program

A safe and healthy excercise program is multi-faceted, sometimes requiring new clothing and shoes, learning new exercises, and establishing a new routine, to name a few. This section describes the following 12 elements:

- Professional Evaluation and Guidance
- Physiologic Changes Associated with Exercise
- Exercise, Clothing and Shoes
- How Often to Exercise
- Exercise Intensity
- Program and Progression Plan
- Warm-up and Cool-down
- Aerobic Exercise: A Walking Program
- Flexibility and Stretching Exercises (Yoga or Pilates)
- Logging Behavior Changes
- Avoiding Exercise Program Drop-out

Professional Evaluation and Guidance
I strongly recommend that when beginning an exercise program, you be evaluated and guided by a professional with knowledge of sports medicine. The providers most effective at exercise prescriptions are either licensed exercise physiologists or trained sports medicine nurse practitioners, medical doctors, or physical therapists who will probably work in collaboration with your primary care provider. The goal is to make sure your cardiovascular and muscular skeletal systems can tolerate increased activity and still provide excellent health.

You should consult a licensed exercise support person for a minimum of six months when beginning a new exercise program. They can be a vital component for exercise success and will:

- provide your exercise prescription
- guide your exercise progress
- deliver whatever exercise education is necessary to improve fitness
- encourage you in times when exercise motivation is low

Exercise Warning Signs

Before beginning an exercise program, learn some important exercise warning signs. Stop exercise immediately and seek medical care if you experience any of these symptoms:

- palpitations (irregular or rapid heartbeat)
- sudden increases in your stress levels
- disorientation or vision disturbances
- nausea or vomiting
- sudden clamminess and perspiration
- chest pains, aches, or pressure
- shortness of breath
- dizziness
- upset stomach

To determine the optimal exercise program for you, consider getting an evaluation for any of the following areas that are relevant to you:

- complete health history
- evaluation of current lifestyle
- supplement use
- psychological questionnaire
- dietary evaluation
- exercise history
- physical exam—all systems
- weight
- blood pressure
- heart rate
- strength test
- flexibility test
- BMI (body mass index) (see Chapter 17)
- body composition test (see Chapter 17)
- routine lab testing
- advanced genetic cholesterol tests (see Chapter 3)
- EKG

- VO2 max test
- cardiovascular test
- stress test

The above evaluations are highly recommended and may include some other screening tests as well.

Evaluating Your Overall Health

When you evaluate your overall health, you need to consider your current psychological health, cholesterol levels, inflammatory markers such as elevated C-reactive protein, fibrinogen, Lp-PLA2, glucose levels, insulin levels, Apo E genotype, and your body composition. Medical screening is strongly advised, including a full physical, with special attention to the body's energy, metabolism, and musculoskeletal and cardiovascular system. Until you have been completely examined and clinically evaluated, you will not know your level of risk for any potential or existing disease process—low, medium, or high risk. When evaluating body composition, it is very important to consider the human body's blood chemistry at the same time because an abnormal body composition can produce abnormal blood chemistries.

Physiologic Changes Associated with Exercise

There are many different types of physical exercise; they can be grouped into three general categories: aerobic (cardiovascular), anaerobic (strength training), and flexibility. Each yields different physiological changes in the human body. Performing these different types exercises daily, as determined by your Apo E genotype, changes the body's chemistry and affects the human cell in a positive way, by building better human tissue and yielding improved first cell health, tissue health and lastly organ health. This translates into improved health effects, not only on the physical body, but also the mind, and the spirit.

Aerobic Exercise

Aerobic exercise increases a persons heart rate and sustains the heart rate for a specific amount of time. Cardo-respiratory endurance exercising is a specific type of aerobic exercise that has the capacity to carry out large muscle, active, higher intensity exercises for longer time periods. Cardio-respiratory exercise is directly dependant on the condition and functioning state of the respiratory, cardiovascular, and muscular skeletal system. Walking, bike riding, running, and swimming are examples of aerobic exercise.

Physiological changes that occur with aerobic exercise include:

- increased maximal cardiac output
- increased blood volume and ability to carry oxygen
- reduced workload on the heart for any given sub-maximal exercise intensity
- increased blood supply to muscles and ability to use oxygen
- lower heart rate and blood pressure at any level of sub-maximal exercise
- lower resting systolic and diastolic blood pressure in people with high blood pressure
- increased HDL cholesterol
- decreased blood triglycerides
- reduced body fat and improved weight control
- improved glucose tolerance and reduced insulin resistance

Anaerobic (Muscular Strengthening and Endurance) Exercise

Anaerobic exercise increases and sustains a person's heart rate for short periods of time. This type of exercise refers to the capacity of the muscular system's movement and performance ability. Muscle strength or weakness is directly related to the maximum power or force that can be created by a specific muscle or group of muscles. Muscle endurance is the performance of a muscle contraction being repeated multiple times to satisfactorily produce muscle stress or fatigue, thereby producing a state of maximum voluntary contraction for a tolerated period of time. Weight lifting repetitions and sprinting are examples of anaerobic exercise.

Physiological changes that occur with anaerobic exercise include:

- improved flexibility
- decreased risk of musculoskeletal injury
- increased musculoskeletal performance
- improved postural stability/decreased risk of falls
- decreased muscle soreness with activity
- decreased risk of lower back pain
- improved muscle coordination

Flexibility Training

Flexibility training gives the body a greater range of motion (ROM) to move. This type of exercise refers to the body's ability to move a joint and all related tissue connected to a specific joint—tendons, ligaments, muscles, etc. Joint movement has a specific capacity of movement referred to as a range of motion or (ROM). Human flexibility is dependent on multiple factors—hormone levels, bone structure, joint capsule distensibility, size, length, strength of ligaments, muscles. Age and gender also play an important factor, especially in muscle strength and distensibility.

Physiological changes that occur with flexibility training include:

• improved flexibility
• decreased risk of musculoskeletal injury
• increased musculoskeletal performance
• improved postural stability/decreased risk of falls
• decreased muscle soreness with activity
• decreased risk of lower back pain
• improved muscle coordination

No matter where you are in your life—young or old—take time each day to move your body. If you devote as little as 10 minutes to moving your body, it will respond in health and happiness. Note that the best type of movement and exercise program for you can only be determined when you know your Apo E genotype.

Exercise, Clothing, and Shoes

Clothing and footwear should be correctly sized and comfortable. Dress according to the weather and temperature. If you think the temperature could change during your exercise session, dress in layers. Personally, I like to dress as warm as possible in the beginning phases of my exercise session and shed clothing as I go.

With every type of activity, having the proper equipment is important to reduce your chances of injury. Have your exercise specialist or a good podiatrist evaluate your natural foot position. This ensures that you get the correct type of shoe for your feet. Some shoe stores offer a foot evaluation, but I would go to a person who is well educated in exercise and exercise shoes.

How Often to Exercise

This needs to be determined by you, your Apo E genotype, and your exercise specialist. However, the new general recommendation is to 30 to 60 minutes of moderate physical activity four to seven days a week. Start with five to 10 minutes a day and slowly work up to the 30 to 60 minutes.

Guidelines for Beginning an Exercise Program

Start slowly: Consider very low intensity exercises that you can gradually increase in intensity, with time. Walking and swimming are among the best exercises to begin a program. Not everyone has access to a pool, but everyone has access to walking.

Schedule exercise time: Exercise needs to be part of your schedule. If you wait for free time to just show up, it is likely your exercise program will never happen. Why? Because we always have something else we can do. Ask any busy person. Exercise should be on the same priority level as taking a shower or eating a meal. You must make time for movement.

Stay focused on what you want: Time, family, weather, and work can all be barriers to a regular exercise routine. Recognize the problems that you know will get in the way of a routine exercise program and develop a plan to overcome them. Do not allow anything to come between you and what you want to accomplish.

Consider a support system: Having a support system in place to encourage you in your daily exercise is extremely helpful. It is part of the exercise prescription. Your support person can be a medical professional, a spouse, family member, friend, or co-worker. Choose someone you feel comfortable with and whom you know will help you over the difficult times. Choose support people who already have good health-promoting habits in their lives—or who want to develop them with you!

Exercise Intensity

The exercise intensity of an activity or movement indicates how much power or force is used in performing that exercise. The intensity of an activity determines how much, and what type, of fuel is needed to provide the energy required for that exercise.

Fuel Needs

As we saw in Chapter 3, the body utilizes two types of fuel—short-term and long-term.

- Anaerobic exercise uses carbohydrate or fast, immediately available, short-term fuel.

- Aerobic exercise requires a constant supply of oxygen and a combination of fuels, first carbohydrate, then fatty acids and glycerol (fat)—a longer-term fuel. The amount of fuel used depends directly on the demands on the heart to pump and deliver oxygen and fuel. Aerobic exercise has a positive effect on the circulatory system. In fact, it has a beneficial systemic effect on the whole body if the body is properly fueled. Aerobic activities are best when practiced for extended periods of time—say 30 minutes or more—and use the large muscles in the lower part of the body (buttocks, thighs), which have an excellent whole body effect. As we age or as the body becomes more or less fit, the demands on the heart for oxygen and fuel change.

• Yoga or stretching at low intensities utilizes glucose for fuel, and some more high-intensity forms of yoga will start utilizing fat for fuel as long as a heart rate is maintained at an aerobic level.

These three types of exercise have different effects on the human body's chemical state and the way it uses fuel. The body adapts to both aerobic and anaerobic exercise by producing more or less of different enzymes inside the muscle, which utilize either blood glucose or fat for fuel. If you are an active aerobic exerciser and not a weight/strength exerciser, your body will produce aerobic enzymes in your muscles instead of the anaerobic enzymes, and vice versa. My goal is to provide an exercise guideline for your Apo E genotype. I will update this information as new research becomes available.

Calculating the Appropriate Heart Rate

Here is a general formula to help determine a general target heart rate. You can use this calculation if you cannot gain the information with a VO2 max testing method (see below).

220 minus your age = your maximum heart rate,
then, depending on fitness and current levels of exercise,

For example:
220 - 40 years = 180 (a 40 year old's approximate maximum heart rate).
or
220 - 60 years = 160 (a 60 year old's approximate maximum heart rate).

Then multiply by 60 percent or 85 percent to get your estimated maximum heart rate. Use 60 percent if you are just beginning to exercise, and gradually increase to 85 percent as your stamina increases.

For example:
60% heart rate
220 - 40 years = 180 x 60% = 108
220 - 60 years = 160 x 60% = 96

85% heart rate
220 - 40 years = 180 x 85% = 153
220 - 60 years = 160 x 85% = 136

Calculating the Appropriate Heart Rate

Keep in mind that this "target heart rate" is a general guideline that focuses on the general population, rather than a specific individual's ability. Again, I recommend that you work with a medical professional trained in exercise physiology who can give you a personalized exercise prescription and program.

An exercise physiologist will probably use a testing method called "VO2 max." This test can give you a far more specific measurement of your body's ability to exercise by measuring how fast your body uses oxygen while exercising.

As you exercise in your currently tolerated Apo E zone for a given amount of time—days and weeks, your body will adapt, and its internal fuel-consuming enzymes will grow to a higher level, increasing your exercise tolerance level as long as the same amount of exercise is carried out every 48 hours.

The Apo E Exercise Zone Scale

Studies show that our own personal estimate of effort, or *our own view of how hard we are exercising,* is highly correlated with our actual heart rate and oxygen consumption during exercise. This means we should pay more attention to our inner warning mechanisms to guide our bodies during an exercise session. If a certain type of exercise feels too difficult, it probably is. If you have not exercised in a long time, you are not conditioned to have the muscle engine capacity to tolerate or perform the exercise type or pace of someone who exercises regularly for extended periods. The beginning exerciser may rate a given exercise as "very hard," but after you have been performing the same exercise for a longer period of time and have developed your muscles, you may find the same level of exercise fairly light. Your experience of the effort used in doing any particular exercise is directly related to your intra-muscular exercise equipment.

The Apo E Exercise Zone Scale shown below can be adapted to every possible level and type of fitness. Following this scale will help you begin to trust your inner exertion abilities, instead of an external generalized formula. Beginning exercisers are instructed to walk one mile at their own pace. After they have completed the exercise they can look at the exercise zone scale and evaluate at what level they were exercising. Did they feel as if they were exercising at Zone 7 or was it at Zone 2? If they were at Zone 2, they need to pick up the pace a little until they feel they are operating in the moderate zone for them—not too easy and not too hard. In my experience, most people don't know what their correct zone is and tend to overdo it when they start out. Their rating for Day 1 is probably going to be a Zone 6 or even a Zone 7. Learning to pace themselves at about Zone 3 or 4 is an important first stage of an aerobic exercise program.

Exercise Zone Scale

Zone 1	Zone 2	Zone 3	Zone 4	Zone 5	Zone 6	Zone 7
Very, Very Easy	Very Easy	Fairly Light	Somewhat Hard	Hard	Very Hard	Very, Very Hard

Exercise Effort Level

When exercising ask yourself, "How do I feel?"
Rate your current exercise level.
What exercise zone are you currently exercising in?

• Are you exercising too hard?

• Are you exercising too light?

• Are you exercising just right?

Exercise Effort Level

Use the Apo E Exercise Zone Scale, where appropriate, to answer the following questions:

• What is my current level on the exercise zone scale?
• Am I exercising within my current prescribed zone?
• When I exercise, am I asking myself, "How do I feel?"
• Does my exercise feel too hard?
• Does my exercise feel too easy?
• Am I making exercise progress?

Consider the following general guidelines:

- When exercising you should be able to carry on a conversation.
- You should have easy, regular breathing, and not be gasping for air.
- You should not feel exhausted during or after exercising.

Table 12.1: Macronutrients Used for Each Recommended Exercise Plan				
	Exercise intensity (% MHR)[a]	Heart rate range	% of carbs[b]	% of fat[c]
Apo E 4/4 75% aerobic, 25% anaerobic	60-65	120-125	35	65
	65-70	130-140	40	60
Apo E 4/3 75% aerobic, 25% anaerobic	60-65	120-125	35	65
	65-70	130-140	40	60
Apo E 4/2 50% aerobic, 50% anaerobic	70-75	140-150	50	50
	65-70	150-160	65	35
Apo E 3/3 50% aerobic, 50% anaerobic	70-75	140-150	50	50
	75-80	150-160	65	35
Apo E 2/3 55% aerobic, 45% anaerobic	70-75	140-150	50	50
	75-80	150-160	65	35
	80-85	160-170	80	20
Apo E 2/2 55% aerobic, 45% anaerobic	70-75	140-145	50	50
	75-80	150-160	65	35
	80-85	160-170	80	20

a.   Exercise intensity as defined by a percentage of maximum heart rate.
b.   The percentage of recommended carbohydrate intake that is used during exercise.defined by a percentage of maximum heart rate.
c.   The percentage of recommended fat intake that is used during exercise.

Type of Muscle Fibers

Muscle is the body's engine and makes up about half of all body composition. Muscle is composed of three main types of muscle fiber.

Type I: Slow-contracting fibers use the body's aerobic metabolic pathways.

Fuel used: Glucose first and then free fatty acids

Type II: Faster-twitch fibers use anaerobic metabolic pathways.
Fuel used: Glucose

Type III: Intermediate-twitch fibers use both aerobic and anaerobic metabolic pathways.
Fuel used: Equal balance of glucose and free fatty acids

Different Apo E genotypes have different dominant types of muscle fibers that prefer different types of fuel:

Apo E 4 dominant in muscle Type I

Apo E 2 dominant in muscle Type II

Apo E 3 dominant in muscle Type III

Garbage In-Garbage Out—Again

This is so important that I'll remind you again what happens when a person has eaten excessive inflammatory fats from saturated and trans fat sources that are now stored in the body's cells. When you begin an exercise program to reduce body fat, *you are now asking your body to mobilize and use these stored inflammatory fats as fuel.* This can elicit an inflammatory response and you may need medical support until the excessive stored trans and saturated fats have cleared from your body, which can take up to 9 to 18 months.

Program and Progression Plan

An exercise program consists of three phases, each having different goals. Each phase builds on the previous one, with the end result being a healthy physical body:

Initial Conditioning Phase
- Duration: 4-6 weeks
- Goal: increase frequency (sessions/week)

Improvement Conditioning Phase
- Duration: 7-11 weeks
- Goal: increase the duration (minutes/session)

Maintenance Conditioning Phase
- Occurs after 12-24 weeks of regular exercise
- Goal: maintain the exercise regimen (and your cardio-respiratory fitness)

Life long exercise behaviors usually can be maintained if continued more than 24 weeks.

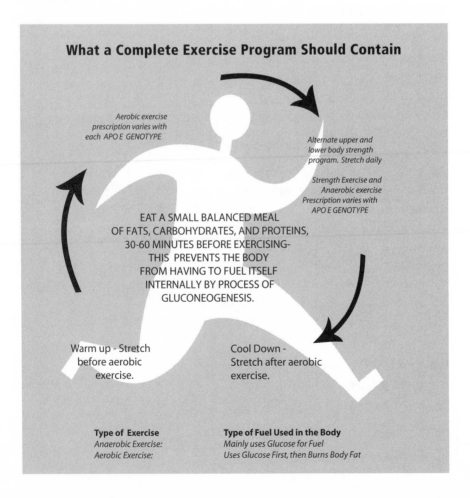

What a Complete Exercise Program Should Contain

Aerobic exercise prescription varies with each APO E GENOTYPE

Alternate upper and lower body strength program. Stretch daily

Strength Exercise and Anaerobic exercise Prescription varies with APO E GENOTYPE

EAT A SMALL BALANCED MEAL OF FATS, CARBOHYDRATES, AND PROTEINS, 30-60 MINUTES BEFORE EXERCISING- THIS PREVENTS THE BODY FROM HAVING TO FUEL ITSELF INTERNALLY BY PROCESS OF GLUCONEOGENESIS.

Warm up - Stretch before aerobic exercise.

Cool Down - Stretch after aerobic exercise.

Type of Exercise
Anaerobic Exercise:
Aerobic Exercise:

Type of Fuel Used in the Body
Mainly uses Glucose for Fuel
Uses Glucose First, then Burns Body Fat

Warm-up and Cool-down

Warm-up and Stretching

Preparing for exercise is important at any age and fitness level. The key to preventing exercise injuries is to warm up beforehand. This helps increase blood flow to the muscles, including the heart; ligaments and tendons are less likely to tear or be strained if they're warmed up first. A warm-up includes a slow increase of activity to help increase blood circulation. Some of my very sick patients with chronic arthritis actually go into a hot tub or spa to warm up and stretch, and I have noticed that Apo E 4s like to warm up the same way.

Flexibility is a must when performing any exercise. Flexibility training teaches your ligaments and tendons to stretch and retract appropriately, which helps prevent injury to the muscles and fractures to the bones. After your warm-up, stretch slowly, without forced bouncing movements, and hold each stretch for 20 to 45 seconds. Never stretch to the point of pain.

The stretching exercises can be either static or dynamic. Static stretching involves slowly stretching a muscle to the point of mild discomfort and then holding that position for an extended period of time. Dynamic stretching involves the active stretching of the muscles by slow, controlled movements through the full range of motion.

You can stretch as part of your warm-up and cool-down routines, and even between resistance training sets or exercises.

Cool-down

The cool-down period provides a gradual recovery from the aerobic (endurance) phase and includes exercises of diminishing intensity. Static stretches are more appropriate to the cool-down since they help muscles to relax and increase their range of motion. Cool-down should consist of the following:

- 5 to 10 minutes of low-intensity, aerobic-type activity (to decrease body temperature and remove waste products from the working muscles)
- 5 to 10 minutes of static stretching exercises (to increase range of motion)

Flexibility Training Prescription

Stretching exercises should include three or four exercises for the major muscle groups of the upper and lower body. Start slow. If you are only able to do these exercises once, then do them only once. Don't overdo any exercise because over-exercising leads to injury. Increase the amount of exercise as you can tolerate it.

Stretching Exercises[13]

Improving Your Flexibility

Stretching exercises give the human body freedom of movement to do the things you need to do in your daily life.

Hamstring Stretch

For the back of thigh muscles

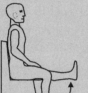

- Sit sideways on a flat hard surface.
- Keep one leg stretched out on surface, toes pointing up.
- Keep other foot on the floor.
- Straighten back.
- Hold stretch 10-30 seconds.
- To feel a greater stretch, lean forward from your hips.
- Repeat 5 times on each side.

Calf Stretch

For the lower leg muscles—with knee straight and knee bent

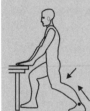

- Stand with hands supported on a table, arms outstretched and elbows straight.
- Keeping your knee slightly bent, toes of the other foot slightly turned inward, step back 12-24 inches and place foot flat on floor. Stretch is felt in the calf muscle.
- Hold stretch for 30 seconds.
- Repeat with each leg up to 5 times.

Ankle Stretch

For the front ankle muscles

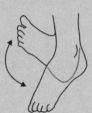

- Sit toward the front edge of a chair and lean back, using a cushion to support your back.
- Stretch your legs out in front of you.
- With your heels on the floor, bend your ankles to point feet toward you then away from you.
- Hold the position for 2 seconds.
- Repeat up to 5 times.

---

13   The following boxes contain exercise information adapted from The National Institute on Aging, U.S. Department of Health and Human Services (HHS).

Triceps Stretch

For the back of upper arm muscles

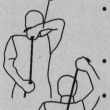

- Hold one end of a cloth in one hand.
- Raise and bend that arm to drop towel down back. Keep your arm in this position, and continue holding onto the towel.
- Reach behind you with your other hand and take hold of bottom end of towel with other hand.
- Move hand higher up towel, which also pulls your other arm down. Continue until your hands come close together or touch.
- Repeat on each side up to 5 times.

Wrist Stretch

For the wrist and hand muscles

- Place hands together (see picture).
- Slowly raise arms as far as you can, keeping hands flat against each other.
- Hold stretch for 30 seconds.
- Repeat up to 5 times.

Quadriceps Stretch

For the front of thigh muscles and knees

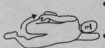

- Lie on your side on the floor, your hips aligned one directly above the other.
- Place your head on your hand.
- Bend knee that is on top.
- Reach back and grasp leg or heel.
- Slowly pull leg until you feel a stretch in the front of thigh.
- Hold stretch for 30 seconds.
- Repeat up to 5 times with each leg.

Double Hip Rotation

For the hip and thigh muscles

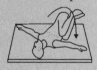

- Lie on your back on a flat surface, knees bent, feet flat.
- Keep shoulders flat.
- Keeping knees bent and together, slowly move legs to one side as long as it feels comfortable.
- Hold stretch up to 30 seconds.
- Return legs to upright position.
- Repeat on each side up to 5 times.

Single Hip Rotation

For the pelvic and inner thigh muscles

- Lie on your back on a supportive surface, knees bent and feet flat on the surface.
- Shoulders should remain flat throughout the exercise.
- Lower one leg slowly to side, keeping the other leg and your pelvis in place.
- Hold stretch for up to 30 seconds.
- Repeat for each leg up to 5 times.

Shoulder Rotation

For the shoulder muscles

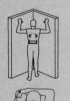

This exercise can be performed standing upright or lying on the floor.

- As floor exercise: stretch arms out to side. Shoulders and upper arms remain flat on the floor.
- As standing exercise: With elbows bent and hands turned toward wall, let your arms gently roll backwards from the elbow until you feel a stretch.
- Hold stretch up to 30 seconds.

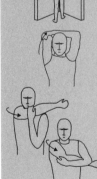

- With your arms bent at the elbow, slowly lift your arms up again. Then let your arms slowly roll forward, remaining bent at the elbow.
- Hold stretch for up to 30 seconds.
- Repeat up to 5 times.

Neck Rotation
For the neck muscles

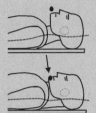

This exercise can be done standing or on the floor.
* Move your neck slowly from side to side.
* Hold stretch for up to 30 seconds on each side. Place your head in a comfortable position when moving your head forward or backward. In addition keep your knees bent and back comfortable during this exercise.
* Repeat up to 5 times.

Strength Exercises

Exercise either the upper or the lower body—not both—every day.

Arm Strengthening
Strengthens the shoulder muscles

Arm exercises can be performed sitting or standing.
* If sitting, sit on an armless chair with your back well supported by the chair–feet remain on the floor.
* Hold hand weights straight down by your sides, with palms facing inward.
* Slowly raise both arms to your side, as high as you can move toward shoulder height.
* Hold lift for 1-2 seconds
* Slowly lower arms to beginning resting position. Relax.
* Repeat as tolerated, up to 15 times.

Floor Lift
Strengthens the abdominal and thigh muscles

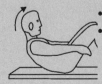

* Slowly lift the upper body as seen in the picture.
* Repeat as tolerated, up to 15 times. Rest in between repetitions.

Biceps Curl
Strengthens the upper-arm muscles

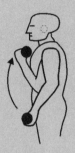

This exercise can be performed either standing or sitting.
- Keep feet flat on the floor, shoulders even.
- Hold hand weights straight down at your sides, with palms facing inward.
- With an intentional slow movement, bend one elbow, lifting weight toward chest. (Turn palm to face shoulder while lifting weight.)
- Hold lift for 1-2 seconds, then slowly lower the arm to resting position.
- Repeat as tolerated on both arms up to 15 times.

Plantar Flexion
Strengthens the ankle and calf muscles

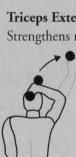

- Stand straight, feet flat on the floor, holding onto a support.
- Slowly raise heels off the floor onto tiptoes, as high as you can go. Hold for 1-2 seconds.
- Then lower heels back to the floor.
- Repeat up to 15 times.

Triceps Extension
Strengthens muscles in back of the upper arm

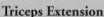

Support your arm with your other hand throughout the exercise.
- Sit with your back supported.
- Keep feet flat on floor with shoulders even.
- While holding a weight in your hand, raise active arm above your head, toward the ceiling, palm facing in.
- Support your active working arm, below the elbow, with your non-working hand.
- Slowly bend raised arm at the elbow, bringing hand weight toward same shoulder.
- Slowly straighten arm toward ceiling.
- Hold your lifting arm for 1-2 seconds.
- Repeat up to 15 times with each arm.

Knee Flexion

Strengthens the back of thigh muscles

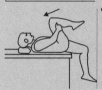

This exercise can be done standing up or lying down.
- Gently bend one knee toward chest, without bending waist or hips. Hold the stretch for 1-2 seconds.
- Lower leg down, then rest.
- Repeat with both legs up to 15 times.

Hip Flexion

Strengthens the thigh and hip muscles

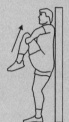

This exercise can be done standing up or lying down.
- Slowly bend one knee toward chest, without bending waist or hips. Hold position for 1–2 seconds.
- Slowly lower leg back down, then rest.
- Repeat for each leg up to 15 times.

Shoulder Flexion

Strengthens the shoulder muscles

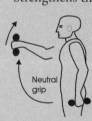

- Sit in an armless chair with your back supported by back of the chair.
- Keep feet flat on floor even with your shoulders.
- Hold hand weights straight down at your sides, with palms facing inward.
- Raise both arms in front of you (straight elbows, palms upward) to shoulder height. Hold position for 1 second.
- Slowly lower arms to sides, then rest.
- Repeat with both arms 8-15 times.

Knee Extension

Strengthens the front of thigh and shin muscles

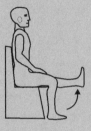

- Only the balls of your feet and toes are resting on the floor. Place a rolled towel under knees, to lift your feet, if desired. Place hands on your thighs or on the sides of the chair.
- Extend one leg in front of you as straight as possible.
- Flex foot to point toes toward ceiling. Hold for 1 to 2 seconds.
- Slowly lower leg.
- Repeat with each leg up to 15 times.

Side Leg Raise

Strengthens hip and thigh muscles

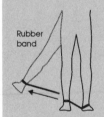

Rubber band

Use weights or strengthening band for this exercise.
- Stand behind a chair, feet 6-12 inches apart.
- Facing forward and using a chair for balance, slowly lift one leg 6-12 inches out to side. Keep your back and legs straight and hold position for 1-2 seconds .
- Lower leg, pause and then repeat with other leg.
- Start with few repetitions, then slowly increase to 10-15.

Aerobic Exercise: A Walking Program

Walking is an excellent form of aerobic exercise. I chose walking because it is a very flexible activity. Regardless of fitness level, walking is something nearly everyone can do.

Aerobic exercise is a continuous movement at a moderate intensity level so that your lungs and heart can provide enough oxygen to prevent lactic acid from building up and creating anaerobic conditions (no oxygen) in your cells. Each of us has our own unique aerobic level depending on how fit we are. If you are out of shape, you do not have much aerobic capacity in your muscles that pull in the fuel used by aerobic exercise—oxygen and free fatty acids. This type of exercise uses glucose first, then switches over to fat—the long-term fuel—for sustained periods, which makes aerobic exercise the fat-burning exercise for the body.

When preparing for aerobic exercise it is extremely important to warm up slowly and stretch the muscles, ligaments, and tendons that will be used during the session. This prevents injury and ensures a productive exercise program. A walking program has many benefits, such as:

- It's free.
- It's available to nearly everyone.
- No equipment is needed.
- It's convenient.
- No training needed, unless you are 9 months to 1 year old.
- You can change the pace whenever needed.
- It's flexible; walking can be increased to a jog or run or decreased to a slow, gentle pace.

Use the Progressive Exercise Schedule on the next page to help you plan and follow a regular exercise program. As you get to week 6, you might want to refer back to page 138-140 and review the information about each of the conditioning phases.

Progressive Exercise Schedule

Week 1

EXERCISE ACTIVITY	Stretch	Warm-Up Walk	Aerobic walk	Cool-Down & Stretch	Strength Exercise	Total Time
DAY 1	5 min	5 min	5 min	5 min		20 min
DAY 2	10 min					10 min
DAY 3	5 min	5 min	5 min	5 min		20 min
DAY 4	10 min					10 min
DAY 5						0
DAY 6	10 min					10 min
DAY 7						0

Week 2

EXERCISE ACTIVITY	Stretch	Warm-Up Walk	Aerobic walk	Cool-Down & Stretch	Strength Exercise	Total Time
DAY 1	5 min	5 min	5 min	5 min		20 min
DAY 2	10 min					10 min
DAY 3	5 min	5 min	5 min	5 min		20 min
DAY 4	10 min					10 min
DAY 5	5 min	5 min	5 min	5 min		20 min
DAY 6						0
DAY 7						0

Week 3

EXERCISE ACTIVITY	Stretch	Warm-Up Walk	Aerobic walk	Cool-Down & Stretch	Strength Exercise	Total Time
DAY 1	5 min	5 min	5 min	5 min		20 min
DAY 2	10 min					10 min
DAY 3	5 min	5 min	5 min	5 min		20 min
DAY 4	10 min					10 min
DAY 5	5 min	5 min	5 min	5 min		20 min
DAY 6						0
DAY 7	10 min					10 min

Progressive Exercise Schedule

Week 4 (initial conditioning phase)

EXERCISE ACTIVITY	Stretch	Warm-Up Walk	Aerobic walk	Cool-Down & Stretch	Strength Exercise	Total Time
DAY 1	5 min	5 min	5 min	5 min		20 min
DAY 2	10 min				10 min	20 min
DAY 3	5 min	5 min	5 min	5 min		20 min
DAY 4	10 min				10 min	20 min
DAY 5	5 min	5 min	5 min	5 min		20 min
DAY 6	10 min					10 min
DAY 7	5 min	5 min	5 min	5 min		20 min

Week 5 (initial conditioning phase)

EXERCISE ACTIVITY	Stretch	Warm-Up Walk	Aerobic walk	Cool-Down & Stretch	Strength Exercise	Total Time
DAY 1	5 min	5 min	5 min	5 min		20 min
DAY 2	10 min				10 min	20 min
DAY 3	5 min	5 min	5 min	5 min		20 min
DAY 4	10 min				10 min	20 min
DAY 5	5 min	5 min	5 min	5 min		20 min
DAY 6	10 min				10 min	20 min
DAY 7	5 min	5 min	5 min	5 min		20 min

Week 6 (initial conditioning phase)

EXERCISE ACTIVITY	Stretch	Warm-Up Walk	Aerobic walk	Cool-Down & Stretch	Strength Exercise	Total Time
DAY 1	5 min	5 min	15 min	5 min		30 min
DAY 2	10 min				10 min	20 min
DAY 3	5 min	5 min	15 min	5 min		30 min
DAY 4	10 min				10 min	20 min
DAY 5	5 min	5 min	15 min	5 min		30 min
DAY 6	10 min				10 min	20 min
DAY 7	5 min	5 min	15 min	5 min		30 min

Progressive Exercise Schedule

Week 7 (improvement conditioning phase)

EXERCISE ACTIVITY	Stretch	Warm-Up Walk	Aerobic walk	Cool-Down & Stretch	Strength Exercise	Total Time
DAY 1	5 min	5 min	20 min	5 min		35 min
DAY 2	10 min				10 min	20 min
DAY 3	5 min	5 min	20 min	5 min		35 min
DAY 4	10 min				10 min	20 min
DAY 5	5 min	5 min	20 min	5 min		35 min
DAY 6	10 min				10 min	20 min
DAY 7	5 min	5 min	20 min	5 min		35 min

Week 8 (improvement conditioning phase)

EXERCISE ACTIVITY	Stretch	Warm-Up Walk	Aerobic walk	Cool-Down & Stretch	Strength Exercise	Total Time
DAY 1	5 min	5 min	20 min	5 min		35 min
DAY 2	10 min				10 min	20 min
DAY 3	5 min	5 min	20 min	5 min		35 min
DAY 4	10 min				10 min	20 min
DAY 5	5 min	5 min	20 min	5 min		35 min
DAY 6	10 min				10 min	20 min
DAY 7	5 min	5 min	20 min	5 min		35 min

Week 9 (improvement conditioning phase)

EXERCISE ACTIVITY	Stretch	Warm-Up Walk	Aerobic walk	Cool-Down & Stretch	Strength Exercise	Total Time
DAY 1	5 min	5 min	25 min	5 min		40 min
DAY 2	10 min				10 min	20 min
DAY 3	5 min	5 min	25 min	5 min		40 min
DAY 4	10 min				10 min	20 min
DAY 5	5 min	5 min	25 min	5 min		40 min
DAY 6	10 min				10 min	20 min
DAY 7	5 min	5 min	25 min	5 min		40 min

Progressive Exercise Schedule

Week 10 (improvement conditioning phase)

EXERCISE ACTIVITY	Stretch	Warm-Up Walk	Aerobic walk	Cool-Down & Stretch	Strength Exercise	Total Time
DAY 1	5 min	5 min	25 min	5 min		40 min
DAY 2	10 min				15 min	25 min
DAY 3	5 min	5 min	25 min	5 min		40 min
DAY 4	10 min				15 min	25 min
DAY 5	5 min	5 min	25 min	5 min		40 min
DAY 6	10 min				15 min	25 min
DAY 7	5 min	5 min	25 min	5 min		40 min

Week 11 (improvement conditioning phase)

EXERCISE ACTIVITY	Stretch	Warm-Up Walk	Aerobic walk	Cool-Down & Stretch	Strength Exercise	Total Time
DAY 1	5 min	5 min	30 min	5 min		45 min
DAY 2	10 min				15 min	25 min
DAY 3	5 min	5 min	30 min	5 min		45 min
DAY 4	10 min				15 min	25 min
DAY 5	5 min	5 min	30 min	5 min		45 min
DAY 6	10 min				15 min	25 min
DAY 7	5 min	5 min	30 min	5 min		45 min

Week 12 (maintenance conditioning phase)

EXERCISE ACTIVITY	Stretch	Warm-Up Walk	Aerobic walk	Cool-Down & Stretch	Strength Exercise	Total Time
DAY 1	5 min	5 min	35 min	5 min		50 min
DAY 2	10 min				20 min	30 min
DAY 3	5 min	5 min	35 min	5 min		50 min
DAY 4	10 min				20 min	30 min
DAY 5	5 min	5 min	35 min	5 min		50 min
DAY 6	10 min				20 min	30 min
DAY 7	5 min	5 min	35 min	5 min		50 min

Progressive Exercise Schedule

Maintenance Weeks _____

EXERCISE ACTIVITY	Stretch	Warm-Up Walk	Aerobic walk	Cool-Down & Stretch	Strength Exercise	Total Time
DAY 1						
DAY 2						
DAY 3						
DAY 4						
DAY 5						
DAY 6						
DAY 7						

Strength Training

Strength training causes the muscles to adjust to the stress or resistance placed upon them. If you stress a muscle with anaerobic exercise, the body will accommodate with additional strength in that muscle. Strength training increases a person's consumption of short-term fuel because it creates an increase in the enzymes that use glucose. More muscle equals more muscle enzymes, which in turn equals a higher metabolism, glucose need, and fuel use.

There are two types of strength exercises:

• weight resistance (such as sit-ups, push-ups)

• machines or free weights

If you are new to strength exercise, consider first using only your body weight as a resistance to accomplish the specific movement. This helps you prevent injury as you increase your fitness level. After you become stronger, you can incorporate free weights and then move to a weight machine.

Important: For each strength training session, begin with a warm-up and stretching session as described above. At the end, cool down slowly to allow the body to gradually come back to a normal movement level. The heart rate should be allowed to gradually decrease to help balance blood delivery and prevent blood pooling or possible fainting.

A Patient's Story: James

James, 38, was a determined exerciser: 40 to 50 minutes of hard bike riding every morning, an hour of aerobics plus strength training at lunch, and more riding in the evening. But until he had chest pains and shortness of breath one day during a bike ride, he had never suspected he had coronary artery disease.

After a screening stress test with his primary care doctor produced more chest pain during the test, James was referred to a cardiologist, who immediately placed a stent in his coronary artery to open up his artery and help clear the blockage. Shortly afterward, James returned to his usual exercise routine and continued his strict low-fat diet, following the typical advice for such patients. He was also referred to me for additional care, but did not appear for his appointment.

Within five weeks of the first stent being placed, James again experienced chest pains and shortness of breath. His cardiologist discovered that coronary plaque had already overgrown the stent, once again blocking the coronary artery and causing chest pain. So James had a second type of stent inserted.

Frightened about the poor condition of his health at such a young age, he kept his next appointment with me. He clearly wanted to know why he had such aggressive heart disease and what he could do to stop or reverse it. He had never had any significant health problems before the chest pains began, but his medical history revealed a strong family record of heart disease at early ages, which had been the motivation behind his extreme exercise routines. His daily caloric intake was on the low side, and it was split between only breakfast and dinner; he rarely ate anything in between, which left his body with insufficient fuel for a good part of the day. His main source of protein was meat, and he ate little in the way of good fats. With his intense exercise routine, he had only 7 percent body fat. With a happy marriage and an enjoyable job, his only real source of stress was his heart condition.

A complete cholesterol test showed his total cholesterol, LDL, HDL, and triglycerides well within normal numbers, thanks at least in part to the statin medication he had begun taking after the chest pains began. But after I evaluated all 13 different types of cholesterol, we discovered he also had an abnormally high amount of what are called small dense LDL particles. These very tiny particles of bad cholesterol slip through artery linings twice as fast as the larger LDL particles and encourage artery inflammation—this was most likely the reason for his artery disease as well as the rapid re-blockage around the first stent. He also had a trait called LDL pattern B, which also encouraged his artery disease. Finally, James's gene test revealed him to be Apo E 2/3. This is a gene type that does not seem to do well with a very low-fat diet. Taken together, all these traits combined to produce a rapid growth in his heart disease.

We looked at James's risk factors and his behaviors, including diet, exercise, and work, as well as his personal mission and life's journey, including what he could learn from this experience. Then we created a plan to address his entire being—body, mind, and spirit, plus his physical environment. He had begun exercising so often and so hard and drastically reducing his fat intake because he feared dying at a young age from heart disease, as many of his relatives had done. He believed this to be a logical path to follow, based on his doctor's recommendations and the generalized advice in the media. Unfortunately, it was the wrong path for him.

James was very anxious and nervous about having two occasions of chest pain and having two stents inserted in such a short time period and wanted to prevent another episode. So in addition to the proper diet and exercise for his genotype, along with necessary medication, we focused on the ultimate outcome for his total health, defining that as a healthy physical, psychological, and spiritual body with no diseases whatsoever. We also explored the positive factors of his experience and what he might learn from it all. I explained some effective tools for relieving his stress and anxiety, including meditation, prayer, yoga, and a relaxation breathing technique he could do anywhere, anytime.

Finally, we reviewed James's plan of care, and he said he had already begun to feel better, knowing he could improve his health. He was ready to begin his new lifestyle, in partnership with three main support people: his primary care doctor, his cardiologist, and me, his integrative medicine provider. He would be the judge of all our advice. Feeling as if he had some control over his life once again, James now felt hopeful and determined to follow his clear plan of action. Within a very short time, he felt much better and more energetic. Lab tests showed that all his cholesterol numbers improved.[14]

Flexibility and Stretching Exercises (Yoga or Pilates)

You may be reluctant to start exercising regularly because it involves pain, strain, special equipment, other people to work out with, or travel. If this is true for you, then a gentle form of exercise called yoga may be just the approach you need to get started on the road to overall fitness. Yoga not only focuses on the alignment of your outer body but also encourages awareness of your inner self. It can be very restful to the mind as well as something to stretch and strengthen the body.

The word "yoga" means union. It is a discipline that seeks to unite the body, mind, heart, and spirit. It consists of a series of physical postures along with breathing exercises that are easily learned. Regular practice increases flexibility, strength, balance, grace, breath control, endurance, and overall health and integration of mind, emotions, and body. The exercises also provide special stimulation of the endocrine glands and thus promote a rebalancing of your energy. Many people experience a greater serenity about life in general, as well as improved circulation, a firmer, trimmer body, and less illness.

You are advised to move slowly and with concentrated awareness, to avoid strain or pain, and to coordinate your breath with your movements. Yoga exercises can be done almost anywhere. It helps to wear loose clothing to make stretching easier, and to have a mat or cloth under you, something that marks this spot as your yoga practice space. You can teach it to yourself simply by following a book or set of instructions, although a trained teacher is highly recommended, especially as you advance into more difficult postures.

---

14 *ADA's Nutrition and You: Trends 2002 Survey.* Survey results are based on telephone interviews with a nationally representative sample of 700 adults conducted inn April 2002 by Wirthlin Worldwide. The survey has a confidence interval of plus-or-minus 5 percent in 95 out of 100 cases.

Here is a simple yoga posture called the Lion: Inhale deeply, then forcefully exhale through your mouth. While exhaling with mouth wide open and eyes wide and staring, thrust out your tongue and stretch arms down with fingers stiff and spread tautly apart. Hold the breath for a few seconds. Then close your mouth and inhale deeply through the nostrils, expanding the abdomen. Exhale again slowly through your nostrils and relax. Repeat three times.

Yoga classes are widely available, as is a popular westernized variant, called Pilates (Puh-LOT-eez). If a book or DVD is not enough for you, check your local community bulletin board. Be aware that yoga comes in many flavors, some much more strenuous than others, so sample as many as you can and pick your favorite.

Logging Behavior Changes
What Is a Health Log?
A health log is a tool designed to help you establish and follow a new behavior. The behaviors most frequently observed with these kinds of logs are exercise and eating patterns, fluid intake, and sleeping patterns, though they may also support new behaviors ranging from personal hygiene to a spiritual practice. Logging your daily thoughts about whether you are embracing or struggling with the new behaviors can help you sustain your new behaviors.

Research has shown that keeping a health log is an extremely important part of a person's success with developing a new behavior or changing an established behavior. Some of the best Olympic athletes, triathletes, cyclists, swimmers, and runners keep detailed records of their daily performance that includes not only their physical performance but also a psychological component—their thoughts and feelings.

Getting a Logbook
Logbooks are available in most bookstores or on the Internet. I have always enjoyed going to my local bookstore to find a new logbook. For me, the cover can be important. If I like it, I'm more apt to use my logbook. And because my logbook helps me record all my thoughts and behavior changes in one place, I am able to refer to my positive changes when I need encouragement.

General Exercise Log
You can create a general log to document the type of exercise you are doing. You will log the amount of time you spent exercising, your beginning heart rate and your mid-exercise target heart rate, and how you felt before and after exercise (rating 1–10).

Now lets look at two examples of logging—one for a walking exercise and one for a nutritional change.

Pedometer Program Log

The Pedometer Log on the next page is for those who would like to keep track of their progress with a walking program, by counting the number of steps taken during an exercise session. If such a program is of interest, you will need to use a walking pedometer to be able to keep track of your steps.

A pedometer is a little machine about the size of a cell phone. It is usually worn on a waistband or belt and counts the number of steps a person takes by measuring body movement. Some pedometers are simple tools that just measure steps. Some are a little more complex and can track steps, calories, and distance walked. I am not sure how accurate the calorie count and distance tracking are, but they sure are fun to use. A pedometer can be worn during a given exercise session or worn all day.

A goal is to walk as many steps as you can in the beginning. For example: 400 steps. Then slowly increase your steps on a daily basis to 410, 425, and so on. Once you have finished your exercise session, log your steps on an exercise log sheet or in your exercise journal.

My patients have a lot of fun with the Apo E Gene Diet Pedometer Program. School children especially love pedometers; they become very excited about getting in their quota of steps during the day.

Pedometers are available for purchase in many stores. However, they vary in quality, so invest in one that will last. In addition, consider buying a pedometer with a safety strap; pedometers are famous for ending up in the toilet. You can go to our website www.ApoEGeneDiet.com for some information about our online pedometer program.

Pedometer Program Log

NAME: MONTH:

	Steps:	Steps:	Steps:	Steps:	Steps:	Notes:
MON	Goal:	Goal:	Goal:	Goal:	Goal:	
	Steps:	Steps:	Steps:	Steps:	Steps:	
TUE	Goal:	Goal:	Goal:	Goal:	Goal:	
	Steps:	Steps:	Steps:	Steps:	Steps:	
WED	Goal:	Goal:	Goal:	Goal:	Goal:	
	Steps:	Steps:	Steps:	Steps:	Steps:	
THU	Goal:	Goal:	Goal:	Goal:	Goal:	
	Steps:	Steps:	Steps:	Steps:	Steps:	
FRI	Goal:	Goal:	Goal:	Goal:	Goal:	
	Steps:	Steps:	Steps:	Steps:	Steps:	
SAT	Goal:	Goal:	Goal:	Goal:	Goal:	
	Steps:	Steps:	Steps:	Steps:	Steps:	
SUN	Goal:	Goal:	Goal:	Goal:	Goal:	

Your Food Log

Use the Sample Food Log below to log your food log your food and fluid intake for seven days using a new sheet for each day. Write in the type, amount, and time you ate the food. This will help you see whether you are missing meals or successfully supporting good eating habits.

Sample Food Log

FOOD LOG	Sunday		Monday		Tuesday		Wednesday		Thursday		Friday		Saturday	
	Food	Amt	Food	Amt	Food	Amt	Food	Amt	Food	Amt	Food	Amt	Food	Amt
Breakfast														
Morning Snack														
Lunch														
Afternoon Snack														
Dinner														

Avoiding Exercise Program Dropout

Many people who begin an exercise program drop out within the first few days, weeks, or months. Even regular exercisers, on occasion, have to triumph over obstacles that can prevent them from staying with a regular exercise program. Stopping or taking a break from exercise is normal—this is the body's natural break time. Fortunately, an exercise support system can keep these breaks from becoming permanent.

People who *do not* get advice from a licensed exercise physiologist or certified sports medicine professional may set unrealistic goals for themselves. They may try to do too much too quickly and often become frustrated or injured, at which point they give up. In fact, the major causes of people giving up their exercise program are frustration, being overwhelmed, and not having first been through a pre-planning exercise process.

Exercise and movement are basic to life. The human body needs to move, and move often. This is simply a part of our genetic and physical makeup. Just because our lifestyles have become more sedentary in recent years doesn't mean our bodies no longer require lots of movement to be healthy. We didn't always have the supermarket where we could buy our food. Once, we had to work really hard to grow and produce our own food, or at least walk to buy it. Moving our bodies every day to just eat and survive was much more common even 50 years ago than it is today. Unless you are extremely active in your work or leisure (with an activity, such as extreme sports), consider doing your body a favor by exercising regularly.

Chapter Thirteen

HEALTHY FOODS
AND OTHER NUTRIENTS

It's common to think that our bodies grow until a certain age, then stop. But in reality, the human body is in a constant state of growth and repair. To best handle these tasks, the body should receive an optimal diet from optimal food sources. This means that our food choices in both the macronutrients (big foods) and the micronutrients (smaller nutrients) should not only follow a general guideline, but should also be tailored for our Apo E genotype. For example, we should receive a certain percentage of the macronutrients of fat, carbohydrate, and protein based on our particular Apo E genotype. However, nutrition experts say that some foods are beneficial for everyone. Here are some of the foods that I suggest you consider when adding new foods to your diet. Enjoy!

Apo E Gene Diet Top 15

Below are the healthiest 15 foods and drinks according to many nutrition experts. The Apo E Gene Diet also recommends them for many reasons, including heart protection, phytochemical content (which may help reduce cancer risk), high fiber, low glycemic load (which helps to regulate blood sugar levels), cancer protection, nutrient density, great taste, versatility of food type in cooking, and good fat content, to name only a few benefits. This section will tell you more about some of them, but know that they are all healthy, delicious, and good for you.

- avocado
- broccoli
- extra virgin olive oil
- green tea
- red grapes
- whole soy
- garlic
- berries
- dark chocolate
- flaxseed
- whole grains
- tomatoes
- fresh water (100% clean)
- nuts (walnuts, almonds, for example)
- wild fish (Alaskan sockey salmon, for example)

Water

About 70 percent of the human body is made up of water. Most of this is found in the body's muscles, bones, blood, and lymph. Water is an essential body component, involved in every function, including regulating body temperature, assisting in respiration, transporting nutrients, circulation of all body fluids, absorption of nutrients, and waste removal from cells. A good daily intake of water is essential if your body is to function optimally, and it needs to be spread over the course of the day, since it is being continually lost through many bodily functions. It is difficult to give an exact recommendation of how much water you require each day, since individual needs differ and the external environment also plays a big role in the body's fluid requirements. A general guideline is six to eight glasses each day, although there seems to be no research to support these figures (and the custom of people carrying bottled water everywhere was perhaps was just good marketing from the bottlers).

Even more important than quantity is quality. The water you drink needs to be as pure as possible. If you drink water from a source that has cell-damaging chemicals in it, the result will be high cell stress and this, in turn, can give rise to cell and tissue damage and disease. This is particularly important for the Apo E 4s, as this genotype has very low tolerance for toxic chemicals.

Tap water run through a good filter is often of better quality than water obtained in bottles, is one-tenth the cost, and is far less costly to the planet than the huge costs of manufacturing the plastic bottles (made from dwindling petroleum supplies), transporting them (more petroleum), and finally hauling them to landfills when they are not recycled (and many are not). In addition, the plasticizers in plastic bottles can leach into the water inside, with unknown future health effects, so carry your water in glass bottles whenever possible. Daily doses of leached plastic are not good for anyone and especially not good for the Apo E 4s.

Water quality can vary greatly, and when you find what you think is a pure source, have it tested by an independent lab. If your water does not get an A+ result, consider installing a water filter. Remember, toxic substances chronically interfere with the normal processes of the body and can cause disease. The body can tolerate an occasional imbalance or interference, but when it becomes chronic, the body becomes overwhelmed and then sick.

Chlorine and lead are the two most common toxic contaminants in water. While chlorine kills bacteria and viruses in water, it is also not healthy for human cells. It may increase the risk of heart disease and has been linked to some kinds of cancer and birth defects. Lead is particularly damaging for fetuses, infants, and children—and probably for everyone else, since it can result in organ damage and stunt nervous system growth. Water with more than 10 parts per billion of lead is a health risk.

Mercury is also toxic to the developing brain and nervous system of an unborn fetus, but currently research is very limited on mercury's chronic effects on adults, especially on effects resulting from the levels now found in most seafood.

Other toxic contaminants in drinking water may include, but are not limited to, micro-organisms (viruses, bacteria), disinfectants, heavy metals, fertilizers, pesticides, herbicides, a host of other inorganic and organic chemicals, and radionuclides (or low levels of naturally occurring radioactive contaminants). Some experts also view fluoride as a toxic chemical, but consensus is lacking, so I suggest you educate yourself about fluoride, especially if you are an Apo E 4.

Dr. Andrew Weil suggests that if you use tap water for drinking or cooking, let your kitchen faucet run for three to five minutes every morning to flush out the lead that can concentrate there. In short, your drinking water should be pure, with no toxic additives.

Garlic: Our Aromatic Friend

Garlic is a very interesting plant. A cousin of the lily, it contains a substance called allicin that is the active ingredient in garlic's distinctive flavor and smell. The aroma is released only when the garlic clove skin is broken, allowing an enzyme called allinase to react with the odorless compound alliin, which creates the familiar allicin.

The use of garlic has been traced back to ancient times, as long ago as 4000 years, when it was used not only for cooking but also for a multitude of health benefits by the ancient Egyptians, Greeks, French, and Romans. Today, most cultures use garlic in cooking. People either love it or dislike it—or it dislikes them.

Garlic is the subject of considerable, ongoing research to evaluate its potential health benefits, particularly relating to cancer, cardiovascular disease, and viral infections. Although garlic's ability to improve health by reducing cholesterol has not been substantiated, early studies have shown some anti-platelet and circulation-improving qualities.

I recommend that you eat garlic in your food, or take a small serving of fresh garlic, each day. By keeping the amount small, you can reap the benefits while avoiding the distinctive (some might say overpowering) smell. If you are taking any anti-clotting or blood-thinning medicines such as Coumadin, check with your medical provider before increasing your garlic consumption significantly.

Including garlic in your daily intake can be easy and delicious. Here are a few of my favorite dishes to which garlic can be added easily:

- soups
- roasted potatoes with olive oil
- roasted chicken and turkey with herbs and citrus juices
- tomato-based soups and pasta dishes
- salad
- roasted vegetables
- stir-fry fish and vegetables dishes
- omelets, scrambled egg white or egg substitutes, and egg dishes
- roasted red pepper salsa

These are just a few. Be creative and add garlic to your favorite recipe. Who knows, you may end up liking garlic ice cream.

The Mysterious Mushroom

Most everybody knows what a mushroom is. Some of the oldest varieties can be found growing in circular patterns called fairy rings, which even today can be found right next to Stonehenge, in southern England. When I was a child living in Cornwall in the south of England, the common button mushroom grew wild in the fields behind our home. These little fungi held a mysterious, almost magical presence for me. I would go out with my family to pick mushrooms together, and we would clear the field of these little white buttons one day, only to find just a short time later that they had grown back. As a child, this fascinated me. Later on, it was especially interesting to learn there is an entire world of mysterious mushrooms that hold immense health benefits just now being discovered by the Western medical community, even though the Eastern world has known about them for centuries.

Simply described, the mushroom is a fast growing, spore-producing fungus that gains its food from anything that is decaying. There are many types of mushrooms—ranging from the delicious and nutritious to the exotic and deadly varieties. Leaving the toxic ones behind, mushrooms can benefit our health in very powerful ways by:

- stimulating the immune system
- helping fight and resist viral diseases
- helping treat certain cancers
- lowering cholesterol levels

Mushrooms provide the following nutrition:

- fiber
- protein
- vitamins (niacin, B12, Vitamin C, thiamin, biotin)
- minerals (phosphorus, selenium, potassium, iron)

I see an exceptionally exciting use of mushrooms in the medicinal arena, as well as in the culinary arts. My advice is to keep your mind and palate open to new and interesting ideas for fungi and mushrooms. The mushroom is proving to be very versatile and can be easily grown by anyone, practically anywhere: outdoors, indoors in natural or controlled climate environments. They just might improve your health while at the same time adding a delicious complement to your next omelet or pasta dish. An excellent resource for mushrooms is at www.fungi.com.

Consider eating all mushrooms cooked. The following varieties hold positive health benefit.

- shiitaki (lentinula edodes)
- oyster mushrooms (pleurotus ostreatus)

- nameko Mushroom (philiota nameko)
- lion's mane mushroom (hericium erinaceus)
- enokitake mushrooms (flammulina populicola)

Tea Therapy

Tea is a popular beverage in many countries, ranging from England, Scotland, and Australia to China, Japan, and India. Although not yet as popular a beverage here in the United States, a growing number of tea drinkers are taking advantage of recent research regarding tea's potential health benefits. In ways similar to red wine and chocolate, entire food industries are built around tea. The formal Japanese tea ceremony dates back to the early 1600s. Having grown up in Scotland and England, I have been a tea drinker for most of my life, so I was very excited when I learned that this familiar beverage might also provide a positive effect on good health.

Tea's health benefits are due to:

- an antioxidant effect that helps decrease general body inflammation
- a reduction in blood clotting in the arteries and improvement in artery-lining health
- a decreased heart attack risk, with as little as three 8-oz. cups of tea per day

These positive effects come from catechins—extremely powerful antioxidants, specifically polyphenols and bioflavonoids—that seem to be very beneficial to the human body and may help counter the effects of aging and chronic disease.

The most popular teas today come from a plant called the *Camellia sinensis*. Originating in ancient China, this tea became popular in England in the late 1700s, and teahouses there became social gathering places. *Camellia sinensis* produces most varieties of tea, ranging from the common black and Oolong teas, the lesser-known white teas, to the now-famous, highly beneficial green teas. The difference in color comes from how the leaves are processed: dried leaves become black tea, lightly steamed leaves produce green tea, and leaves picked very early and left unprocessed become white tea. If you are looking for a tea packed with an exceptional punch of antioxidant, you may want to try green tea or the new varieties of white tea. Decaffeinated tea has also been shown to yield health benefits.

One other benefit of tea drinking is the relaxation that comes from taking a break to sip this warm, delicious beverage. Tea drinking definitely produces relaxation in both the mind and the body. Does this come from the tea itself or the relaxing behavior related to drinking it? I believe it's a combination of both.

Take a Tea Break

Compare drinking your tea from a plastic or paper cup to sipping hot tea from an English bone china cup or iced tea from a Scottish or Irish cut-crystal glass—it's an experience well worth having. You may not have time to sit down with friends for an hour every afternoon for an English high tea with a sultana scone, fresh fruit, jam, and Cornish clotted cream, but you could take a 10- or 15-minute tea break (remember the fine china!) and have a small snack. (In fact, the Apo E Gene Diet recommends morning and afternoon snack breaks.) Take this personal reward of quiet time to reflect on your life or to chat with a friend. Bring some flowers into your day to add some beauty to your surroundings. It doesn't take much effort to bring the elegant quality of the past to the busy world of today. Happy tea sipping! I will think of you and send you positive energy for making a positive cultural change as I sip my tea from my English teacup each morning and afternoon. Remember: focus on what you want!

If you would like to search for your own special china tea cup, here are some famous English china and crystal companies for you to explore.

Spode	www.spode.co.uk
Wedgwood	www.wedgwood.com
Royal Doulton	www.royaldoulton.com
Waterford	www.waterford.com/index.asp
Edinburgh Crystal	www.edinburgh-crystal.co.uk

A few years ago I had the pleasure of participating in an old, very spiritual Japanese tea ceremony with a type of tea called Matcha, which I had never had before. Matcha has a very organic taste, which many of us in the West are not used to. A Japanese colleague of mine, Yoshihiro Hotta, MD, performed the tea ceremony and then shared his experiences of other tea ceremonies.

This beautiful cultural experience can bring a renewed spirit and quality to a common beverage that many of us indulge in every day. The next time you get ready to drink your hot green or black tea, think about the centuries of culture behind just this one plant and feel some peace of mind as you sip it, knowing that your steaming drink will have positive effects on your health.

Ginger

The Latin name for ginger is *Zingiber officinale*. Its main beneficial ingredient is gingerol. Ginger provides many health benefits, the main one being its exceptional anti-inflammatory properties.

I've always liked ginger. As a child I enjoyed ginger pieces and also ginger cake and biscuits, and homemade non-alcoholic ginger beer. I can still remember seeing the homemade ginger brew in thick, old-fashioned bottles sitting in the parlor of our old country home, lined up against the cold, damp, cob walls for what seemed like forever. Once it was ready to drink, the ginger flavor was unforgettable.

I have been recommending ginger to my patients for many years. It is a very effective supplement for its anti-inflammatory properties and excellent flavor. I suggest adding ginger to Asian food such as stir-fry and wok dishes, as well as to fresh fish, sauces, salads and cold foods, fresh fruit, and cooked vegetables. Consider adding ginger to hot tea and iced drinks, and if you are adventurous, consider making some homemade ginger beer. Explore the use of ginger in your daily cooking and see if the delicious flavor of ginger could bring a touch of pizzazz back to your food or your (non-alcoholic) beer drinking!

Ginger Beer Recipe

Ingredients

2 oz. ginger root	8 pints water
1 1/4 oz. cream of tartar	10 oz. brown sugar
1 packet yeast	Up to 2 whole lemons can be added if you like

Directions

Boil 8 pints of water. Add all ingredients to a large pot and mix well. Let sit for 24 hours. Bottle and allow to sit in a cool room for a few weeks to brew.

Dark Chocolate

Oh, for the love of chocolate! Did you ever dream a medical practitioner would encourage you to eat chocolate? Well, it's true, I do recommend it, since chocolate is proving to have some excellent health benefits.

Made from the seeds found in the pods of the *Theobroma cacao* plant, chocolate can be fun to give and fun to receive. For a long time, we have connected chocolate to happy occasions such as Valentine's Day, anniversaries, birthdays, Halloween, and other fun events. Dark chocolate seems just right for a romantic gift (and the addition of a dozen long-stemmed red roses can't hurt!). Yet sometimes eating chocolate leaves us feeling guilty because we know we're not supposed to eat candy. Today, unfortunately, chocolate is often highly processed and mixed with many unhealthy products.

But the more natural form of chocolate—cocoa, or cacao—has many beneficial qualities for protecting health. Certain forms of pure, dark chocolate with more than 70 percent cacao and less sugar provide benefits from flavonoids, just as tea does, including antioxidant effects and improving vascular and artery quality and blood platelet or cell stickiness (this last is a quality shared with red wine). Milk chocolate or white chocolate (which is not chocolate at all) do not provide these benefits.

For me, the balance of sipping hot tea while nibbling a piece of well-made, dark chocolate has magical properties—which could be why there is so much research being done to find out more about chocolate. It shows such promise for promoting health that The National Center for Complementary and Alternative Medicine at the National Institutes of Health is conducting studies regarding chocolate and how it can improve blood pressure and insulin resistance. So far, the research is telling us to include a wide variety of flavonoid-rich foods in our diet every day—including some high-quality dark chocolate.

Soy—An Excellent Food, with Cautions

Soy is a legume that contains a high-quality protein as well as isoflavones, which may protect against breast cancer, prostate cancer, menopausal symptoms, heart disease, and osteoporosis. Soy also contains a fat, but a type that does *not* seem to cause inflammation in the body unless processed. Therefore, I recommend eating only soy *protein* from its whole food sources—soybeans (edamame), tofu, tempeh, and soy milk—while avoiding any and all processed soy foods.

Processed soy food can come in many forms, including flour, oil, protein powders, soy concentrates, and the soy isolates added to many processed foods. The soy processing industry has become a multibillion-dollar business, but since we do not yet know the effects of eating excessive amounts of soy protein, there appears to be cause for concern. Meanwhile, with recommendations about how much soy to eat ranging from a lot to a little, I think it's reasonable to eat only moderate amounts of soy and only from the natural whole food form.

Soy also contains a natural substance called phytoestrogen, which is shown both to reduce your risk of cancer or increase it, and for this reason also, soy remains a controversial source of protein for many. While I think soy protein has great health benefits, it may take a while to learn to like it and adapt to the taste. I recommend first adding a small amount of a soy into a recipe, then trying a soy dish as your main protein source.

A note about soy milk: It often includes a thickening agent called carrageenan, which is derived from red seaweed. Carrageenan is in all sorts of foods, especially dairy products and toothpaste. It has been connected to gastrointestinal ulcerations and cancer, so my recommendation is to consider avoiding soy milk made with it. Brands of soy milk that *do not* contain carrageenan include homemade soy milk, Trader Joe's Organic Unsweetened, Westsoy, and Organic Vitasoy. Not all Vitasoy flavors are carrageenan-free—check the label.

A Patient's Story: Jeff

In early 2004, Jeff, 54, went to his primary care physician about an elbow problem, and during the visit he mentioned he hadn't had a cholesterol test in two years. His doctor sent him to me for those tests, and he had blood drawn for the standard cholesterol panel—total cholesterol, HDL, LDL, triglycerides—as well as for testing the subclasses crucial to understanding someone's entire cholesterol story. Jeff had known about this additional testing, but his doctor had never recommended it.

Jeff's results were substantially the same as they were two years earlier. While he said he was pleased, I was concerned: Even though his total cholesterol, HDL, and LDL were in line, his triglycerides and many of the cholesterol subclasses were outside the healthy range. Along with these warning signs, he was 45 pounds overweight, had been controlling his high blood pressure with medication for 15 years, and also taking three drugs to lower his cholesterol. His diet consisted of lots of red meat and fast foods, with very few fruits and vegetables. He said he worked out "once or twice a week" and used wine to relax in the evening, usually three or four glasses, but sometimes more.

I knew from Jeff's medical history that his father had died of a heart attack at age 59. He said his father had been overweight all his life, smoked cigars, loved to eat steaks, never exercised, and was always stressed from running his business. Furthermore, his father's mother had died at a young age as well. Given all these indicators of poor health, I asked Jeff if he thought he could make some changes to improve his health.

"Sure, but why?" he asked.

I showed him some information about heart attacks and explained how they happen, explaining in detail the subclasses of cholesterol and how important they are to health. As his interest grew, I suggested a total program that included healthy changes to his diet, a better exercise program, readjusting his cholesterol medications, and the addition of several vitamins and minerals. Perhaps with fears of an early death in mind, Jeff agreed to this program, and in order to help him make the correct changes, he also accepted an appointment with a dietician and a physical therapist. I also gave him some books to educate him about this entire process: *Before the Heart Attacks* by Dr. Robert Superko, *8 Weeks to Optimal Health* and *Healthy Aging* by Dr. Andrew Weil, and *The Power of Intention* by Dr. Wayne Dyer.

Most importantly, though, Jeff also had a genetic test to determine his Apo E genotype. This would be the guide to his new nutrition and exercise program, which he understood was not a temporary "diet" but a new way of living that he could follow for the rest of his life.

Jeff eagerly embraced his new program, accepting my recommendations of sample meals and new foods, many of which he had never tried or heard of, and some of which he said "sounded downright weird," like soy milk. Accepting his program as a challenge, he plunged in and found that soy milk, especially the vanilla flavor, was "quite good." And when his extreme enthusiasm led to his being called the "food police," he discovered that "harmony requires flexibility."

"I've learned to like tofu and soy milk," he said, "but it's not something I brag about to my golfing buddies."

Jeff lost more than 45 pounds in 18 months, despite a few ups and downs. Since he is given a body composition test (determining lean mass vs. body fat) every six weeks, he knows what he has to do to build muscle and keep the fat off. His exercise program was designed by a physical therapist and is modified frequently as he progresses. He works with a personal trainer since that keeps him motivated; otherwise, he admits that he tends to do the exercises he likes and drop the ones he's not so fond of. Now in a stable workout routine, Jeff gets his cardio exercise on an elliptical machine for 40 minutes and also weight trains an additional 30 to 45 minutes, five days a week. As a former couch potato, he now looks forward to his workouts. "If I miss a session, I just don't feel the same that day," he said.

When his weight first began to go down as he increased his exercise, Jeff's blood pressure dropped, and dropped low enough so that he felt dizzy and had less energy. His cardiologist recommended cutting the dosage of his blood pressure medicine in half, but the problems continued even after a month of less medication. Then Jeff's primary physician told him to stop the medication completely, which Jeff did. When his cardiologist learned about this six months later, he wasn't comfortable with Jeff's decision, so Jeff agreed to have his blood pressure checked in another six months, at which time the cardiologist would make a decision about the medication. Jeff passed the test and has been off the medication ever since while maintaining normal blood pressure. He still takes niacin and a cholesterol medication because of a gene trait not connected to his diet or Apo E genotype.

In Jeff's own words:
"I am struck by the changes I have made and the results I have achieved. It's only now that I have made these changes that I can appreciate what they have done for me. They are based on integrated medicine, taking care of the whole person. The blood tests were the beginning, and certainly they pointed us in the right direction as far as medication was concerned, but without the lifestyle changes and the professional help that I received to make those changes, I do not believe I would have achieved the results that I have achieved so far. I am still making progress, still learning, still succeeding, and still failing, but it's been a great journey and one which I hope to continue with for the rest of my life."

Smart Foods

Smart foods, sometimes called functional foods, are a subclass of nutrients called phytonutrients. Phytonutrients provide not only nutrition but also biologically active compounds with significant protective and health enhancing qualities.

Research on these phytonutrients is ongoing, and focuses on determining the true function of these beneficial nutrients. Do they support the immune system? Do they reduce inflammation? Do they protect human cells against immune system triggers such as allergens or viral and bacterial infections? Does their function extend beyond the immediate cell response, to protect against long-term processes such as inflammation in the cardiovascular system and the precursors of cancer? We don't know for sure yet, but I believe we will find that these phytonutrients play a much bigger role in supporting the immune system than we have given them credit for in the past.

Key Types of Phytochemicals and Phytonutrients	
Phytochemical	Food Sources
Alpha-linolic acid	whole soy, flaxseed and walnuts
Carotenoids	tomatoes and tomato sauce
Flavonoids	most berries, pears, apricots, tomatoes, onion, red cabbage, pinto and black beans
Curcumin	Indian curry powder, mixed spice, turmeric, cumin
Capsaicinoid group	peppers (hot chili peppers), capsaicin is the active ingredient
Isothocyanates	spinach, kale, broccoli, cauliflower, cabbage
Indoles	brussels sprouts, turnip, horseradish
Isoflavones	soy, flaxseed, grains, beans and peas
Lignans	seeds and grains
Phenols	spinach, kale, broccoli, cauliflower, cabbage, brussels sprouts, peppers, tomatoes, celery, parsley, soy, oranges, limes, lemons, whole flaxseed, grains, most berries
Terpenes	herbs, citrus and red cherries

Alcohol—Good or Bad?

Is alcohol harmful or protective? Alcohol consumption is a controversial subject in medicine today because it has shown both positive and negative properties. Medical research on red wine has shown *some* positive cardio-protective effects, mainly an increase in HDL, the good cholesterol. However, this has led some medical providers to make blanket assumptions and statements about alcohol that patients can translate as, "Drink alcohol—it's good for your heart, so drink it and drink it often."

But let's stop and think about this for a minute. First of all, if there is a "good" amount for daily alcohol intake, it is a moderate amount—not all you can drink. The American Heart Association's definition of moderate alcohol consumption is no more than one drink per day for women and no more than two drinks per day for men, where one drink equals 12 oz. beer, 5 oz. wine, or 1.5 oz. distilled spirits. In addition, what about a person who has glucose intolerance, insulin resistance, or diabetes, and is on two or four medications, or has very high triglyceride levels? A person with any one of these should stay away from alcohol, yet I have known practitioners to tell these patients to drink it because it's good for them. When I look at these patients' medication lists, I see statin therapy (LDL cholesterol-lowering medication), Niaspan (a slow release form of niacin), Vitamin B3 (*reduces* LDL cholesterol and *raises* HDL cholesterol), diabetic medicines, and sleeping pills, all of which can make alcohol consumption dangerous. The benefits in these cases do not outweigh the risk. People taking cholesterol medications especially need to avoid alcohol because combining these medications with alcohol can cause serious harm to the stomach lining, liver, and kidneys. Even so, I've seen many patients who take high doses of cholesterol medication and also drink alcohol, with their doctor's permission—a dangerous mistake in my view.

So once again we see that a blanket health recommendation can't possibly apply to every individual. Alcohol has been shown to raise LDL cholesterol in all Apo E genotypes, and I see LDL increase even more in the Apo E 4s. Alcohol raises *all* cholesterol levels, as well as triglyceride levels, which have been shown to raise the most dangerous types of cholesterol (LDL). The only Apo E genotype that shows a promising effect from alcohol is the Apo E 2/3, but this genotype has a sensitivity to triglycerides with simple carbohydrates, and alcohol can elevate triglyceride levels.

I recommend that a patient with any active disease *not* drink alcohol. However, if you are in very good health and drink alcohol in a moderate fashion, here is a list of some positive effects of consuming small to moderate quantities:

- relaxation and stress reduction
- pleasurable taste
- romantic associations
- increase in HDL good cholesterol
- tannins, flavonoids, and antioxidants in wine
- possible increase in nitrous oxide production, potentially widening and improving flow in arteries
- potential improvement of antioxidant defense system
- reduction of platelet stickiness

Could the negative effects of alcohol outweigh the positive effects? Its negative effects include:

- immediate absorption into the circulatory system, causing rapid rises in triglycerides, blood sugar, and insulin, and reduction in reaction times (dangerous if driving)
- increased blood sugar levels even more quickly in diabetic and insulin-resistant people
- worsened diabetes
- increased "bad" LDL cholesterol in certain Apo E genotypes by as much as 300 percent
- hindered calcium metabolism and bone growth

With wine, is it the ethyl alcohol component that gives the benefit, or is it something in the grape juice? Grape juice alone has been shown to lower the risk of developing blood clots that may lead to heart problems. In addition, research has identified the antioxidant catechin as a major antioxidant in grapes, and catechin from grapes remains in a person's bloodstream more than four hours after consumption—longer than the alcoholic variety.

While there are lots of good qualities to alcohol when used wisely, it pays to think carefully when it comes to alcohol consumption.

Sodium in the Diet

Sodium—salt—is a must-have chemical element essential for good health. In the body, it is mainly found in the fluids around the cells—the blood and lymph. Sodium is very important for regulating fluid balance, and without it nerves and muscles do not function. With too little sodium, the body loses its ability to incorporate other major nutrients and cannot hold an adequate water-to-mineral balance. But when sodium intake exceeds what the body can handle, the kidneys have to work harder to remove it. A sustained buildup may cause the body to hold extra fluids in the blood and around the cells, which can contribute to a higher blood pressure from excess water retention.

Sodium is found naturally in many foods, and most of us, especially those with high blood pressure, should not consume more than 2400 mg. a day. However, the average American now consumes between 4000 and 10,000 mg. of sodium daily! Most of this excess sodium generally comes from eating too much processed food, which now makes up a large part of the average diet in the Western world. These foods nearly always have high levels of salt, partially because salt is a good, cheap preservative. In addition, the sodium used in these foods has had some tasty, valuable substances removed from it, with the salt and its preservative qualities restored afterward.

Many people think that the more "natural" forms of salt—rock salt or sea salt—are more healthy. Not really: sodium chloride is sodium chloride, regardless of its form. One excellent benefit of The Apo E Gene Diet is that the natural, whole, unprocessed foods it recommends are naturally low in sodium. A daily intake of unprocessed foods like fruits, vegetables, and plant proteins or fats contains far less than the recommended maximum of 2400 mg. sodium.

How well can you adjust to a low sodium, whole-food diet after eating highly refined foods for a long time? Quite well, if you shift your diet gradually; your taste buds may go into shock if you attempt a rapid change. If 6000 mg. per day has been your average intake, you can gradually lower it to 5000 mg. per day by the end of the first week, continuing down to 4000 mg. the following week, then to 3000 mg., reaching a goal of 2000 mg. per day by the end of the first month. The goal is to slowly make changes you can live with, while enjoying this new nutritional recommendation for the rest of your life.

A good place to start reducing sodium levels is by reading the labels for the sodium content in the foods you eat. Choose products labeled "sodium free," "low sodium," or "unsalted." In addition, the following general guidelines will help you make the transition from high sodium foods to natural whole foods:

- Buy fresh vegetables, poultry, fish, and lean meat.
- Use herbs, spices, and salt-free seasoning blends in cooking and at the table.
- Cook rice, pasta, and hot cereals without salt or preservatives.
- Remove all instant or flavored rice, pasta, and cereal mixes with added salt.
- If buying frozen or canned foods, choose those with labels that say "no salt added".
- Avoid all foods with preservatives.

In addition, cut back on frozen dinners, mixed dishes like pizza, packaged mixes, canned soups or broths, and salad dressings, choosing instead low sodium versions of:

- canned organic soups
- dried soup mixes
- organic bouillon
- canned vegetables and organic vegetable juices
- condiments like catsup and soy sauce
- crackers and baked goods
- snack foods like chips, pretzels, and unsalted nuts

Note: Rinse canned foods, such as water-packed tuna or vegetables, to remove some of the salt.

Micronutrients

As their name says, micronutrients are necessary only in very small amounts to help the body run its normal functions. Mainly vitamins and trace minerals (micronutrients) help maintain the structure of the body, as well as regulate many internal processes. They can be obtained from a balanced and varied diet of whole foods, which, in today's world, can be difficult to obtain. When an optimal diet is not available, I recommend a high-quality daily multivitamin.

An important factor in aging is deterioration at a cellular level. As we age, the efficiency of our cells decreases, with the effect that our body operates at one-half to one-fourth of the energy it had in its younger days. Fortunately, a regular intake of micronutrients from whole food can help prevent this inner-cell deterioration.

The brain is the most important organ affected by aging, since it consumes more energy than any other organ of the body. An energy deficit in the brain and central nervous system affects the activities of all the organs throughout the body, as well as mental acuity and mood. This could be a key factor for diseases such as Alzheimer disease. It is possible that a regular, balanced supply of micronutrients from fresh fruits and vegetables, whole foods, and daily supplemental vitamins and minerals can be a huge benefit.

Choosing Dietary Supplements or Vitamins

How do you choose multivitamins and minerals? How do you know which is the best one for you? The supplement industry is a fast-moving, multibillion-dollar operation not regulated by any government agency. While some products are very high-quality and provide honest supplementation for a fair price, others are supercharged by gimmicky marketing schemes that play on the promise of extreme health claims.

Reputable supplements can be a very good insurance policy when you're not eating an optimal diet, but you need to understand the risks and benefits of any supplement. This is not easy. Supplements are not regulated, most medical providers are inadequately trained in their use, and the research is limited. So if you are going to purchase a vitamin, you may want to do a little research yourself. The best policy is education.

Talk to an integrative medical provider trained in the field of dietary supplementation. Ask questions of anyone recommending a particular supplement. Ask what type of training they have had, and their qualifications for recommending a certain vitamin or botanical supplement. These products are not harmless. The incorrect dosage of supplements can cause problems. Choose a formulation designed, selected, and approved by a team of trained experts (not just one person) and manufactured under strict quality control.

Check whether the ingredients are tested both prior to and after manufacturing to ensure the content and doses are correct. All should be free of any preservatives, artificial colors or flavorings, and non-essential additives. Avoid products connected to money-making pyramid schemes.

The American Medical Association has a very strict policy regarding products that practitioners sell for profit in their exam rooms, so be wary of providers who do so. Also be aware of medical practitioners endorsing a product for profit. If a practitioner makes a recommendation, be sure ethical practices are considered first.

Chapter Fourteen

SHOPPING AND DINING TIPS FOR HEALTH

I grew up in the small town of St. Austell in the south of England. Most of the local merchants had their shops and markets on the town's main streets, but they were nothing like the shopping areas we have today. The closest shop resembling a supermarket was the local market house, with small stalls where local tradesman sold their goods. Every type of food was represented, and I can still remember many of them: Butchers with different types of meat, a baker, Cornish pasty shop, dairy, fish, green grocer, hardware, wood and coal shop, flower shop. My favorite was The Sweet Shop, which had the best sweets you could have imagined—licorice, fruit gum, and dolly mixture, (a kind of soft, fruity candy). My grandmother seemed to know everyone, and I usually didn't mind going shopping with her since I was allowed to buy sweets and sit on the steps of the market house watching the people come in and out.

Those days, and those kinds of shops, are long gone. In the "old days," people knew where their food came from and what it contained. This began to change in the early 1900s in the United States with the appearance of the large self-service stores called supermarkets, which now have become massive food suppliers. Often, they do not hold the intention of providing the best, most nutritious, high-quality whole food of the past. Luckily, specialty food markets have begun to reappear, and many supermarket chains are adding organic products and other healthy foods to their shelves in response to consumer demand.

Due to all the changes in food growing and manufacturing practices, we must now pay attention to how our food was grown—for example, with pesticides or not? Is it a "genetically-modified organism" (GMO) or not? We must also pay attention to how it was processed and prepared. This section shows you how to choose your food wisely no matter where you shop or dine out. Not everyone will have the wide variety of choices that comes with living in California, but you can learn how to choose a supermarket or a restaurant wisely.

Common sense tells us that we need good, clean, appropriate food in order to provide our bodies with the building blocks of good health. We cannot possibly expect to remain healthy if we are not providing all the proper nutrients our bodies need. Remember that grocery store managers want to stock the products you will buy, so ask them to carry healthy products you don't already see on their shelves. Chances are, many other people who are also becoming more health-conscious want the same products. If you want to buy organic foods, then ask for them and tell your friends to ask as well. If you want to avoid genetically modified food, ask your grocer if a particular food has been modified in that way (although it may not be possible to tell, since there is currently no government regulation that requires the labeling of GMO foods). If you want meat and chicken grown without hormones or antibiotics, or fruits and vegetables grown without pesticides, ask for them. Don't buy foods with preservatives and additives. Finally, if you don't know what's in a food product, don't buy it. Grocery stores will stop carrying products that no one buys.

In the end, it is up to each one of us to make healthy and intelligent choices about the foods we buy and eat. You might consider buying locally grown food in season. Buying from local organic farmers usually means purchasing products from people who put a great deal of effort into supplying their customers with high-quality herbs, spices, fruit, vegetables, eggs, poultry, and meats.

It is up to each of us to make healthy and intelligent choices regarding to the food we purchase and consume.

Restaurants

Eating out is very commonplace in today's world. There are many reasons why this is true, but the most common is probably convenience, stemming from lack of time. Anyone who has cooked a meal from scratch knows how long it takes to prepare and cook even a basic home-cooked meal, beginning with deciding what to eat, shopping for the food, cooking it, eating the meal, and then cleaning up afterwards. Many families in America just do not seem to have the time to do all this anymore and, as a logical substitute, they eat in restaurants more often.

In addition, restaurant food tastes good. The average person is not a chef, and it's difficult to compete with great-tasting food prepared by a talented chef. Keep in mind, however, that the intention of most chefs is not generally focused on maximizing the customer's health but rather on presentation of good-tasting food, so that customers will return. More and more chefs are becoming health-conscious, but even they may still wish to slip a little something into the food that tastes great but is not especially good for the customer.

Here's an example of that. I once attended a presentation in Arizona with Dr. Andrew Weil and Rosie Daley, Oprah Winfrey's chef. Both of them were in very funny form. As Daley was demonstrating how to prepare a heart-healthy dish, Dr. Weil sat in the audience, making an occasional comment. Every so often, Daley would share the contents of a recipe and then add, "If you want this dish to taste really good, add some real butter." She would look at Dr. Weil, who would reply, "Or not. It's delicious enough without the butter. Don't listen to Rosie." The audience loved these friendly disagreements, but keep in mind that even the best chefs who work closely with the best practitioners of integrative medicine are still focused on making food taste good and are therefore tempted to use not-so-healthy ingredients.

On the Menu: Nutritional Confusion

As a practitioner of integrative medicine, I have seen that one of the most powerful tools for reducing and alleviating disease is the diet. People are often reluctant to try this nutritional medicine because they've been utterly confused about diets and nutrition, thanks to what they see in the media. They ask, "What is the most popular diet of the day? Is it low-fat, high-fat? Low-carb, high-carb, high-calorie, low-calorie?" In addition, many people are satisfied with their diets and see no need to change, regardless of their current health status. And many people who eat frequently in restaurants and enjoy it, do not realize that they have lost control over what goes into the food they're eating.

This confusion is not surprising. The so-called experts can't seem to agree on the best diet for good health, so how can the average person have a hope of understanding? People tend to give up on a healthy diet after convincing themselves they have no time to understand the nutritional value of what they are eating. Nevertheless, a good start is to think positively and then, if you eat out a lot, acknowledge that restaurant meals do count. Start with a little education from a reliable source. The most unreliable nutritional information is usually the most accessible, particularly from ads (beware of infomercials touting health or diet products!) but also from articles in popular magazines and newspapers, the Internet and TV. On the other hand, the most reliable sources require some time and commitment to uncovering the research. First, educate yourself. Seek out trusted, evidenced-based information from a reliable source, such as a trained integrative medicine provider who has been well trained in all fields of medicine, including MDs, doctors of osteopathy, nurse practitioners, or physician's assistants. Then, focus on a commitment to visiting health-conscious restaurants and ordering healthful meals there.

Another factor in healthy eating is to become a food detective, both when you're grocery shopping for yourself and when eating out. You may find it easier to eat out if you screen the restaurant's menu beforehand to find out if you can stick to your recommended diet. Locating healthy food choices for your Apo E genotype may not be easy at first, but learning about macronutrients and how they affect you can be good for your health. Remember that what is on your plate and goes into your body becomes your body.

You should limit or even avoid certain foods, except perhaps on your birthday, which, you should note, happens only once a year. You can splurge occasionally, but, like many of my patients, you might find that changing to a healthy diet means your stomach may no longer appreciate a splurge, thanks to all the positive changes the body makes when fed the right diet.

Foods to avoid in a restaurant (and elsewhere):

• rich sauces, including butter, cream, hollandaise, and béarnaise

• fried foods—pan-fried or deep-fried

• braised cheese, au gratin, or scalloped dishes

• hashes

• potpies

One way to begin establishing your new nutritional habits when eating out is to get comfortable asking questions about the menu and how the food is prepared, and then making special requests that fit your diet. Most restaurants understand that many of their patrons have become more health-aware, so the chef and staff are making more efforts to accommodate their requests. You can request that the server ask the chef how foods are prepared (the server probably will not know without asking), and you can also ask that your selection be prepared the way you want it done.

When I order in a restaurant, I want to have a meal both healthy and delicious, so I often do both of those things—which is when my family wishes they could crawl under the table and disappear. But since I'm paying for the meal and understand that the restaurant staff most likely doesn't care about my health, I simply ask for what I want to eat. In most restaurants, you can put together a healthy meal by doing the following:

- Order steamed, broiled, roasted, poached, or dry-broiled preparations.
- Choose red and stock-based sauces.
- Ask for salad dressing "on the side" and use sparingly.
- Try lemon juice, vinegar, olive oil, or buttermilk dressing as a low-fat alternative.
- Trim all visible fat from meat and the skin from chicken before eating.
- Hold off on the butter and margarine; use avocado instead.
- Practice portion control (many restaurants now serve one person with enough food for four people).
- Stay away from foods described as large, jumbo, supreme, king-sized, double, or triple.
- Order one 5-lb. lobster (hold the butter, bring the lemons) with lots of salad and veggies for the entire table.
- Search out smaller descriptions: petite, regular, small, single, appetizer, children's portion.
- Don't be tempted by offers of more food for less money.
- Share menu items with your dining partner.

Most importantly, if you are not served what you ordered or it was not prepared to your specifications, send it back to the kitchen. As a patron paying for the food you want, you have the right to send back any food not prepared according to your request. The kitchen of a busy restaurant is fast-paced, and a special meal request can get lost very quickly, so if your entrée comes to the table smothered in sauce that you requested on the side, it might simply have been an oversight. You can usually remedy this situation by politely asking your server to take it back and replace it with the correct item.

Also, be aware that many food portions in restaurants are getting larger and larger these days—much larger than healthy portion sizes. For instance, the recommended portion of steak is 3 to 5 oz., but the average petite filet in a steak restaurant today can be anywhere from 10 oz. to 18 or even 20 oz. Wow! Unless you're a lumberjack working in the frozen country up north and burning 12,000 calories a day, that's too much food to stuff into your body. What are you going to do with all that meat? Grow another arm?

I had to chuckle recently when I was ordering in a restaurant. I asked the server about the size of the lobster tail, and he replied, "They range from 2 lbs. to 5 lbs." Who on earth could eat 2 lbs., not to mention 5 lbs., of lobster at one meal? Needless to say, I did not order the lobster or the butter sauce. Remember: In order to eat less, you must order less.

Mindful Dining: Setting a Table Fit for a King and Queen

In these hectic times, eating nothing, or grabbing something on the go, are the two choices often facing us. Not eating when you need to is not healthy, but there is also a difference between consuming food and dining. Eating, ingesting, food intake, consumption, dining, snacking, eating on the run, fast food, convenience foods, and food "to go" are just some of the many descriptions for the modern culinary experience. As you can see, most of the latter descriptions are about saving time. For many of us, gone are the days of eating at home, or packing a small parcel of food prepared at home to take with us on a journey. In the not-so-distant past, there were few restaurants and no fast food outlets, and the home-prepared meal was about all that was available. Home cooking was an art and displayed daily. Many times the meal served was a cherished event, especially the evening dinner, because it was a family's main social activity centered on a pleasurable dining experience.

Learning from Our Past

For many centuries, food preparation has been a primary activity in the center of daily life. Sometimes, it was also a major form of entertainment. It may have begun with the hunt of the day, which many times supplied the main dish.

Collecting flowers and vegetables from the garden or hothouse and afternoon walks down to the local farmhouse or shops to get milk, meat, cheese, or eggs were all part of the meal preparation experiences of the past.

The English trend of entertaining with afternoon tea at 3:00 started in the late 1700s, when dinner typically was served from 7:00 to 8:30. Because people grew hungry during the long stint between lunch and dinner, it became common to serve a light afternoon snack with tea. Anna Marie Stanhope, Queen Victoria's lady-in-waiting, later began the practice of inviting friends for tea and is often credited with turning this practice into a social event for many middle and upper class households.

As the popularity of afternoon tea grew, the English china pottery industry began with the discovery of English china clay. This led to the growth of the china pottery industry by William Adams & Sons, Spode, Wedgwood, Denby, followed by such artistic delights as Edinburgh and Waterford crystal glasses and England's famous Sheffield sterling silver cutlery.

Formal gatherings that revolved around this afternoon tea, as well as the evening meal, became an established pattern, and the tea and dinner table were transformed into an art form. Eventually this major form of entertaining evolved into more of a family tradition. My family followed this tradition as I grew up in Cornwall, where afternoon tea had taken on cultural as well as economical importance. Besides being the home of the copper and tin mining industries and a strong and vibrant fishing industry, Cornwall is the major source of English china clay and is home of the high-class Cornish Cream Tea, "The Best Cream Tea Event in all of England."

The fashionable cultural event of the daily "high tea at three" included displaying your beautiful English bone china tea service with aromatic English teas in warmed china teapots. Exhibit plates were used to display and present dainty cucumber and watercress sandwiches and an array of Cornish pilchards or herrings on toast. There were Cornish buns and sultana scones, topped with wholesome local fruit jam and, of course, a mountain of unwholesome—but we didn't know that back then—Cornish clotted cream. This culinary experience was laid out on a white linen tablecloth, with fresh linen napkins and silver spoons, knives, and forks. In the center of the table was usually a small bouquet of delicate wild flowers. I can still remember fresh strawberries and cream, hot cross buns and jam—all culinary delights of Cornwall.

This formal, festive feasting, a great part of the English culture, spread around the world. It influenced some of the early Americans' traditions, encouraging, for example, an iced version of tea. Sadly, today's fast-paced lifestyle has diminished the once daily ritual of high tea gatherings to something done only on a special occasion.

Today, most people are so busy they rarely find the time to experience some of these wonderful aspects of dining together that I knew so well as a child. There is no time to stop, reflect, and enjoy our family and friends, even our possessions. The attractions of the past's romantic dining experiences included the time spent with friends and family, savoring the food, not to mention the ritual of preparing the food and setting the table, and collecting roses from the garden or wildflowers from the meadow. Compare the elaborate dining experiences of the past to the dining experiences of today's fast-paced world. Today, there aren't many times that we bring out the good china, the special silverware, and the extra-nice crystal for a meal—maybe Thanksgiving, Christmas, and a birthday or two. It is no longer a daily ritual.

Many people still enjoy preparing a fine meal for a gathering of friends and families, complete with the excitement of a beautiful table laden with delicate china, sparkling crystal, shiny silver, and fresh white linens, but it is difficult for most of us to find the time to do this. In many households, daily meals have changed from home-cooked to fast food, complete with plastic containers, forks, knives, spoons, and paper or plastic cups with straws. Even I resort to fast food choices once in a great while. However, I know that the common dining experience can change, and with a little effort, a rich cultural tradition can return to our lives.

Here are some suggestions to enhance your dining experience:

- Light a candle on the table while eating breakfast in the morning.
- Put a flower in the vase to lift your spirits while drinking that cup of coffee or tea.
- Bring a flower home or to work for your table or desk.
- Choose a china cup instead of a paper version.
- Choose a crystal glass bowl instead of a plastic container.
- Take a minute before eating to give thanks with a song, grace, or even 10 seconds of silence.
- Most of all, remind yourself that you and your family are worth the effort.

Families are connected through tradition and stories, which can help build trust and communication between their members. If you usually eat out, consider skipping the restaurant tonight. Cook dinner at home together. If you already cook dinner for your family, consider making this time together even more special. Leave the paper napkins in the drawer tonight and use cloth, or surprise the children by asking them to put flowers on the table. Light a candle, or use the china a little more often. And please, turn off the television. For those moms and dads who have little children, invite them to join you in setting the dinner table as if you were kings, queens, princes, and princesses. Imagine and talk about what it was like back in the "olden days" when family and friends entertained each other. The children will probably love it. They seem to always want to know the stories of the world, and the best people to tell them these stories are their moms and dads.

My husband and I often serve a mysterious dinner on the floor in our home for our children, under a rainbow of multicolored toile that serves as a magic Eastern desert tent. At a dinner such as this, your family can discuss past traditions, dining, and culture. You can also explore how to bring a little tradition into your family life today. If there are small children present, conversation may center on fairies, pirates, kings and queens—Robin Hood, King Arthur and his knights, or even Cinderella. You might want to use a little book I wrote for a school children's program called the *Cornish Fairy-Pixie Conference*. It is set in medieval Cornwall and contains artwork to guide children in a fun walking exercise and a diet program using a pedometer for each child and posters that can be put on the wall.[15] And consider some simple whole food meals you can make at home. You can find lots of great books in your library or bookstore, even for "quick and easy" whole food preparation. Begin with planning even one meal at home each week. If you can engage a friend in becoming a food detective, you can share the great recipes you each discover, or even get together to prepare a healthy meal each week. A little planning like this can help immensely with the long-term goal of better nutritional intake and enhanced health.

15   For a copy of this book, write to: The Harvest of Hearts Program
       4165 Blackhawk Plaza Circle, Suite 125
       Danville, CA 94506

       All proceeds go to "The Harvest of Hearts Program," which educates children and their parents about the benefits of healthy nutrition and exercise.

※

Chapter Fifteen

THE HARMONY OF MIND, EMOTIONS, BODY, AND SPIRIT

I think, therefore I am.
—René Descartes

Does the way we think change our physical body? Are our mind, emotions, and body connected, or are they completely separate entities?

The 17th-century French philosopher and mathematician, René Descartes, contemplated the philosophical question of how the world seemed to him, versus what the world actually was. He asked questions such as:

- Who am I?
- Where do I come from?
- What do I really know?
- What can I be certain of?

What Descartes concluded was, "I think, therefore I am." He thought: I am thinking, so my mind is real. We have physical bodies, we can touch the physical body and the world; therefore, our bodies are also real.

Reductionism theory emerged from this philosophical thinking process. It was based on the cognition that because we can actually see and measure the physical body, it is truly real. Medicine was on its way to full-fledged separation of mind, emotions, and body, as it focused on the physical realities of "If I can see it, or touch it, I know it is real." Since the mental, emotional, or spiritual aspects of the physical body could not be touched, felt, or understood, they did not exist, at least to the world of medicine. Hence medicine took the responsibility for the care of the physical body alone, and the mind, emotions, as well as the spirit and soul, were given to the church for safekeeping.

This separation was not necessarily a bad thing, because it enabled medicine to focus on the physical realities of the body, which it could witness, dissect, measure, and weigh. As a result, medical scientists made amazing discoveries in the physical world of physiology, anatomy, microbiology, molecular biology, genetics, biochemistry, and pharmacology. Medicine thought it had arrived— until quantum physics entered the picture in the early part of the 20th century. As medicine caught up with physics, however, the discoveries of quantum physics threw many previously held "facts" about the physical universe out the window. It showed that there was much more to understanding and treating the body than had been thought. Quantum physics defies description, even among the quantum physicists themselves, but an idea can be gotten from a popular movie, "What the Bleep Do We Know?"

Additionally, the work of Hans Selye, MD, who uncovered the mechanisms of stress in the human body in the 1940s, laid the groundwork for what we now recognize as the intricate connection between the mind and the physical body. Medicine can no longer view mind, emotions, and body as three separate entities.

The power and potential of understanding the connections between the mind and body are quite incredible—*whole-body health involves caring for the mind, emotions, and spirit as well as the body.* With that in mind, I want to present a new perspective on how to both view and approach your health—and your life.

The bottom line is that the human body doesn't function on the physical level alone. It also functions on psychological, emotional, environmental, energetic, and spiritual levels. The way you think and feel, the state of your environment, and your relationship to spirit *all* impact—influence and shape— your physical body, all the way through to your cells and genes. Quantum science has proven this, and clinical medicine is now using this knowledge with patients, recognizing there is more to treatment than handing out pills and performing surgeries.

Have you ever asked yourself:

- How does my mind influence my physical body?
- How do my emotions influence my physical body?
- Does my environment influence my mind?
- Does my environment influence my emotions?
- Are my mind, emotions, and body connected, or are they three separate entities?

While a single theory rarely provides the whole answer, advances in science and technology have enabled us to understand more than ever before. Some of the answers to our questions regarding the power and potential of the mind-emotion-body connection can be found in the fields of psychoneuroimmunology and neuroendocrinology. From these disciplines, we know that certain thought patterns produce beneficial or harmful body responses, and that these in turn can produce corresponding positive or negative physical outcomes or states of health. This is real clinical science that we can apply to our lives, to bring us better health, joy, and happiness.

Perhaps one day we will be able to answer the question, "What is a thought made of?" Once we have a complete understanding of our physical selves, perhaps we can apply what we've learned to a deeper understanding of how thoughts affect the physical body. Possibly, one day, we can join the three arenas of mind, emotions, and physical body, and view them working interdependently as a whole, instead of as separate entities. This will enhance our efforts to be of service to humankind through science and medicine.

Evidence of the Mind/Emotion/Body Connection

Let's look at some common human experiences that typically produce negative or positive thinking states, and what research tells us about the chemicals the body produces in response to them. Here are some "negative" human experiences:

- loss of a loved one through death
- divorce or separation
- depression
- loneliness
- chronic stress

The negative thinking states typically associated with these experiences have been shown to reduce the immune system's ability to fight disease. If we perceive the world as stressful, we will continue to produce stress hormones generated by negative feelings. Here are some "positive" human experiences:

- fulfilling personal relationships and social support structures
- fulfillment of your life's work
- humor and laughter
- guided imagery
- hypnosis
- relaxation techniques
- meditation
- aerobic activity and exercise

The positive states often associated with these experiences increase your number of white blood cells and other immune factors such as your T-cell count, elevate endorphin levels, and promote healing and a feeling of well-being.

If we evaluate patients who report being happy and content in their lives and contrast their immune functions with those of patients who are chronically stressed, unhappy, or depressed, we find that the disconnected, unhappy patients are sicker. So we can use the mind/emotion/body connection to improve our health and prevent disease. It is useful to classify the different states of awareness available to us to see how each influences—even governs—our brain and central nervous system.

Levels of Awareness

The following model was adapted from many sources (it also correlates to the seven chakras, see page 215) using seven levels of awareness that we, as humans, may operate on. As you read through these, consider which is the level or levels you operate on most of the time. An awareness of each level can be of use in helping you define who you are, and what you want.

First Awareness Level: Fight-Flight-or-Freeze Response

The fight-flight-or-freeze response is an acute survival reflex mechanism that was programmed into our brains for millions of years. The oldest part of our brain on an evolutionary scale is called the "reptilian brain." This response is a necessary component for the survival of all animals with a central nervous system. Life-threatening events produce a specific type of acute stress response or chemical chain reaction in the body. These adrenal stress hormones are responsible for shutting off all non-necessary body systems and focusing on the systems essential to our survival, such as the brain, heart, and lungs.

We do not have to think about anything to generate this response. It just happens. Thanks to this response, people have found themselves able to perform amazing things they ordinarily could never have accomplished, such as lifting a car to save another person or running faster than they had ever imagined possible.

While primitive humans often had to fight for food or survival and to flee from danger, modern humans rarely encounter actual life-threatening events. This doesn't stop activation of this inner-body protective warning system, however, and our brains are often imagining situations from the past or future that seem like they are life-threatening but aren't.

The freeze component of this response has been largely suppressed by our "civilization." When other animals have survived a life-threatening experience and are emerging from the freeze state, they literally shake it off. We humans tend to not do this, and that suppression of the unshaken-off fear remains in our bodies. It is now implicated in many post-traumatic stress conditions (PTSD), with stress being stored in parts of the brain and body.

Second Awareness Level: Spontaneous Action Response
The second level of awareness is the reaction response—an adaptation of fight-flight-or-freeze that evolved because the human mind, by using intellectual processing, concluded that we do not always need to fight or flee a situation of potential negativity or danger. If a situation is not really life-threatening, we could theoretically avoid the intensity of the fight- flight-or-freeze response by using a different response: a controlled reaction response. This response can be calculated to fit our needs based on our personality's ability, positive or negative, to be expressed with a kind, mean, or indifferent demeanor.

The fight-flight-or-freeze reaction is still with us. We know that responses to stress can come in many forms—as severe as a full-fledged panic attack, as gentle as what we call butterflies fluttering in the tummy, or even a hot flash. It also can be as silent as an elevated blood pressure reading. All are expressions of the fight-flight-or-freeze survival mechanism.

Today we know a great deal more about the environment produced by chronic stress within the body on a daily basis. Chronically stressed bodies produce a chain reaction response, with stress hormones, glucose, and fat being dumped into our bloodstreams. Today we know that these reactions are generated by the negative thinking states engendered by certain experiences.

Should we, could we, be using our mind in a different way? Should we be modifying how we view and react to the world? If your answer is yes, be aware that some of our reactions to life are difficult to change because they are learned behaviors, usually ingrained into our cellular chemistry at an early age. Receptor sites in the body feed off the chemistry generated by this stress response. Interestingly, if we do not feed those receptor sites we can actually experience a withdrawal from not having them filled—the same as a drug addict on cocaine or heroin would experience, but not as strongly. This can make personal change more difficult than we might hope it would be.

Third Awareness Level: Calming Awareness Response

This tranquil response coincides with not having to work hard to survive, hunt, fight, or sleep all of the time. It arises when human beings have time to rest, think about, and reflect upon life's ever-changing challenges. When humans have time to do all of that, they evolve into higher functioning beings.

Some people might choose to classify this state as meditation, prayer, analytical thinking, or contemplative problem solving. How does this level relate to us in today's highly technological environment? In a chronically stressful life, few of us have the time or space to engage in reflection and questioning—we revert to the unconscious older patterns. And yet, it's more important than ever to reclaim this state if we are to develop and sustain a healthy, balanced life.

The bottom line is, don't be a caveman. Strive to step out of that primitive, reptilian brain, spontaneous reaction and gain some tranquil time for yourself where you can explore some of your own questions. Questions such as "What do I want out of my life?" "How are my relationships going?" "Am I doing in my life's work?" Shift yourself from the caveman mentality and focus on you and what you want.

Although it sounds simple, it's not always easy. Women, for example, tend to get lost in their husband's and children's lives, but some women are not cut out for a life of laundry, children, dishes, and household chores. On the other hand, men tend to focus on bringing in the income and providing for the family's needs outside the home. To you both, I recommend taking a day off—or as much time as possible—to re-evaluate your work and duties to focus on your desires. By searching deep within yourself for what you really need and want, you might be amazed by what you find. The next time you are performing your regular tasks, whether around the house or where you work outside the home, slip into your intuition within a restful state and ask, "Do I like my life the way it is? Is this what I imagined doing with my life?"

Fourth Awareness Level: Instinctive Response

Instinct, intuition, sixth sense, and one's source of spiritual intelligence can create higher thoughts than the rational mind is capable of generating. Instinctive intuition is not the same as rational thought. It is more of a knowing without knowing how you know it: you can somehow feel it, sense it.

To answer the question, "Do we know we have a physical body?" we must do as René Descartes suggested and move into that spiritual, nonphysical essence of our being that we may sense but cannot see. Here we can connect with an experience of higher knowing—an orientation of knowing that something is so, even though we may not know how or why we know. At the same time, this state is not a feeling of gaining or losing; it is just "what is"—the instinctive, intuitive knowing that something is right or correct.

Maybe some people can get to this level of knowing, but can you? The answer is an unequivocal yes. The fact is, you already have it inside of you, and you do not need to find what you already have. You just need to set the intention to use it. To do so, I suggest you do a breathing exercise or enter a silent state within yourself and ask your instinctive intuition to be activated and heightened. Then, ask a question. You will get an intuitive reaction, no matter what question you ask. To experience this is a powerful feeling, and the attempt has never failed me.

Fifth Awareness Level: Imaginary Response

This is the imaginative or visionary state. This is where you actually begin to know what is needed to generate what it is you want to manifest. This state evolves naturally when you are in sync with the purpose and mission of your life journey. I know this because I have been doing this visualizing my entire life, though I may not have always been totally aware of it.

My experience has shown me that once I become aware of what I want to manifest, the universe seems to show up with exactly what I need. You too, will have an intuitive feeling that this—whatever it is you are drawn to manifest—is right for you. Sometimes others' intentions try to push you off your original mission, but it is up to each of us to stay true to our mission. If you are focused and keep tapping into what you truly desire in your life—what feels good and right for you—you will manifest whatever it is you choose.

Sixth Awareness Level: Innovative Response

At this level, you can gain an understanding that you can create something not currently present in your reality. I have had this experience in my life and have created many things I have never seen before. To understand that you can create something by recognizing the components that must go into it and then create that something of your own intention is the creation response level in action. It doesn't have to be anything fancy at first, but just knowing that this creative process and response is possible is very important.

With every creative process, we need spirit. You and your creative spirit need to be engaged if you are to create whatever it is you want. Spirit brings together the pieces.

Let's say you want to build or create something—a song, a book, a cake, a dress, or even a company. What do you need? Break the end product down to find what the whole is comprised of—many parts, many ingredients? But even having these, it takes the will and the intention to put those parts together to be able to make the dress, cake, song, or book. Once you actually take your desire and put something together, it is unique, it is your creation. You can say, "Well, lots of people make cakes or books or dresses, even companies," but it may never have been done by you in your way with your particular viewpoint. Focus on your mission, your awareness, your life, your creation. You are important and your desire to build something is also important. Function at your own level of creativity. Believe that you count as a creator in this world—because you are one.

Seventh Awareness Level: Spiritual Response

The spiritual response is being aware of a higher source of spiritual "something." No matter how we paint this higher "something," if we reach this spiritual response level, we ask some foundational questions of the universe. Most of us who experience this level at some point in our lives come to realize that we have a higher spirit level or higher divine source. We don't experience it as we do other, more physical levels; it's a completely unique experience and goes back to the foundation of creation where "the making" of something comes from spirit. This process goes all the way back to those fundamental questions that our French philosopher René Descartes asked: "Who am I? Where do I come from?"

We can ask the same of everything around us. Where do all the different varieties of cakes, songs, and businesses come from? Where do all the butterflies, birds, and flowers come from? Fundamentally, from the same place all other creations come from, but when you break down those creations into parts and follow them back to their source, you still come up with the same question and same sort of an answer. You can't have the physical development of a pie, cake, or business without a spiritual wanting or desire to create.

So ultimately I do not think we know the answer to Descarte's questions because the source of formation is beyond our own understanding. We clearly do not have enough information to gain a cognitive understanding to answer these questions that were asked hundreds and even thousands of years ago, and are still being asked today. Some would define the starting place of physical formation as "God." Depending on where you live and what culture you live in, or at what time of your life you are in, your definition of the ultimate being or creator will vary. I don't think it really matters, as long as you realize that you do have access to a higher spirit or higher divine source. That belief needs to have importance and belong to you, and only you.

What does all this mean? Review these levels of awareness and try to understand where you operate: Are you operating in the first level of awareness from a fight/flight/freeze response where you are constantly in the protective mode? This is a very stressful response to be living in. If you expend most of your energy trying to survive, not a lot is left for anything creative. If you are able to live beyond the first few levels of awareness, it is a lot easier on your body, and life is more productive, joyful, and creative. Be aware that moving up to higher levels is more difficult for some Apo E genotypes. While no one stays out of the fight/flight/freeze response all the time, the Apo E 2s and 4s seem to have a harder time getting to the higher levels if they are not in balance with their environment.

How Does This All Fit into the Apo E Gene Diet?

We need to have the right nutritional ingredients, based on our genetic makeup, to be able to maintain cell balance and ease in the body. Yet, as we've seen, our bodies do not get nutrition from food alone. The way we think, how we feel about life, and the state of our environment, as well as how we have been trained to deal with the environment around us, all affect this balance.

Depending on the level of awareness from which we're operating at any given time, we may respond with the endorphins of love if operating on Level 5–7, or produce the chemicals of fear in the fight-flight-or-freeze mode of Level 1. Operating at Level 1 requires a large and constant flow of blood sugar, so if you are in chronic state of fear and you are an Apo E 4, your body is constantly producing the stress hormone, adrenaline. This in turn requires more fast-acting glucose fuel, which adds an additional demand for fuel—the body now has to work extra hard and is less able to attend to the growing and healing that occurs when it is supposedly at rest.

Just because you are not eating the correct food and otherwise creating a gene-supportive environment, your body doesn't stop needing the right fuel. The brain will ask the liver to make some fuel (glucose) to feed it, and the body adapts to produce it, feeding itself from itself—becoming its own internal fuel source. That internal fuel production process is hard on the body in many ways, and it can unbalance your body's cells and tissues. This process happens with the all Apo E genotypes but not at the same degree as the Apo E 4s.

Do you have this chronic stress? A typical answer is, "Sure! It's the nature of my work, and I can't change it." If you cannot change your work, can you change how you react to it? Focus on what you can do, not on what you cannot.

When operating on Levels 5–7, as you focus on what you love and make changes to give yourself more of that, you find the world will help you. The more you can practice being on the higher levels of awareness, the more you can create a better life, which goes back to one of the reasons you are reading this book in the first place.

Focus on what you actually want *for you*. Stay focused and directed on your desire and needs. Identify what level of awareness you are operating at most of the time. If you are not happy with this, know that you can change levels. Make it a priority to take some quiet time to make change.

Knowing the levels of awareness you are on plus your Apo E genotype, you can begin to understand if you need to make changes or if you are all right staying at the levels of awareness that are familiar to you.

Of course, this is very dependent on your knowing who you are and what you want. Consider your current level of awareness. Are you going about your life in a state of observation, living in someone else's intention—operating at a Level 1 or 2 of awareness? Or are you living in your own intention—a state of creation at an awareness Level of 6 or 7? You be the judge. We began this process in Chapter 2, but now we will look at this a little more deeply. I believe that who you are now, and how you perceive your state of health and happiness, will be different than when you first began reading this material. Let's see.

Learning Who You Are, and What You Want

Everyone has a natural preference for what they would like to do. Most of us would like to have what we want and get rid of what we don't want. Yet sometimes we seem to argue for our own limitations, coming up with a host of reasons for why we can't have what we want. The fact is, you can have exactly what you want and get rid of what you don't! You can create your perfect life—just the way you want it. Here's how.

First, you need to decide exactly what you want and do not want in your life. If you have never given this any thought, you may have to think about it for some time. You may have been living in other people's worlds and doing what they wanted you to do for so many years that you have never taken the time to seriously think about what it is you actually like, need, or want. I did this for many years, until one day I got smart and said, "No. I don't want that. I want something else in my life."

But while it is easy to say this, actually taking the steps to accomplish the change you want is another matter altogether. Let's look at how you can make it happen.

You need to map out very clearly, on paper, what exactly you want. Then you need to map out just how you will accomplish each goal. You can review your work with a spouse or partner later, but initially you must do this work by yourself. This exercise requires imagination (daydreaming, some might call it), and may involve meditation or prayer. We will look at these more closely in the next chapter. For now, you can get started with the checklist below.

Your map does not have to be perfect the first time around. Initially, you may want to work on naming only a few of the things you want or changes you want to make. Starting small is best; do not try to make too many drastic changes all at once. Your goal can be simple or it can be complex, but putting your plan on paper is very important. Once your plan is set, you can modify and refine any aspect of it that you care to.

Now, let's begin. *If you had all the time in the world and no restrictions on what you did with it, how would you spend your time? If you had endless monetary resources, what would your life be like?*

Ah, wait. I heard you say, "I don't all the time in the world or all the monetary resources." Don't focus on the information of the past. *Focus on the future of what will be.* The task involves mapping your life as *if* you have already accomplished your goals. For now, set your goals on what will be and what you would like it to be—not on what it is not.

Now, I'm asking you to set aside some time to look over some specific areas of your daily life, to consider what is, and what may be, and what would be *ideal, for you.* If you don't know what you want, you're unlikely to get it!

In Your Ideal World

Breakfast and Morning Snack

- In your ideal world, what would your breakfast and morning snack be, with a focus on health?
- Who prepares your food? You or someone else?
- If you are counting on someone else to prepare your food, do they know what you need to maintain good health?
- Are they educated about healthy foods or are they providing what the masses want?

You need to get control of what goes into your meals. Remember that what goes into your body becomes your body. I suggest you be specific in naming your preferred type of:

- fluids
- proteins
- complex carbohydrates
- fruits and/or vegetables
- good fats
- Write in your preference._____

Exercise

What is your preferred type of exercise program?

- stretching
- warm-up
- aerobic—cardiovascular
- anaerobic—strength
- cool-down
- Write in your preferred exercise. _____

When would you most like to exercise?

- morning
- noon
- afternoon
- evening
- Write in your preferred time. _____

Work

- Are you currently doing your life's work?
- What do you currently do in your work or job?
- Rate your work—"1" being you dislike your work, and "10" being the perfect work for you:

Like   Dislike
1   2   3   4   5   6   7   8   9   10

- If you could do any work, what would you like to do?
- How many days a week would you like to work?
- What time would you like your work day to begin and end?

All day—an 8-hour day

7 a.m.–3 p.m.

9 a.m.–5 p.m.

10 a.m.–6 p.m.

11 a.m.–7 p.m.

Morning only

6 a.m.–Noon

7 a.m.–1 p.m.

8 a.m.–Noon

Afternoon only

Noon–4 p.m.

Noon–5 p.m.

Noon–6 p.m.

Afternoon and evening

Noon–8 p.m.

Noon–9 p.m.

Noon–10 p.m.

Evening only

6 p.m.–10 p.m.

6 p.m.–11 p.m.

6 p.m.–Midnight

Or write in your perfect work hours_____

Or do you prefer not to work at all?

- Is your work space all yours or shared?
- Are you comfortable with the noise level?
- Does the space support you in doing your best work?
- What can you do to make it better, now? This may be as simple as placing a photograph of a loved person or place on your desk or as complex as rearranging the furnishings.

Lunch and Afternoon Snack

- What would your lunch and afternoon snack be, with a focus on health?
- Where would you eat it—at home, in a park, a restaurant or fast-food choice?
- With others or alone?

Name your preferred type of:

- fluids
- proteins
- complex carbohydrates
- fruits and/or vegetables
- good fats
- Write in your preference. _____

Home Environment

- What would your ideal home space be like? Consider the size, the furnishings, wether the space is cluttered or uncluttered. Who do you share the space with? Do you have a personal dedicated space just for you? What are the colors like? What are the smells—fresh, or stale? What are the sounds? What about the surroundings?
- Do you care what your home space looks like?
- What would make it very special for you?
- What is just one thing (or two, or three) you could decide to do now that would make it better for you?

Hobbies and Interests

- In your ideal world, what are your favorite hobbies and interests—sports, art, creative development, writing and reading, other?
- How much time do you spend on these?
- When and how do you like to do this?
- With other people or alone?
- How would you most like to do it?

Family

- Ideally, how would you and your family spend your time together?
- Would you spend more or less time with a spouse or partner, children, pets, extended family?

Dinner and Evening Snack

- What would these be, with a focus on health?
- Who would prepare it?
- Where would you eat it—at home, a restaurant, some other special place?
- Alone or with others?

Name your preferred type of:
- fluids
- proteins
- complex carbohydrates
- fruits and/or vegetables
- good fats
- Write in your food preference._____

Evening Activities

- Ideally, how would you spend your evenings?
- Alone or with family, friends, or in group activities?
- What would you be doing?
- Would every evening be similar, or would you set aside some for family, some for friends or personal growth actives, some alone or with someone special?

Perfect Sleep Pattern

- Ideally, what time would you go to bed—and rise in the morning?

- What do you consider the optimal number of hours of sleep for you?

- When does your body want to go to bed?

- If you have difficulty sleeping, do you need to use any medications or natural alternatives?

- Does your sleeping environment nurture you?

  Consider: your bed and bedding, furnishings, lighting, colors, temperature, sounds, scents

- Is it right for you?

- What would your ideal sleep environment and sleeping pattern look and feel like?

Happiness

- Circle your level of happiness on the following scale, with 1 being very unhappy, 10 completely happy.

  Unhappy   Happy
  1   2   3   4   5   6   7   8   9   10

- If you are not happy, why?

- Can you identify some of the reasons you are not happy?

- Create your day, your way, and remember that your happiness is your responsibility and no one else's. You can make changes that will make you healthier and happier, and bring you more peace, more joy.

If you feel you cannot accomplish this alone, consider finding someone to support you. Enlist the help of a friend, family member, doctor, or counselor/ therapist. You can create your *life* and *day* the way you want it to be. *Focus on what you want! Not on something you don't want.*

Now let's look at some practical tools that can support you in manifesting your ideal life.

Chapter Sixteen

TOOLS FOR CHANGE

Now that you know what you want, let's look at some tools that can help you make your dreams come true.

Expressive Arts Therapy

Expressive arts therapy can support you in making the changes—psychological, physical, or spiritual—that you want to make in your life. While psychologists are not totally sure how this process actually manifests the desired changes, it does! Most of my patients really enjoy this expressive arts exercise.

With this exercise, you create a picture or "dream board" illustration of your ideal life. This process assists you in focusing on your innermost needs, desires, hopes, and dreams. It puts you a step beyond just feeling or thinking what your life is going to be like when you have it just as you want it, since it helps you actually see some physical picture or form of what your new life is going to look like. You can create this picture with drawings, words, picture objects, figures, and/or paintings. Make it your very own masterpiece. Are you ready? All you need to do is dream and focus on what you want. See yourself as already having this new object or behavior in your life. Then be thankful for your new life as if you are already living it: Your newfound health, your new exercise program, your healthier eating habits, or healthier relationships.

The goal is to include a drawing or picture of each aspect of your life you want to change. Example 1: If you are currently living in a certain town or home, yet you want to live in another, place a picture of the town or home you want to live in on your picture. Example 2: If you want to start eating healthier foods instead of fast food or poor quality, unhealthy food, add pictures of healthy foods. Example 3: If you want to become more active in your life, place a picture of the activity or exercise you see yourself doing every day. Example 4: If you are unhappy in your job, place a picture of the job you want.

Whatever it is—remember to dream from your heart. My patients have used any and all of the tools below to create their personal collage:

- a large cardboard/paperboard or piece of paper to serve as your blank canvas
- crayons, markers, paints, or pencils
- magazines (with pictures you like)
- scissors to cut out magazine pictures
- sticking tape or glue
- photographs of anything you want to add to your life

Once you have all your tools, have fun and create your new life vision board. Then look at your collage every day and see yourself as already living this new healthier dream life of yours.

Mindful Breathing

Mindful breathing involves using the breath to release stress, calm your nervous system, and focus on what you want. Such a shift enhances your health on many levels, and it is a tremendous step toward realizing your dreams.

Most of us are so busy that we rarely find the time to sit calmly and just breathe. Busy lifestyles create an overly overactive nervous system so such breathing is essential for relaxation, contemplation, and focus. It is important to take even a few minutes here and there throughout the day to simply breath, with the intention of returning to a place of calm and focus within yourself—regardless of what is happening around you. Try it. You may be astounded at the gains you will reap.

Here is a simple anti-stress breathing technique you can try right now. If possible, remove yourself from physically being in contact with the stressor.

1. Sit quietly in a comfortable position.

2. Close your eyes and take one or two deep cleansing breaths. With a slow, regular rate, breathe in through your nose and out through your mouth.

3. Blow out all the air in your lungs through your mouth.

4. Take a deep breath in through your nose, hold it for a second or two, and then slowly exhale all your air through your mouth.

5. Do this same kind of breath three more times.

After you have completed the fourth deep breath, sit quietly for a few minutes and see how you feel. Do you feel less stressed and more peaceful? You can do this exercise again if you would like to feel even calmer, and do it any time you feel stressed or anxious.

Remind yourself to do a stress reduction breathing exercise a few times a day. When you practice this type of breathing, you are guiding and teaching your nervous system to become familiar with how it feels to be in a relaxed state. After practicing for only a few weeks, you can just think about relaxing, and your nervous system will follow in kind. The relaxing biochemistry will follow, and then your body usually will relax immediately if it has become familiar with the practice. Historically, it has taken my patients two or three weeks of doing this exercise just a couple of times a day to gain an automatic response so that when they begin to think about relaxing, their body follows.

Meditation

I used to have a problem with the concept of meditation. Having tried it many times over the years with no formal direction or even a belief in the technique, it seemed to be a waste of time and I saw my efforts as a failure. But one day I was given some basic practical instruction that focused and shifted my mind and energy in a different way, letting me get a positive experience from meditation for the first time. Having been instructed to meditate on a specific intention rather than on a general concept, I suddenly was able to connect with a higher feeling and get some clear direction and insight. Wow, what a difference!

Being the practical person that I am, I now see a real purpose for meditation and do it regularly. I no longer have a vision of a yogi sitting on a carpet for hours, seemingly wasting time. What is the purpose of my version of meditation? While I don't meditate in the same way or for the same reasons that yogis do, my purpose is to get valuable information and insights that help me excel in this journey called life. You do can the same.

I decided to put the "art of meditation" to the test. I chose to write this book as a way of documenting what I was learning on my life journey, but I needed all the help I could get. Meditation gave it to me. Suddenly, out of thin air came the information and direction I needed—more than I could have imagined. I got answers to questions and solutions to difficulties I would never have thought possible. I met people who provided me with content I could add to my own ideas for my book. The help I got was so great, it was as if I had tapped into my own personal computer database—a database with some, if not all, of the answers I needed.

I now have a whole new appreciation for meditation. If I can learn to meditate, you can at least try it. Keep it simple and short to begin with. You don't need any fancy stuff. There's nothing you need to buy—no special mats or clothes to wear. All it takes is you and the universe, relaxed and comfortable.

Practical Meditation with a Purpose

Find a place and time when you can have uninterrupted quiet. You *can't* meditate well in a busy room with people watching TV or any other electronic disturbances (radios, CDs, or telephones). Turn off your cell phone. You need peace and quiet so you can become still and centered.

Sit in a comfortable position. Sitting cross-legged in the middle of a room is not comfortable for me, so I choose to put my body in a comfortable supported position. I most often lie on the ground with a couple of my favorite pillows. When I travel and stay in a hotel, I pull all of those lovely white fluffy pillows off the bed and get all the extra pillows out of the closet. Then, I lie on a sea of soft fluffy pillows and get quiet. You might try relaxing in your favorite chair in a comfortable position. Be sure that your legs and arms are not crossed.

Being comfortable is the key. Make sure you do not have to go to the bathroom. Invariably, once your body begins to relax, the body begins to function more effectively and without fail you end up wanting to go to the bathroom after only a few minutes into your meditation time.

Once you are comfortable, look at your life and focus your thinking on something you would like to change or gain more information about. Here are some examples.

- How can I find an exercise partner to help me be successful in my exercise program?

- I would like some help and guidance with my finances. (Be specific about what you want: I need help paying a bill. I need help accomplishing a little saving each month. I need help to stay within my budget.)

- I would like some direction and help with a relationship.

- I would like to focus on being able to incorporate the right diet into my life.

Keep it simple and be specific, and then see what comes up for you. Remember, this takes practice, so don't expect to become an expert overnight. Use the breathing exercise above to turn off your fast-paced nervous system, which may have been racing all day. When your breathing is smooth and rhythmic, let all negative thoughts that flow into your mind flow right out again. Know that you can't turn off your thoughts, so just let them go once you notice that you're dwelling on something negative. Be prepared for information to flow to you. You might want to have a pen and paper ready so that after your meditation, you can write down the information that comes to you.

The Use of Sound in Meditation

"Om" and "Ah" are two ancient sounds used for meditation. These sounds are from a sacred syllable chanted in Hindu and Buddhist prayers and mantras, and are said to date back as far as 624 BCE. They are connected with creation and joy and are known to encourage information to surface in your conscious mind.

Using sound for meditation is a personal choice. Some people say sound helps; some say it doesn't. I use both the "Om" and "Ah" sounds. I don't decide to use a sound or not—if I start, that's fine, if not, I meditate quietly. Whatever happens at each meditation session is right for you. I have found that using one of these sounds encourages me to focus on creating my own sound and vibration, which brings an experience of clarity and creation.

Meditation and Visualization with the Chakras

The ancient Ayurvedic Hindu tradition, which has successfully taught the art of healing and prolonging life, tells us about chakras (see chakra chart page 215). The chakras are the seven energy centers running from the base of the spine to the top of our head, and each is connected to a major organ.

For your creative meditation exercise, you can begin with an energy-cleansing process to remove negativity and to provide a clear channel for energizing thoughts to enter your consciousness. Visualize energy flowing from the base of your spine and all the way up to the top of your head, then flowing out through the top of your head into the universe. The energy is drawn up from the earth through your first—or root—chakra (at the base of your spine), up along your spine, and out of your head and through the seventh—or crown—chakra.

Does this information all sound a little "out there" to you? It sure did to me—for the longest time. Please consider trying it anyway. At worst you might get really relaxed and go to sleep. At best you could get clear direction and answers to the questions you have. At least try meditation once or twice before dismissing this practice.

Meditation Visualization Chakras Chart

	Crown	Connected with the pineal gland in the brain
	Third Eye	Connected with the pituitary gland in the brain
	Throat	Connected with thyroid gland in the neck
	Heart	Connected with thymus gland and heart in the chest
	Solar Plexus	Connected with the liver and adrenal glands in the abdominal area
	Sacral	Connected with the testes and ovaries in the pelvic area. This is the area of the body where creation occurs
	Root	Connected with the uterus and prostate gland

Guided Imagery

As part of your meditation, you can also try a technique called guided imagery. It can be especially helpful if you find yourself in a situation for which you can find no cause, such as:

- an inability to experience good health
- chronic illness
- recurrent depression
- chronic anxiety
- an inability to heal

I have found guided imagery to be immensely valuable. For example, for many years I had questions about my spiritual health and how it affected my work and my life, and it wasn't until I practiced guided imagery that I finally found answers to many of these questions.

Guided imagery is a form of focused relaxation combined with guided inner exploration. It has been documented to improve a person's health and physical well-being, and it is used to facilitate healing in a variety of illnesses. A very strong body of research is showing us that a high percentage of common medical conditions or problems respond positively to this gentle therapy.

I believe that everyone can benefit from guided imagery whether or not a health problem exists. The intent of guided imagery is making connections between the body, emotions, and mind, using your thoughts and any associated images to encourage relaxation and desired changes in attitude, and producing beneficial changes in behavior.

My first experience of guided imagery was facilitated by a psychologist experienced in the technique. While I was aware that research showed this mode of healing was generating good results, I knew little about the actual practice of it. So, at that time, I did not recommend it to my patients; our appointments were usually so short I was not able to ask all the questions necessary to understand the state of their psychological and spiritual health. However, after studying guided imagery in my integrative medicine fellowship, and experiencing sessions myself, I now have a full appreciation of what it is and the profound role it can play in the healing process. I now highly recommend guided imagery to my patients who would benefit from such a therapy.

Guided imagery supports whole health and healing. It accesses our subconscious, those inner realms where we hold memories of the past in the form of feelings and mental images, which, if negative or blocked, can cause thinking patterns that can obstruct our health. Guided imagery can access much of this stored material and guide the mind to understand the details of an event or occurrence in a way that releases or transmutes any negative associations and replaces these with positive, healing ones.

Guided imagery can be performed with a trained therapist or practitioner. You may also have success using a guided imagery audio CD or tape. While there are many of these on the market today, I highly recommend you choose one that has been developed by a trained guided imagery practitioner. These providers are qualified to guide you in the best possible way. Here are some recommendations that my patients and I have reviewed that have had excellent results:

- Emmett Miller, MD, www.drmiller.com
- Health Journeys, Belleruth Naparstek, LISW, www.healthjourneys.com
- Andrew Weil, MD, and Martin Rossman, MD, CD: "Self Healing with Guided Imagery," available from www.amazon.com
- Andrew Weil, MD, and Jon Kabat-Zinn, PhD, CD: "Meditation for Optimum Health," available from www.amazon.com

Gratitude

An important element in any change process is *gratitude*. Thank your past life and now state that you deserve to move on to a healthier new life. Become grateful for all you have and all that you are going to have. For example, people with chronic illness can see themselves making healthier changes and being grateful for internal natural healing. I recommend that you find an object precious to you, something you can keep with you at all times, into which you can symbolically direct your gratitude. My favorite items for this are a stone I received during the opening ceremony of my integrative medicine program, along with a deep blue, glass-like stone resembling a sapphire given to me by a patient. Both have a very special attraction for me. Find an object that attracts you and holds some special significance. You can then direct the strength of your intention for your new life into this object. When you touch it, the feel of the object will be a reminder of your new behaviors and life you are already living. As you grow with this object, it will become even more valuable as time passes.

A Day with God (or Whoever/Whatever "God" Is to You)

Not everyone believes in the same god or even recognizes that God exists. Some people have no concept of what God is, yet they still have a concept of some higher power. I think it really doesn't matter if you believe in God or not; this exercise can still be valuable to you. If the term "God" interferes with your reading, please substitute any other term you would like.

Here, my entire focus is on positive thoughts. God and the concept of God reside in Love and Light, both positive concepts. I believe we are all here in service to some larger picture, and as part of that, we have an inherent need to create in our areas of interest. Coming to restful awareness and gaining inner direction from this source can be of exceptional value. Yet, if we don't even give ourselves time to stop for one minute and listen to this inner voice or direction from our higher source, we can wander off the path we were born to walk. This method of connecting with a higher spirit of good or God is a form of meditation we can use to listen for that voice.

A Connecting Day with God

Welcome to your day with God. Some of us have never realized our gift or purpose in life. Very few of us take the time to ask for God's help or to listen to the guidance being given us. If you're a person who does not live your life to the fullest, and are not loving what you do and doing what you love, it may be especially important that you consider having "A Connecting Day with God."

Think of it as a day of connecting to an endless river of love and gentle guidance.

So who can benefit from a day with God or a higher spirit? The simple answer to this question is that every one of us needs time to connect in this way. Connecting on a regular basis offers us clear direction for identifying or developing our gifts of creativity and intentionality. Taking a focused day to be with God or your higher spirit, so as to gain vision and direction for your life, is one of the best things you can do for yourself and the people who share your life. It can be a magical day. The experience you can gain from this time is beyond words. It changes you and brings love. You will get answers if you ask your questions. We all have equal access to the same Love. This is not going to be difficult at all. In fact, this will be a very exciting day for you.

Caution: Your experience may vary each time you take the time to connect with God. Have no expectations of what will happen. Enter the experience with an open mind and an open heart. See this time as if you are drifting on a calm open sea, where God is guiding you. It may not turn out to be what you expected, but seek out the underlying gift of the experience, even if you feel disappointed or didn't "get" what you wanted. Sometimes will be more precious than others, but they are all valuable. The important thing is to make it a practice to set aside time for connecting with God and your higher spirit.

Preparing for Your Day with God:
Make a commitment to yourself and to your higher spirit, or God, to spend a day together. Set the date for your day with God. Consider this your special day, but keep it to yourself (for now). Mark it on your calendar and plan for that date. Plan your day with God at least two weeks ahead of time.

Choose the place where you will spend your day with God, somewhere comfortable and where you feel safe. Some examples of places to spend the day are:

- a beach or somewhere near water
- a secluded area in a park
- a scenic area where you have a beautiful view
- a scenic secluded area where you can park your car for the day
- at home, if no one else will be around for the whole day
- a home rented or borrowed or where you can house sit for the day
- a hotel room, with a beautiful view (hang the "Do not Disturb" sign outside)
- a quiet church

Our busy lives have many technological ties that should be avoided during your day with God. Do your best to disconnect yourself, it's just you and God, so:

- Turn off your cell phone and/or pager.
- Turn off the ringer on landline phones.
- Turn off the volume on your answering machine.
- Take no watches or clocks.
- Turn off radio or television.
- Turn off computer or e-mail.
- Make sure no one else is present.

Choose a specific amount of time to spend with God. See if you can designate a large chunk of time. If you can, plan to spend an entire day. To be safe, overestimate the time you need. You do not want to be feeling a need to leave or rush back for any obligation whatsoever.

Write a checklist of things you will need for your day with God. Then, a week before, begin gathering them together.

Nutritional Needs: Plan your nutritional needs for the entire day. Prepare all your food and water ahead of time, so you do not need to spend time preparing anything on your day off. Include:

- plenty of pure, fresh water
- naturally healthy, whole foods with no preservatives or additives
- a simple treat, like a favorite cookie or candy from childhood

Clothing: Consider the temperature of the space you will be in. Plan to bring comfortable warm and cool clothing you can layer if necessary: the old sweatpants and sweatshirt you love so much; your favorite T-shirt with the hole in it; that old cotton dress you have worn 50 times, but is just so special you cannot give it away; that sweater in your closet you just do not want to throw away because it is your favorite—if you want to wear it, wear it. On the other hand, a piece of new clothing you have just bought and want to wear for this special occasion would also be perfect—a new sweater, a comfortable pair of pants. Wear what you feel good in.

Seating: Plan to have something comfortable to sit on. Consider a blanket if you will be sitting outside, or if you think it could be cold.

Money: The cost of the day should be minimal, if anything. Bring only the amount of money you will need for the day.

Medications: Bring any medication you will need during the day.

Supplies: Below are suggestions for supplies you might want to bring with you.

- blank paper, pencil, pen, and a new pack of crayons so you can write down or draw out your thoughts as new insights appear during your day (no cassette recorder or recording devices)
- facial tissues
- a candle and matches if you like
- anything else to help you be as comfortable and focused as possible

Communication and Responsibilities: Inform only the people who really need to know that you are taking the day off and will not be available for the designated amount of time. Designate a contact person whom you can reach should you need to, such as a friend, spouse, minister, or other support person with whom you feel comfortable. Make arrangements for any necessary activities to continue in your absence.

Experience Your Day with God

The day has arrived. Today is your day with God. Waking up and getting started is part of this special day.

If possible, wake before daylight so you can watch the day begin. Dawn can be a magical time. Try to wake up on your own, without an alarm clock. Be present in thought as soon as you open your eyes. Realize today is your Day with God. Get out of bed when you feel you are ready.

Consider a morning prayer or meditation for the day. Take care of your daily hygiene routine for your body. If you had planned to drink and eat now, do so while taking time to thank God for this nourishment. Check to be sure you do not forget anything before you proceed to your destination, whether at home or away.

Think of your day as having no schedule. You are just going to be with yourself and God. When ready, get comfortable and warm. Have all your writing and drawing materials around you.

You may want to light a candle. This is to be a day of relaxation and vision. Most of the time, stress can stop us from seeing what we're supposed to see in our lives, so take some deep breaths to help you relax. Better yet, try the wonderful breathing technique above.

Once you have done this relaxation breathing, you will be in a very comfortable state of mind. Allow your day to unfold as it comes. If you feel you are not connected, ask why. You will know when you need to take a break for food, but be sure not to overeat. If you don't feel like eating, that's okay. If you have ideas coming to you and need to write them down or draw them, do so. Go with whatever comes to you. Any thoughts that come to mind should be the ones you follow. Have a fun, magical, happy experience!

As your day with God—or whatever God is to you—comes to a close, take some time to write down your experience, any insights you gained, and how you are going to use the information you learned. For the next few nights, pay attention to what comes to you. Write down your dreams and thoughts.

Continue to be connected with God or whoever you believe your creator to be, so the journey you have chosen will be a happy and productive one.

Chapter Seventeen

THE APO E GENE DIET PLANS

Now that you have a bag of tools to support you in making the changes you want to make, let's look at the specifics of how you can initiate and sustain any recommended nutritional changes. We will discuss the Apo E Diet is in detail. Remember, this is *based on a comprehensive system of caloric calculation and includes nutritional recommendations based on a person's Apo E genotype. This means that this chapter is only of direct relevance to you when you have identified your Apo E genotype.* The recommendations are part of a comprehensive prevention program, and only you and your medical practitioner can properly evaluate how they apply to you.

Caution: Do not use any of these nutritional recommendations unless you know your Apo E genotype. Only then will you be able to know what plan is right for you. Example: If you are an Apo E 2/3 and you follow an Apo E 4/3 diet, this can cause imbalance within your body. If this is taken to an extreme, and you eat the wrong diet for a long period of time, it can lead to diseases and illness.

The Apo E Gene Supportive Environment—Evaluation Levels

In order to gain an optimum gene-supportive environment for an individual Apo E, these evaluation levels are recommended in addition to testing for your Apo E genotype. Striving for an optimal balance within each level should be your goal.

Evaluation Level 1
- height
- total body weight
- hydration status
- BMI
- individual daily caloric requirement
- body composition: lean mass and fat mass

Evaluation Level 2
- total screening cholesterol panel: sub-fraction cholesterol panel Apo B particle
- homocysteine level, including an MTHFR gene evaluation TSH, thyroid evaluation
- inflammatory markers—fibrinogen, CRP, Lp-PLA2
- insulin level, fasting glucose, HA1c

Evaluation Level 3
- Current disease status 1-10
  (1=high levels of disease; 10=free of disease)
- Ambulatory level status 1-10
  (1=bedridden; 10=no walking limitations)
- Respiratory status 1-10
  (1=poor respiration status;
  10=excellent respiration status)
- Vascular/circulatory status 1-10
  (1=poor vascular status; 10=excellent vascular status)
- Psychological status 1-10
  (1=poor psychological status;
  10=excellent psychological status)
- Family history 1-10
  (1= extensive family history of disease;
  10=no current family history of disease)

The Apo E Gene Diet Plan that's Right for You

Once you know your Apo E genotype, there are three steps to determining The Apo E Diet plan that's right for you.

- Step 1 determines the calories required for daily activities.
- Step 2 determines your body composition.
- Step 3 identifes the Apo E Gene Diet nutritional recommendations for your genotype.

Let's look at these in greater detail.

Step 1: Determine the Calories Required for Daily Activities

I introduced calories in Chapter 5, but now we get into the specific calculations, which are based on two levels:

- Normal body functioning needs—the calories your body requires to sustain your typical body functions such as digesting food, maintaining your circulation, breathing, plus your general daily activity level.

- The additional calories required for an exercise program or athletic activity—calories used over and above those of your normal activities, such as 30 minutes of running, 40 minutes of walking, or 60 minutes of biking.

Below are two methods of determining approximately how much energy—how many calories—your body needs from food each day. The first is a manual method that illustrates the principles behind the calculations. The second is the much more practical automated way it is usually done.

Manual Calculation
The method described below requires no equipment. You simply add together the two separate caloric requirements mentioned above. This provides you with the approximate number of calories your body requires each day, based on your height and weight as shown in the table below. Keep in mind these are approximate calorie counts.

Male Daily Calorie Requirements
Multiply your weight by 10 and add double your body weight.
For example, for a 150 lb. male:
   150 x 10 = 1,500
   2 x 150 = 300
   1500 + 300 = 1800 calories per day

Female Daily Calorie Requirements
Multiply your weight by 10 then add your body weight.
For example, for a 120 lb. female:
   120 x 10 = 1200
   1200 + 120 = 1320 calories per day

   Adding in the activity component for females (chose one):
   Low-level activity (1–2 days exercising/week):
   Multiply your weight by 14 (weight =130 lbs.)
   Example: 130 x 14 = 1820 calories/day.

   Medium-level activity (3–4 days exercising/week):
   Multiply your weight by 16.
   Example: 130 x 16 = 2080 calories/day.

   High-level activity (exercise 6–7 days a week):
   Multiply your weight by 19.
   Example: 130 x 19 = 2470 calories/day.

Bio-Impedance Test
This is one of the most practical methods of determining caloric needs, but it requires taking a bio-impedance test in a clinical setting. The instrument measures your basal metabolic rate, giving you your daily caloric requirements immediately.

What is your basal metabolic rate (BMR)? Your BMR is the amount of energy you require to maintain basic bodily functions. Approximately three quarters of the body's energy is needed to support the metabolic cellular function, which includes activities such as that of the cardiopulmonary systems and maintaining body temperature. The rest is the usual amount needed for discretionary movement and thinking.

A bio-impedance test (see page 228) is one of the most practical methods of determining your daily caloric requirement, but it also evaluates your body composition—the second important factor in determining the right diet plan for you.

Step 2: Determine Your Body Composition—
The Bathroom Scale and Beyond

Everybody is familiar with the most common of human body surveying tools—
the bathroom scale. Few, however, realize that daily "scale jumping" can be
hazardous to your health! You jump on the scale and say, "Yes! I lost five pounds
yesterday! I am healthier today." This assumption may be true, but most likely
it is not. Whether a weight loss is healthy or not depends on what kind of body
component you lost: fat, muscle, or water. A bathroom scale detects only your
total body weight and for this reason a very poor health evaluation tool.

Body Mass Index

Your *body mass index* (BMI, *not to be confused with BMR above*) is a measure of
your body mass related to your height and weight—specifically your weight (in
kilograms) divided by your height (in meters) squared. The BMI is a reliable
indicator of total body mass, which can help in identifying health risks. The
score applies to both men and women with these limits:

• It may overestimate body mass in athletes and others who have a muscular build.

• It may underestimate body mass in older people and others who
have lost excess muscle mass.

The BMI is grouped into classifications as follows:

• underweight = less than 18.5
• normal weight = 18.5–24.9
• overweight = 25–29.9
• obese = 30 or more

Body Composition

We've seen that the bathroom scale gives a very gross idea of your body
composition, telling only how many pounds you weigh. Your body mass index
gives a more refined picture of your body composition by taking into account
height and frame size. Determining caloric needs with a body composition
measurement using a bio-impedance meter gives the most accurate assessment
of body composition. It's a simple, painless, non-invasive test that many medical
providers and exercise physiologists offer.

A body's composition can be defined as lean mass, fat mass, and fluids where:

• lean mass = muscles, bones, tendons, ligaments, skin, etc.

• fat mass = the body's stored fat

• fluids = water, blood, and a host of other fluids like saliva, bile, and cerebrospinal fluid

Two people who weigh 150 lbs. may have a completely different body makeup. One might have too much fat, the other have more muscle and almost no fat. If you eat a balanced diet for your genotype and exercise regularly, chances are you have a normal body composition. If you don't eat a gene supportive-diet, chances are you will have an unhealthy body composition.

A body composition test is a more comprehensive way of assessing health, as it allows us to see the body mass by category. Only when you know the percentage of lean mass, fat mass, and fluids can you determine whether or not you have the correct body composition.

Bio-Impedance—Body Composition Test

A body composition test works on the theory that carbohydrates consist of three water molecules for every carbohydrate, or glycogen, molecule. The more molecules of glycogen you have, the more water you are able to store in your muscles. A great little device called a bio-impedance body-composition testing machine measures how much water you have in your body, based on the bioelectrical impedance of your tissues—fat and muscle conduct an electric current differently, depending on the water content. By using this machine you can find out the fat mass, lean mass, and water contents of your body, and thereby determine the ideal calorie intake for you.

Finding Out if your Body Composition Is Gene Supportive

Here we use BMI and other data, along with your body composition (measured by your provider or at a fitness center) to determine how your body is reflecting the gene supportiveness or unsupportiveness of your environment.

Men should have no more than 16 percent body fat. Women should have no more than 22 percent body fat. A high percentage of body fat indicates you are overfeeding your body for the amount of exercise you are getting, which promotes disease.

Exercise: Finding Your Ideal Body Composition

1. Find and record your body mass index _____
   (from Table 16.2 Body Mass Index, page 227-232)

2. Is your BMI within the normal range of 18.5–24.9? ____Yes ____No.
   If no, is it higher or lower? ____Higher ____Lower

3. Find and record your lean mass range _____
   (from Table 16.1: Lean Mass Recommendation for Males
   and Females).

4. Determine your current lean mass percentage _____
   (from a body composition test by your medical provider or
   exercise physiologist).

5. Is your lean mass percentage within the range in step 3?
   ____Yes ____No.
   If no, is it higher or lower? ____Higher ____Lower

6. Record your fat mass percentage goal _____
   (Men: 16% or less; Women: 22% or less).

7. Determine your current fat percentage: _____
   (from a body composition test by your medical provider or
   exercise physiologist).

8. Is your lean mass percentage under the goal in step 6?
   ____Yes ____No.

This information is valuable in developing your personalized program
for minimizing your risk of disease.

Table 16.1: Lean Mass Recommendation for Males and Females[a]										
Pounds of Lean Body Mass (Frame Size) for Men										
5'5"	5'6"	5'7"	5'8"	5'9"	5'10"	5'11"	6'0"	6'1"	6'2"	6'3"
108-120	110-125	112-129	118-132	122-137	127-145	133-153	137-163	140-168	143-176	145-183
Pounds of Lean Body Mass (Frame Size) for Women										
5'0"	5'1"	5'2"	5'3"	5'4"	5'5"	5'6"	5'7"	5'8"	5'9"	5'10"
70-86	73-89	75-91	78-93	81-96	83-99	86-102	95-105	93-109	95-112	98-119
Recommendation Fat Percentage for Males and Females										
Male	Less than 16% body fat									
Female	Less than 22% body fat									
Recommendation BMI for Males and Females										
Male	BMI based on less than 25 BMI height and weight									
Female	BMI based on less than 25 BMI height and weight									

a.   Based on research by Covert Bailey.

BMI

Height (inches)	19	20	21	22	23	24	25	26	27	28	29	30	31	32	33	34	35
	Body Weight (pounds)																
58	91	96	100	105	110	115	119	124	129	134	138	143	148	153	158	162	167
59	94	99	104	109	114	119	124	128	133	138	143	148	153	158	163	168	173
60	97	102	107	112	118	123	128	133	138	143	148	153	158	163	168	174	179
61	100	106	111	116	122	127	132	137	143	148	153	158	164	169	174	180	185
62	104	109	115	120	126	131	136	142	147	153	158	164	169	175	180	186	191
63	107	113	118	124	130	135	141	146	152	158	163	169	175	180	186	191	197
64	110	116	122	128	134	140	145	151	157	163	169	174	180	186	192	197	204
65	114	120	126	132	138	144	150	156	162	168	174	180	186	192	198	204	210
66	118	124	130	136	142	148	155	161	167	173	179	186	192	198	204	210	216
67	121	127	134	140	146	153	159	166	172	178	185	191	198	204	211	217	223
68	125	131	138	144	151	158	164	171	177	184	190	197	203	210	216	223	230
69	128	135	142	149	155	162	169	176	182	189	196	203	209	216	223	230	236
70	132	139	146	153	160	167	174	181	188	195	202	209	216	222	229	236	243
71	136	143	150	157	165	172	179	186	193	200	208	215	222	229	236	243	250
72	140	147	154	162	169	177	184	191	199	206	213	221	228	235	242	250	258
73	144	151	159	166	174	182	189	197	204	212	219	227	235	242	250	257	265
74	148	155	163	171	179	186	194	202	210	218	225	233	241	249	256	264	272
75	152	160	168	176	184	192	200	208	216	224	232	240	248	256	264	272	279
76	156	164	172	180	189	197	205	213	221	230	238	246	254	263	271	279	287

To find your BMI, select your height in the left-hand column. Move across the line to find your weight. The number at the top of that column is your BMI.

BMI	36	37	38	39	40	41	42	43	44	45	46	47	48	49	50	51	52	53	54
Height (inches)	Body Weight (pounds)																		
58	172	177	181	186	191	196	201	205	210	215	220	224	229	234	239	244	248	253	258
59	178	183	188	193	198	203	208	212	217	222	227	232	237	242	247	252	257	262	267
60	184	189	194	199	204	209	215	220	225	230	235	240	245	250	255	261	266	271	276
61	190	195	201	206	211	217	222	227	232	238	243	248	254	259	264	269	275	280	285
62	196	202	207	213	218	224	229	235	240	246	251	256	262	267	273	278	284	289	295
63	203	208	214	220	225	231	237	242	248	254	259	265	270	278	282	287	293	299	304
64	209	215	221	227	232	238	244	250	256	262	267	273	279	285	291	296	302	308	314
65	216	222	228	234	240	246	252	258	264	270	276	282	288	294	300	306	312	318	324
66	223	229	235	241	247	253	260	266	272	278	284	291	297	303	309	315	322	328	334
67	230	236	242	249	255	261	268	274	280	287	293	299	306	312	319	325	331	338	344
68	236	243	249	256	262	269	276	282	289	295	302	308	315	322	328	335	341	348	354
69	243	250	257	263	270	277	284	291	297	304	311	318	324	331	338	345	351	358	365
70	250	257	264	271	278	285	292	299	306	313	320	327	334	341	348	355	362	369	376
71	257	265	272	279	286	293	301	308	315	322	329	338	343	351	358	365	372	379	386
72	265	272	279	287	294	302	309	316	324	331	338	346	353	361	368	375	383	390	397
73	272	280	288	295	302	310	318	325	333	340	348	355	363	371	378	386	393	401	408
74	280	287	295	303	311	319	326	334	342	350	358	365	373	381	389	396	404	412	420
75	287	295	303	311	319	327	335	343	351	359	367	375	383	391	399	407	415	423	431
76	295	304	312	320	328	336	344	353	361	369	377	385	394	402	410	418	426	435	443

National Institutes of Health
National Heart, Lung and Blood Institute, Bethesda, MD

Step 3: Identifying the Apo E Gene Nutritional Recommendation for Your Genotype

Once you know your Apo E genotype, you can use the information in this section to find the specific recommendations for you.

Detailed Apo E Gene Diet Nutritional Recommendations

Building on my overview of the best nutritional recommendations for each genotype in Chapter 10, I continue here with more specific information about the Big Three needs of each genotype—starting with the 4/4s so as not to play favorites. Note there are different ratios suggested for higher calorie diets.

Apo E 4/4 Nutritional Recommendations
For diets less than 2400 Kcal: fat 20%, protein 25%, carbohydrate 55%
For diets greater than 2400 Kcal: fat 20%, protein 20%, carbohydrate 60%

Carbohydrate: From complex carbohydrates with low glycemic load, regulated by high-fiber content.[16] It is most crucial for this genotype to avoid all refined carbohydrates.

Protein: From plant protein sources as much as possible.

Fat: Lowest fat content requirement. Obtain from monounsaturated and polyunsaturated sources only. Avoid animal saturated fat sources in favor of plant sources, avoid all trans fats.

Food intake timing: For optimal fuel delivery, eat every three hours while awake to ensure an adequate blood glucose level at all times.

Apo E 4/3 Nutritional Recommendations
For diets less than 2400 Kcal: Fat 20%, protein 25%, carbohydrate 55%
For diets greater than 2400 Kcal: Fat 20%, protein 20%, carbohydrate 60%

Carbohydrate: From complex carbohydrates with low glycemic load, regulated by a high fiber content.[17]

Protein: Mainly from plant protein sources, with some consideration to additional protein sources, preferably from an omega-3 fish source.

Fat: Second lowest fat content requirement. Obtain from monounsaturated and polyunsaturated sources, avoiding most all animal saturated fats and staying with plant sources of saturated fat and avoiding all trans fats.

16, 17 Glycemic load is described in Chapter 8. The high-fiber content in this diet helps slow down glucose release into the bloodstream, and if coupled with a small amount of monounsaturated fat from a plant source, stomach emptying is delayed and blood glucose is prolonged and stabilized. Food intake timing: For optimal fuel delivery, eat every three hours while awake to ensure an adequate blood glucose level at all times.

Apo E 4/2 Nutritional Recommendations
Fat 25%, protein 20%, carbohydrate 55%

Carbohydrate: From complex carbohydrates with low glycemic load, regulated by a high fiber content.[18]

Protein: Mainly from plant protein sources, with some consideration to additional protein sources, preferably the omega-3 fish source.[19]

Fat: Needs moderate dietary fat. Obtain from a combination of monounsaturated and polyunsaturated sources. No trans fat.

Food intake timing: For optimal fuel delivery, eat every three hours while awake to ensure an adequate blood glucose level at all times.

Apo E 3/3 Nutritional Recommendations
Fat 25%, protein 20%, carbohydrate 55%

Carbohydrate: From complex carbohydrates with low glycemic load, regulated by a high fiber content.[20]

Protein: Mainly from plant protein sources, with some additional protein sources, preferably an omega-3 fish source, and other animal sources.[21]

Fat: Need moderate dietary fat. Obtain mainly from monounsaturated, polyunsaturated sources[22] with limited saturated fat intake. No trans fat.

Food intake timing: For optimal fuel delivery, eat every three hours while awake to ensure an adequate blood glucose level at all times.

---

18   Glycemic load is described in Chapter 8. The high-fiber content in this diet helps slow down glucose release into the bloodstream, and if coupled with a small amount of monounsaturated fat from a plant source, stomach emptying is delayed and blood glucose is prolonged and stabilized.

19   Keeping in mind that protein and fat usually come packaged together, pay close attention to the recommended serving sizes, and leave an adequate amount of fat clearance time (24–48 hours) in between eating fish or any animal protein with high saturated fat content.

20   Glycemic load is described in Chapter 8. The high-fiber content in this diet helps slow down glucose release into the bloodstream, and if coupled with a small amount of monounsaturated fat from a plant source, stomach emptying is delayed and blood glucose is prolonged and stabilized.

21   A limited saturated fat source can be considered, but pay close attention to serving sizes and leave adequate clearance time (24–48 hours) between consuming fish or animal protein containing saturated fat.

22   Pay close attention to recommended serving sizes and leave adequate clearance time (24–48 hours) between animal fat and protein food intake.

Apo E 2/3 Nutritional Recommendations
Fat 30%, protein 15%, carbohydrate 55%

Carbohydrate: From complex carbohydrates with low glycemic load, regulated by a high fiber content.[23]

Protein: From a combination of protein sources, plant and animal with optimal timing of animal protein clearance, but not any more than once every 24–48 hours. Intake from other animal protein.[24]

Fat: Needs more dietary fat than the above genotypes. Obtain mainly from monounsaturated and polyunsaturated sources with limited saturated and trans fats.[25]

Food intake timing: For optimal fuel delivery, eat every three hours while awake to ensure an adequate blood glucose level at all times.

Apo E 2/2 Nutritional Recommendations
Fat 35%, protein 15%, carbohydrate 50%

Carbohydrate: Greatest need of all genotypes for High-Quality complex carbohydrates with low glycemic load, regulated by a high fiber content.[26]

Protein: From a combination of protein sources, mostly plant sources, but with some consideration to additional protein from the omega-3 fish source, with limited intake from animal protein.[27]

Fat: Needs the most dietary fats of all genotypes. Obtain from monounsaturated and polyunsaturated sources, with limited saturated and trans fats.[28]

Food intake timing: For optimal fuel delivery, eat every three hours while awake to ensure an adequate blood glucose level at all times.

23, 26 Glycemic load is described in Chapter 8. The high-fiber content in this diet helps slow down glucose release into the bloodstream, and if coupled with a small amount of monounsaturated fat from a plant source, stomach emptying is delayed and blood glucose is prolonged and stabilized.
24, 25, 27, 28
A limited saturated fat source can be considered, but pay close attention to serving sizes and leave adequate clearance time (24–48 hours) between consuming fish or animal protein containing saturated fat.

Apo E Menu Suggestion Plans for Each Genotype and Different Caloric Levels

Chapter 19 contains the ApoE Gene Diet sample meal plans, which include suggestions for breakfast, lunch, and dinner meals, as well as a morning and afternoon snack. After you know your Apo E genotype, you can use the sample meal plans to design your personal meal plans. For example, if you are an Apo E 4/3 with a daily calorie requirement of 1800, review the Menu Suggestion Plan for Apo E 4/3—1800 calories.

If you would prefer different food choices for any of the meals listed in the sample meal plans, you can use the Food Exchange List (see page 237-241) and find a replacement food.

About the Food Exchange List

This exchange list is based on a serving size. Remember to stay within your serving recommendations for the day. When selecting a protein food, the serving size can change depending on the food type. For instance, 1 oz. of cooked fish is equal to one serving. You may have 10 servings of protein a day, so be mindful of serving sizes—learn what a serving looks like. With milk-type products (such as skim milk and soy), serving size changes depending on the type of product.

Keep in mind the following to ensure that you design appropriate meals:

• Carbohydrates come from grain, starch, fruit, and vegetable sources.

• Fats come from both plant and animal sources.

• Proteins come from both plant and animal sources.

• Always exchange the same food type so your diet will remain balanced.

   ◆ carbohydrate for carbohydrate

   ◆ fat for fat

   ◆ protein for protein

• When substituting a food, be mindful of the serving size.

• When possible, choose organic and avoid all genetically modified foods (GMO).

• Avoid all foods coming from unhealthy farming practices. Consider buying your food locally; farmers' markets can be a great source of good fresh produce.

Food Exchange List

Carbohydrates

Carbohydrates are the number one energy food source for the body. The single servings listed below are selected because they provide a good variety of shorter-term fuel with low glycemic load (see page 62). With low glycemic load foods, the glucose delivery is lower and slower to the body and is also regulated by its high fiber content because the fiber slows down the digestion so the food is not absorbed too rapidly and therefore doesn't raise blood sugar as rapidly.

Carbohydrates: Fruits

1 cup or 18 grapes
1 cup or 15 cherries
4 fresh apricots or 7 halves dried
1 fresh apple or 4 rings dried
1 medium orange or 2 mandarins/tangerines
½ cup kiwi
¾ cup of blueberries
1 cup papaya/mango/guava/pineapple
¾ cup of raspberries
1 medium peach/nectarine
1 medium plum or pear or ½ large pear
1 ¼ cup melon (watermelon, honeydew, cantaloupe)
¾ cup strawberries
¾ cup loganberries
2 tbsp. dried cranberries or raisins
3 medium prunes
½ banana
1 ½ figs
¾ cup blackberries

Carbohydrates: Vegetables
½ cup cooked, 1 cup raw:
  turnips
  bok choy/leeks
  broccoli & sprouts/broccolini/cauliflower
  carrots/celery
  onions/scallions
  summer squash
  green beans
  asparagus
  artichoke
  brussel sprouts
  radishes
  turnips/rutabaga/parsnips
  eggplant
  English peapods
  cabbage red and white—kohlrabi
  peppers—red, yellow, green/tomatoes
  mushrooms, cooked

1 cup leafy greens such as:
  spinach/mustard greens
  romaine lettuce
  mixed salad greens

Carbohydrates: Grains/Starches
¾ cup plain high-fiber dry cereal
½ cup cooked cereals: oat bran, whole oatmeal
¼ cup low-fat granola
½ small whole grain bagel
1 slice whole grain bread
½ whole grain bun
6-inch whole wheat tortilla
6-inch corn tortilla
½ whole wheat pita
¾ oz. whole wheat pretzels
½ cup whole wheat pasta

$^1/_3$ cup brown rice
½ cup corn, lima beans, peas
3 oz. baked potato (w/skin) waxy type potato
$^1/_3$ cup sweet potato, yam, pumpkin
3 cups plain dry popcorn, no seasonings
7 whole grain crackers (rounds)
3 ginger biscuits (1 serving of recipe)
1 slice angel-food cake ($^1/_{12}$ of a 10" diameter tube)
½ cup beans, non-GMO (black, kidney, lima, navy, white)* count
also as 1 protein

Fats
These suggested servings of fats provide longer-term fuel. Fat is much more complex than carbohydrate. It still contains carbon, hydrogen, and oxygen, but the atoms are linked together in a different chemical bond that takes longer to digest. Fats come as saturated and unsaturated, depending on the type of chemical bond. This makes a big difference in how they interact with our bodies. Also, some fat sources have a greater percentage of fat in them than others. This translates into different amounts per serving size.

$^1/_8$ of an avocado (1 oz)
1 tsp. canola, olive, peanut oil (small amounts only—non-GMO)
8 olives
6 almonds
10 peanuts
4 cashews
4 halves pecans
4 halves walnuts
1 tbsp. sesame seeds
2 tsp. nut butter (peanut, almond, cashew, sesame)
1 tbsp. pumpkin, sunflower seeds
¼ cup purslane
2 tsp. linseed
2 tbsp. flaxseed (ground)
1 tbsp light mayonnaise

Protein
Different protein foods have different concentrations of protein in them. Also, protein has something that carbohydrates and fat don't have—nitrogen from the amino acids. When these are digested and used as fuel in the bloodstream, it is hard on the body because of the nitrogen. They break down to produce a waste product in the liver, called urea, which then has to be cleared by the kidneys.

Protein: Plant Legume Proteins
½ cup beans, non-GMO (black, kidney, lima, navy, white)* count
    also as 1 grain
½ cup soybeans
½ cup legumes—split peas, lentils
1 garden or veggie burger = 2 protein servings
4 oz. tofu/tempeh (non-GMO)

Protein: Egg Proteins
¼ cup egg substitute
2 medium egg whites
1 organic whole egg

Protein: Fish Proteins
1 oz. of cooked fish/seafood:
    black cod
    crab
    halibut
    lobster
    oysters (6)
    salmon
    sardines
    scallops
    sea bass
    shrimp
    trout
    tuna
    herring
    mackerel
    smaller plant-eating wild fish and seafoods

Protein: Poultry Proteins
1 oz white meat, no skin cooked
1 oz. organic chicken, turkey, Cornish game hen, wild: no skin, cooked
1 oz organic non-processed sliced meat, cooked

Protein: Dairy & Soy Proteins
1 cup nonfat milk (from organic source, non-pregnant cows)
1 cup soymilk—(carrageenan free)
½ cup evaporated nonfat milk
1/3 cup dry nonfat milk
1 cup nonfat buttermilk
1 cup nonfat yogurt
1 cup soy yogurt
1 oz nonfat cheese
1 oz low-fat soy cheese
1 oz soy cream cheese
¼ cup nonfat cottage cheese
¼ cup nonfat ricotta cheese
1 cup soy yogurt
1 oz nonfat cheese
1 oz low-fat soy cheese
1 oz soy cream cheese
¼ cup nonfat cottage cheese
¼ cup nonfat ricotta cheese

Build Your Own Apo E Gene Menus

Building your own meal plan is a fun exercise and teaches you how to eat with balance and an understanding of the Big Three, the macronutrients. Use the plate diagram on the next page as a guide to help you determine the correct balance of food servings for each meal. Then use the Food Exchange List on page 237 it to see which foods you can enjoy in each of the Big Three categories.

Review the recommended Apo E Gene Diet for your genotype and calorie level, listed in Chapter 19. Take the total daily servings and divide them into three meals and three snacks. Include items from all food categories in each meal or snack—protein, carbohydrate, and fat. Don't skip any.

Here's an example of a meal plan for a person with an Apo E 4/4 that requires 1400 Kcal per day.

Apo E Gene Diet

4/4 1400 Kcal

Serving considerations per day (be mindful of serving sizes):

Carbohydrates
6 servings grain/starch
8 servings fruit and vegetable

Protein
7 servings fish or plant protein

Fat
3 servings anti-inflammatory fat
2 servings desserts or evening snack

Beneficial fun foods containing essential calories, carbohydrate, protein, and fat.

When you have determined your particular Apo E Gene Diet, complete the Apo E Gene Diet Build Your Own Meal Plan chart on page 244.

Apo E Gene Diet
Macronutrients – Big Foods from Your Plate to Your Cells©

Protein

for growth
and repair

Fats (anti-inflammatory)

long-term fuel

Carbohydrates (grains and starches)

short-term fuel
regulated by
fiber

Carbohydrates (fruits and vegetables)

short-term fuel

© MACRONUTRIENTS – BIG FOODS - FROM YOUR PLATE TO YOUR CELLS©

Apo E Gene Diet™ Build Your Own Meal Plan

Breakfast

Protein Animal/Plan	Carbohydrates Grain/Starch	Carbohydrates Fruit/Vegetable	Fat

Morning Snack

Protein Animal/Plan	Carbohydrates Grain/Starch	Carbohydrates Fruit/Vegetable	Fat

Lunch

Protein Animal/Plan	Carbohydrates Grain/Starch	Carbohydrates Fruit/Vegetable	Fat

Afternoon Snack

Protein Animal/Plan	Carbohydrates Grain/Starch	Carbohydrates Fruit/Vegetable	Fat

Evening Dinner

Protein Animal/Plan	Carbohydrates Grain/Starch	Carbohydrates Fruit/Vegetable	Fat

Supper

Protein Animal/Plan	Carbohydrates Grain/Starch	Carbohydrates Fruit/Vegetable	Fat

Chapter Eighteen

PLANNING AND SUPPORTING YOUR NUTRITIONAL CHANGE

Factors that will support you in making the desired nutritional changes include:

- making changes in a mindful and organized manner
- avoiding making too many changes at one time
- education—knowing why you should change your diet
- knowing how to accomplish nutritional changes related to taste

Let's now look in a little more detail at the final point.

The Sense of Taste and Nutritional Change

Taste is one of our most powerful senses, providing a direct chemical connection from the outside world to our nervous system. Many of us were taught that there are four basic tastes: salt, sour, bitter, and sweet. However, there are two more: umami, which is described as a sort of robust or "meaty" taste, and fat, which researchers are beginning to discover has a taste of its own, although it hasn't yet been adequately described. Each taste category produces its own chemical response in the tongue, delivered to the brain via our taste receptor cells, called papillae, found on the surface of the tongue and the olfactory (smell) system. A host of chemical changes occur in this process, and the different tastes result from the brain receiving different signals from the various foods.

Our taste system has a direct connection to the brain and alters brain chemistry as a result. When a food is eaten frequently, the brain and nervous system get used to a certain level of taste because of the chemistry that taste experience produces. When taste experience changes very quickly, the nervous system responds by producing a different chemical experience. So sudden taste changes can be a difficult adaptation for the nervous system. This is why you need to make food taste changes slowly—the slower, the better.

When you make taste changes, give your nervous system time to adjust to the new chemistry that is produced, or the shock on the nervous system will insist that you go back to the old taste. Bottom line: make changes to your diet slowly.

A Patient's Story: Janet

When Janet came to see me the first time, she was taking eight medications every day. She had chronic body pain, some joint pain, deep fatigue, migraines, and diarrhea 12 to 14 times a day. Her cholesterol was also dangerously high. During the previous few years, she had seen many doctors and undergone extensive testing to find a diagnosis, yet no one could provide a definitive reason for her condition. Eventually, she was given a diagnosis of suspected fibromyalgia with arthritic tendencies and chronic diarrhea. She was prescribed eight different drugs and, even though she hated taking any drugs at all, found that she needed them all just to function each day.

Janet's gastroenterologist had worked with me on several other cases and suggested that she see me. He thought I could help with her cholesterol problem as well as her diet, to see if making some dietary changes would reduce or relieve her chronic illnesses. Believing she had nothing to lose, Janet made an appointment with me.

I did a full physical and an extensive medical history, plus a full blood chemistry evaluation and recommended an Apo E gene test. Her total cholesterol was 304, her LDL was 214, and her Apo E genotype was 4/4.

I asked Janet to begin keeping a diet log, and it revealed that she often fasted for an unhealthy 12 to 16 hours at a time and that the foods she did eat were extremely inflammatory—the standard American diet, or SAD, loaded with animal fat, trans fat, and too many simple carbohydrates. Janet said she loved eating "good, hearty, American food," but with an Apo E of 4/4, which cannot tolerate a high fat diet nor long periods of time without adequate food, it was producing high levels of inflammation in her body, which were responsible for her debilitating symptoms.

We discussed all the findings and together developed a plan so Janet could begin making slow dietary changes. Despite its dangers, she loved her current diet and had been eating it for years, so it was best she make small changes each week. This way, her system would not be shocked by the changes, and her taste system would adjust slowly, which meant she would be more likely to continue with the new plan designed around her Apo E 4/4.

Janet's dietary changes went very well from the start. After just two weeks, her diarrhea decreased from 12 to six times daily; after four weeks, it was cut in half again. Her migraines had decreased, and her chronic pain was reduced to only three areas in her body instead of all over. She was thrilled with such rapid results—but they were only the beginning.

Once she underwent cardiovascular screening and was cleared to begin an exercise program, Janet started a low intensity aerobic exercise program. She soon felt so good, she began working out at a higher intensity, but immediately her pain level increased. She couldn't understand why this should happen when she had been improving so well.

I explained the reason to her. When we exercise for a long time or at high intensity, we burn up fat stores—long-term fuel—in the body, which are built over time from the foods we eat. Janet's body was storing old inflammatory fuel from her former poor eating habits, and so when she bumped up her exercise intensity, those inflammatory fats were released from storage, causing her pain to return as they circulated through her body. Once she cleared these poor quality fat stores from her body, I told her, she would no longer feel the inflammatory response when she performed higher intensity exercise. So, I recommended that she drop her exercise intensity to the original levels prescribed for her and begin taking a ginger supplement, which would help reduce inflammation. Once again, Janet felt much better.

Even though she still had a long way to go, Janet was motivated enough by her positive results to continue slowly making dietary changes and exercising at the appropriate levels for her. It just takes time, and she understood that, happy that she had finally found a way back to health.

Personal Nutritional Change Process

There are a multitude of ways to implement changes in your usual routine. In an earlier chapter, we looked at several tools for change that you might want to draw on at this point. Do you already have a favored technique that works well for you? If so, this is the best way for you to make a change in your diet. If not, take a minute and think back to a time when you made a lasting change in some part of your life. Think about how you accomplished that change. If you have never been able to sustain a change over a reasonable period, speak to others who have. When you have some ideas, you may want to fill out your own Personalized Nutritional Change Plan Form, shown below. Remember, this is for you, not for anyone else. No one does things quite like you, so stay focused on you. Family and friends love to give advice, and while you may want to carefully review their advice, accept only what feels right to you, and let the rest go. Remember the only person who can make the right change and choice for you—is you.

Nutritional Change Plan Form					
	Old Behavior	New Behavior	Food Change	Protein	Carb.	Fat
Week 1 Breakfast						
Week 2 Breakfast						
Week 3 Morning Snack						
Week 4 Morning Snack						
Week 5 Lunch						
Week 6 Lunch						
Week 7 Afternoon Snack						
Week 8 Afternoon Snack						
Week 9 Dinner						
Week 10 Dinner						
Week 11 Evening Snack						
Week 12 Evening Snack						

Making Nutritional Change

The following recommendations will help you more successfully implement nutritional changes:

- Focus on what you want, such as a healthier diet or more energy.
- Start with "The Big Progressive Clean Out" of all those kitchen cabinets, the pantry, and the refrigerator. Clear out all those inflammatory and disease-causing foods you have been eating, especially the processed foods.
- Fill out a Personalized Nutritional Change Plan Form (page 249).
- Look up your Suggested Menus by Genotype and Caloric Level beginning on page 257.
- Make a list of all the healthy foods you are going to eat in the future.
- See the Food Exchange List (see the Food Exchange List page 237-241) for protein choices, carbohydrate starches, fruits and vegetables, and good fats.
- Go to your local store and replenish your kitchen with a supply of healthier foods.
- As you begin to incorporate new foods into your diet, go slowly— see the following section on how to make changes week by week.
- Keep a log of your current daily food intake.

If you like, fill out your own schedule with the Build Your Own Meal Plan (see page 244). Think about how you are going to accomplish this process in your own way. My advice is to get help from an Integrative Medicine practitioner trained in nutrition, exercise, stress reduction, and behavioral change, or some other a support person.

Supporting Nutritional Change

When making nutritional behavior changes, most people get excited and want to make changes rapidly. Don't. If your personality is fast and furious, take a deep breath and ask yourself to slow down so you can make this change last a lifetime. Remember, it is best to make changes slowly. The human body does not like hasty changes—especially with respect to nutrition and food. Your body is currently used to one level of taste, and it can become physically shocked with too rapid a change, just like it can be shocked with a big psychological change. It also needs time to adapt to any emotional changes that may go along with the new diet.

You need to give your body time to get used to the changes. So go slowly and gently. For example: If your body is accustomed to consuming four sodas every day, and you suddenly don't drink those sodas, the body will respond to the subsequent chemistry change immediately. Blood glucose, insulin, and cortisol levels all shift, as do the nervous system and blood vessels, from the drop in the caffeine, sugar, and fluid. To suddenly stop drinking sodas can seem like a good thing to do, but the big shift it causes in body chemistry can generate a negative reaction for the body. It works much better to make changes over a period of time. I would suggest moving, week by week, from four sodas a day to three, then two, then one, and in the meantime trying other drinks in their place. This is the kinder way of doing things.

An important point about this change process can be to understand why you drank four sodas a day in the first place. Many people love soda. It is a fun drink, but it is not a good beverage for a healthy body. So identify the reason why you were drinking it in the first place. Was it because soda was all that was available, or was it purchased by the person in your family who does the grocery shopping? Was it because you had access to free sodas at work, or do you just love the bubbles in soda? For me, I can tell you it's the bubbles—I love drinks with bubbles in them. If soda weren't so negative to my health, I would drink it a lot more. However, I switched to soda water with a little fresh-squeezed lime or lemon juice—this still gives me the bubbles plus some extra vitamin C. Take the time to understand what you eat and drink, and why. It will help you with your changes.

Making Nutritional Change

You can start with any meal in the day. However, most people do best if they start with breakfast and slowly work the diet change into other meals throughout the day.

Separate your food intake into six meals. This alone is a lot of change to accomplish all at once, but this is how I have seen change work most effectively with my patients:

Meal 1 Breakfast

Meal 2 Morning snack

Meal 3 Midday lunch

Meal 4 Afternoon snack

Meal 5 Dinner

Meal 6 Evening snack

Week 1: Stop skipping breakfast (if you did).
Make a change in your breakfast meals only. Identify one to two new breakfast meals from your Apo E Gene Diet suggested meal plan and add them to your food intake. Begin eating a correct serving size of breakfast. Possibly, try a new cereal or milk.
Reading: Review information on food safety and how to read a food label, at http://www.vm.cfsan.fda.gov/~dms/foodlab.html (this information is constantly being updated; stay current)
Journal: Log your changes in your journal.

Week 2: Continue changing the breakfast foods by trying another cereal, fruit, milk or soy milk.
Reading: Begin to practice reading a food label, in the store and at home.
Journal: Log your changes in your Journal.

Week 3: Continue with these changes to breakfast, and add one or two morning snacks from your Suggested Menus by Genotype and Caloric Level (pages 257-325).
Morning: Add to current behavior changes.
Snack: Identify morning snacks from your suggested menus.
Begin eating a small snack from your suggested menus.
Journal: Log your changes in your Journal.

Week 4: Continue changing the morning snack by adding one or two additional morning snacks from your suggested menus.
Morning: Identify another morning snack from your menu plan to try. Keep in mind snacks that taste good and are convenient. Stay with serving sizes.
Reading: Review benefits of green tea (see page 168) and consider the value of flowers in your day. Next time you are doing your shopping, stop and smell the flowers. Most supermarkets have a flower section.
Journal: Log your changes in your Journal.

Week 5: Focus on lunch by adding one or two changes from your lunch food suggestions. Add to last week's successes by making another change to your nutrition. Try a fruit you have never tried before. Pick from your suggested menus.
Reading: Review section on carbohydrates, Smart foods, and micronutrients (see pages 175-180).
Journal: Log your changes in your Journal.

Week 6: Continue changing your lunch by adding one or two foods from your suggested menus. Consider changing an item of your lunch. For example, instead of white bread choose a whole grain bread.
Reading: Review section on phytochemicals (see page 176).
Journal: Log your changes in your Journal.

Week 7: Focus on afternoon snacks by adding one or two items from your suggested menus. Consider snacks that taste good and are convenient for your lifestyle. If you are a business person and are often in long meetings, it is reasonable to request afternoon refreshments. You will be surprised how most people welcome the snack break. Make sure you order healthy snacks that will benefit your meeting by providing high-quality foods. Good nutrition provides good thinking.
Reading: Review section on fats (page 103). Continue and refine the content of your diet by adding "good fats" into your diet. Try a different fat you have never tried before from your suggested menus.
Journal: Log your changes in your Journal.

Week 8: Continue changes by adding one or two more different afternoon snacks from your suggested menus. Consider snacks that taste good and are convenient. Continue to refine the content of your diet. Add new proteins. Try a protein you have never tried before. Pick from your suggested menus.
Reading: Review section on protein (see page 81).
Journal: Log your changes in your Journal.

Week 9: Focus on dinner by adding one or two dinner foods from your suggested menus to your evening meal.
Reading: Review Shopping in the Supermarket. Read the section on water. Continue to refine the content of your diet. Add improved fluids to your diet. Review the amount of fluids you are drinking and your water source. Evaluate the caffeine content of your diet. Review your alcohol intake—pros, cons. Different teas—pros, cons.
Journal: Log your changes in your Journal.

Week 10: Continue changing the dinner meal by adding one or two more dinner foods from your suggested menus. Begin by making a change of a food type. If you have been used to eating excess portions, decrease portion sizes to those recommended. If you are eating in a restaurant, try to order the foods you have on your suggested menu plan. Example: If you want to eat fresh fish, ask for it to be grilled or broiled with olive oil.

Reading: Review section on eating out (see page 185). Also consider reading the section on glycemic load vs. glycemic index (see page 78).

Journal: Log your changes in your Journal.

Week 11: Continue changing the dinner meal by adding one or two supper snack foods from your suggested menus. Add in a small snack at this time.

Grocery store assignment: Ask your supermarket store if they sell organic or genetically modified foods. Look at the convenience foods, such as frozen dinners, natural packaged food, organic convenience foods, and preservative-free foods. Check your recommended diet plan to see whether these foods will help you.

Journal: Log your changes in your Journal.

Week 12: Focus on evening snack by adding snack foods from your suggested menus. Most of us feel that the evening snack is a meal to skip. However, these calories are important calories and nutrients to carry you through the night. Try not to skip your evening snack. Make those foods count.

Add to last week's successes by making another change: Identify three restaurants that will make changes for you with a specific menu item. Have the sauce on the side. With a salad, get the dressing on the side. Identify a restaurant that serves fresh fish and vegetables. Identify those restaurants willing to share and discuss food ingredients on the menu, such as the fats they use in the preparation of food. Find restaurants that have a wide selection on the menu.

Now you have really begun to make changes, let's focus on *when* you eat. Adjust the time when you eat so you are able to get enough food in at the right time.

Reading: Review section on water (see page 164).

Journal: Log your changes in your journal.

Weeks 13–20: Continue changing by adding new foods to all meals. Make changes with meals eaten in restaurants and takeout foods.
Journal: Log changes in your Journal.

Keep in mind that eating needs to fit in with your lifestyle. Consider what to eat in the following situations:

- getting up in the morning
- during commute time
- arriving at work or school
- morning workload (do you need to make time to eat during the morning?)
- morning breaks
- lunchtime (how convenient is preparing, buying, or bringing your lunch?)
- afternoon workload
- return commute time
- evening

Diet Change Plan Summary
The following list summarizes the things to include in your plans for making dietary changes:

- Read about protein foods and what you can consider for your Apo E genotype.
- Learn about carbohydrate foods you can consider for your Apo E genotype.
- Learn about the right amount and type of fat you can eat for your Apo E genotype.
- Focus on your own dietary recommendations, suggested menus by genotype and caloric Level, and learn how to transition to the new food recommendations.
- Understand your diet and why it has been prescribed. It is important, so review the details for your Apo E genotype.
- See individual dietary guidelines.
- Begin nutritional changes by slowly adding in new items to your current eating plan—focusing on making changes to breakfast during first few weeks.

- Then while continuing the changes made to breakfast, add a morning snack for about 1–2 weeks, and so on.
- Continue your diet changes.
- Focus on making changes to your lunch for 1–2 weeks.
- Focus on making changes to your afternoon tea/snack for 1–2 weeks.
- Focus on making changes to your dinner for 1–2 weeks.
- Focus on making changes to your evening snack for 1–2 weeks.

Go slowly! Enjoy experimenting with your new foods and the recipes. This way you will learn how to eat well for life. To be able to help you make these changes, we encourage you to enlist the aid of a partner or a support person for this process. I have added a support person checklist and process—see support person section (see page 71).

Chapter Nineteen

THE APO E GENE DIET
SAMPLE MEAL PLANS BY GENOTYPE
AND CALORIE ALLOWANCE

As you plan your daily menus, keep in mind that most foods are a combination of the Big Three macronutrients—protein, carbohydrate, and fat. It is very rare that a food contains only one nutrient. Do your best to combine and balance your food. Foods typically break down into the following macronutrients:

- fruit contains mostly carbohydrate (with plant fiber)
- some foods, such as beans, contain a mixture of protein and carbohydrate
- dairy foods contain mostly protein, fat and some carbohydrate
- most animal protein contains protein and animal fat
- most plant protein contains a more dilute protein and good anti-inflammatory fat

The following sample meal plans are organized by genotype and then listed by KCALs per day. Each meal plan includes meals for four days.

Suggested Diets
* = see recipe

APO E GENE DIET
4/4 1600 KCAL DAY 1
Serving considerations per day.
(Be mindful of serving sizes.)

Carbohydrates
6 serving portions of grain/starch
7 serving portions of fruit and vegetable

Protein
10 serving portions fish or plant protein

Fat
4.5 serving portions anti-inflammatory fat

Breakfast
1 slice whole grain toast
1 tbsp. organic nut butter
1 medium orange
1 cup nonfat milk
Fluids: water and hot matcha tea
Apo E high-quality multivitamin

Morning Snack
¼ cup whole grain granola
½ cup yogurt

Lunch
2 slices whole grain bread
1 tbsp. organic olive oil mayonnaise
3 oz. baby shrimp
Lettuce and sliced tomato
1 oz. avocado
Lemon ice water*

Afternoon Snack
¼ cup nonfat cottage cheese
½ cup carrots
½ cup cherry tomatoes
Fluids: water and white tea

Evening Dinner
3 oz. wild organic salmon
3 oz. Pam's baked potato with skin
   (1 serving)
2 tbsp. tomato salsa cream (¼ serving)
1 tbsp. chives
1 cup steamed broccoli
1 whole grain bread
¹/₈ avocado
Fluids: water with lemon and fresh mint

Supper or Evening Snack
1 serving chilled strawberry pottage
½ cup nonfat ice cream
Fluids: water and chamomile herbal tea

APO E GENE DIET
4/4 1600 KCAL DAY 2
Serving considerations per day
(Be mindful of serving sizes)

Carbohydrates
5 serving portions of grain/starch
8.5 serving portions of fruit and vegetable

Protein
7 serving portions fish or plant protein

Fat
2 serving portions anti-inflammatory fat

Breakfast
½ cup nonfat cottage cheese
½ banana
½ organic whole grain bagel
½ tbsp. local organic honey
Fluids: water and hot lemon
   mint green tea
Apo E high-quality multivitamin

Morning Snack
½ medium apple
½ tbsp. nut butter

Lunch

1 whole grain pita bread
Shredded lettuce and sliced tomato
2 oz. fresh crab
1 oz. low-fat soy cheese, shredded
2 tbsp. nonfat Caesar dressing
Fluids: orange sparkling water*

Afternoon Snack

1 serving carrot and cucumber yogurt salad
4 whole grain crackers
Fluids: 1 cup green lavender mint tea

Evening Dinner

Shiitake mushroom and spinach lasagna
    (¾ serving)
1 tbsp. parmesan cheese
1 slice rustic whole grain bread
1 cup steamed spinach
Fluids: chamomile tea with essence of
    rosehips and lemon

Supper or Evening Snack

3 diet raspberry ginger biscuits (cookies) (1
    serving)
1 cup nonfat milk

APO E GENE DIET
4/4 1600 KCAL DAY 3

Serving considerations per day
(Be mindful of serving sizes)

Carbohydrates

9.5 serving portions of grain/starch
4 serving portions of fruit and vegetable

Protein

9.5 serving portions fish or plant protein

Fat

6 serving portions anti-inflammatory fat

Breakfast

Scrambled egg whites or ½ cup egg
    substitute
1 slice whole grain oat flax toast
$1/_8$ of an avocado
1½ oz. fat-free cheese
½ cup tomato salsa cream (1 serving)
Fluids: water and yerba tropical fruit green tea
Apo E high-quality multivitamin

Morning Snack

¼ cup nonfat cottage cheese
½ cup blueberries
Fluids: white and mint tea*

Lunch

¾ serving tofu salad
¾ cup grapes
¾ cup nonfat milk
Fluids: iced lemon water—hot green
    raspberry ginger tea

Afternoon Snack

Trail mix: $1/_8$ cup almonds, $1/_8$ cup
    cranberries/raisins, and ½ cup low-fat
    granola
Fluids: Japanese matcha tea*

Evening Dinner

Grilled teriyaki tuna (3 oz. raw tuna with 1
    serving teriyaki sauce)
$1/_3$ cup black beans
Green salad (1 cup spinach, $1/_3$ cup cherry
    tomatoes, $1/_3$ cup cabbage, $1/_3$ cup
    shredded carrots)
Organic fat-free salad dressing, 1 tsp. olive oil
Sparkling lime juice water*
Fluids: hot decaf peach green tea

Supper or Evening Snack

¾ cup strawberries
1 serving angel food cake ($1/_{12}$ cake that is
    10" diam. tube)

APO E GENE DIET
4/4 1600 KCAL DAY 4
Serving considerations per day
(Be mindful of serving sizes)

Carbohydrates
6 serving portions of grain/starch
10.5 serving portions of fruit and vegetable

Protein
8 serving portions fish or plant protein

Fat
4 serving portions anti-inflammatory fat

Breakfast
1 serving Scottish oats
1 cup nonfat milk
Fluids: water and hot green tea
Apo E high-quality multivitamin

Morning Snack
¼ cup organic whole grain granola
1 cup nonfat soy yogurt (Nancy's brand-
    www.nancysyogurt.com)

Lunch
1 whole grain pita bread
3 oz. water packet tuna
1 tbsp. fat-free ranch dressing
Lettuce, onions, and tomatoes
Fluids: hibiscus sparkling water

Afternoon Snack
1.5 oz. low-fat cheese
½ cup organic grapes
Fluids: hot ginger green tea*

Evening Dinner
Vegetable spaghetti (¾ of a serving)
1 tbsp. grated soy cheese
1 serving organic green salad

Supper or Evening Snack
3 small lemon ginger biscuits (1 serving)

APO E GENE DIET
4/4 1800 KCAL DAY 1
Serving considerations per day
(Be mindful of serving sizes)

Carbohydrates
11.5 serving portions of grain/starch
5.5 serving portions of fruit and vegetable

Protein
10 serving portions fish or plant protein

Fat
2.5 serving portions anti-inflammatory fat

Breakfast
1 slice whole grain oat flax toast
½ tbsp. honey
½ cup blueberries
½ cup soy milk
Fluids: water and hot Japanese green tea
Apo E high-quality multivitamin

Morning Snack
½ cup cherries
¾ cup cottage cheese or yogurt

Lunch
1 serving vegetarian tacos
½ cup tomato salsa cream (1 serving)
Fluids: 1 cup low-fat soy milk and lemon
    ice green tea*

Afternoon Snack
1 serving sultana carrot ginger coleslaw
4 oz. whole wheat pretzels
½ cup cherry tomatoes
Fluids: apple spiced green tea

Evening Dinner
3 oz. wild grilled halibut*
3 oz. Pam's baked potato with skin*
3 tbsp. plain yogurt
1 tbsp. chives
1 cup steamed broccoli

½ slice whole grain bread
$^1/_8$ of an avocado
Fluids: water with lemon and fresh mint

Supper or Evening Snack

Chilled strawberry pottage (1 serving)
½ cup frozen yogurt
Fluids: water and chamomile herbal tea

APO E GENE DIET
4/4 1800 KCAL DAY 2

Serving considerations per day
(Be mindful of serving sizes)

Carbohydrates

3.5 serving portions of grain/starch
12.5 serving portions of fruit and vegetable

Protein

11 serving portions fish or plant protein

Fat

2 serving portions anti-inflammatory fat

Breakfast

Scrambled eggs (½ cup egg substitute)
¼ cup tomato salsa cream (½ serving)
1 slice whole grain toast or whole wheat tortilla
½ tbsp. organic honey
Fluids: water and ginger green tea
Apo E high-quality multivitamin

Morning Snack

1 serving sultana, carrot, ginger coleslaw
1.5 oz. soy cheese

Lunch

1 serving tofu salad
1 medium apple
1 cup nonfat milk
Orange sparkling water*

Afternoon Snack

1 serving carrot and cucumber yogurt salad
5 whole wheat crackers

Evening Dinner

Grilled lemon Pacific Rim ginger trout (3 oz.
   cooked trout with 1 serving soy ginger sauce)
3 oz. Pam's baked potato (1 serving)
1 cup Mevagissey ratatouille (2 servings)

Supper or Evening Snack

Apple blueberry crumble (½ serving)
Vanilla custard (1 serving)

APO E GENE DIET
4/4 1800 KCAL DAY 3

Serving considerations per day
(Be mindful of serving sizes)

Carbohydrates

9.5 serving portions of grain/starch
10.5 serving portions of fruit and vegetable

Protein

12 serving portions fish or plant protein

Fat

4 serving portions anti-inflammatory fat

Breakfast

2, six-inch corn tortillas
¼ cup egg substitute
1 ½ oz. fat-free cheese
½ cup tomato salsa cream (½ serving)
Fluids: water and hot orange China green tea
Apo E high-quality multivitamin

Morning Snack

½ cup nonfat cottage cheese
1 cup blueberries
Fluids: white and mint tea*

Lunch

2 slices whole grain bread
3 oz. shrimp or crab
Onions, tomato, and lettuce
1 tbsp. organic fat-free mayonnaise
Fluids: sparkling iced lemon and fresh mint
   water (consider using a crystal glass)

Afternoon Snack

Trail mix: ¼ cup almonds, ¼ cup cranberries/ raisins, and ½ cup low-fat granola
Fluids: decaf matcha tea*

Evening Dinner

1 slice multi-grain bread
Lime and tomato grilled sea bass (use 3 oz. cooked sea bass and 1 serving or ½ cup tomato salsa cream)
½ cup black beans
Organic mixed green salad (1 serving)
Fluids: sparkling lime juice water and hot decaf peach green tea*

Supper or Evening Snack

1 cup strawberries
1 serving angel food cake (¹/₁₂ of a 10" diam. tube)

Lunch

1 whole grain pita bread
4 oz. water packet tuna
1 tbsp. fat free ranch
Lettuce (romaine), spring onions, and tomato
Fluids: hibiscus sparkling water

Afternoon Snack

1 oz. soy cheese
½ cup organic grapes
Fluids: hot ginger green tea*

Evening Dinner

Vegetable spaghetti dinner (1 serving)
1 tbsp. organic grated soy cheese
Green salad (1 serving)

Supper or Evening Snack

3 small ginger biscuits (1 serving)

**APO E GENE DIET
4/4 1800 KCAL DAY 4**
Serving considerations per day
(Be mindful of serving sizes)

Carbohydrates
7 serving portions of grain/starch
12 serving portions of fruit and vegetable

Protein
11 serving portions fish or plant protein

Fat
3 serving portions anti-inflammatory fat

Breakfast

1 serving Scottish oats
1 cup nonfat milk
Fluids: water and hot vanilla white tea
Apo E high-quality multivitamin

Morning Snack

¼ cup whole grain granola
1 cup nonfat yogurt with ½ cup berries

**APO E GENE DIET
4/4 2000 KCAL DAY 1**
Serving considerations per day
(Be mindful of serving sizes)

Carbohydrates
5.5 serving portions of grain/starch
9 serving portions of fruit and vegetable

Protein
10 serving portions fish or plant protein

Fat
5 serving portions anti-inflammatory fat

Breakfast

Scottish oatmeal (1 serving)
¹/₈ cup raisins/cranberries
1 cup nonfat milk or soy milk
Fluids: water and hot matcha green tea
Apo E high-quality multivitamin

Morning Snack

Granola mix: ¼ cup low-fat granola, 8
chopped walnuts, and ¹/₈ cup dried apricots
¾ cup nonfat yogurt

Lunch

Vegetarian tacos (1.5 servings)
California tomato salsa cream (1 serving)
½ medium apple
Fluids: 1 cup nonfat or skim milk and
lemon ice green tea*

Afternoon Snack

Black bean soup (½ serving)
¼ cup cherry tomatoes
Fluids: apple spiced green tea

Evening Dinner

4 oz. baked trout
3 oz. Pam's baked potato with skin (1 serving)
1 ½ oz. nonfat cheese
1 tbsp. chives
Mevagissey ratatouilee (1 serving)
Fluids: water with cucumber, lemon and
fresh mint

Supper or Evening Snack

½ cup low-fat chocolate frozen yogurt
Fluids: water and chamomile herbal tea

**APO E GENE DIET
4/4 2000 KCAL DAY 2**

Serving considerations per day
(Be mindful of serving sizes)

Carbohydrates

8.5 serving portions of grain/starch
7.5 serving portions of fruit and vegetable

Protein

13 serving portions fish or plant protein

Fat

2 serving portions anti-inflammatory fat

Breakfast

1 whole grain bagel
2 medium egg whites
½ banana
½ tbsp. honey
Fluids: water hot mint green tea
Apo E high-quality multivitamin

Morning Snack

½ cup cherries or cherry tomatoes
½ cup nonfat cottage cheese
8 whole grain crackers
1 cup hot green tea (don't forget to
consider a bone china cup)

Lunch

1 slice whole grain bread
1 garden or veggie burger
Lettuce and tomato
1 tbsp. organic fat-free mayonnaise
1 ½ oz. low-fat soy cheese
4 green or black olives
¹/₈ of an avocado
1 cup nonfat milk
Fluids: orange sparkling water* (definitely
consider a crystal glass)

Afternoon Snack

Fresh fruit Shake to Go (¾ serving)

Evening Dinner

Grilled Ahi tuna with black beans (4 oz.
cooked ahi tuna with ½ cup black beans)
1 slice whole grain oat flax roll or bread
Mevagissey ratatouille (1 serving)
Fluids: iced or hot black currant China
green tea

Supper or Evening Snack

3 small ginger cookies*
1 cup nonfat milk

APO E 4/4 2000 KCAL

APO E GENE DIET
4/4 2000 KCAL DAY 3
Serving considerations per day
(Be mindful of serving sizes)

Carbohydrates
7.5 serving portions of grain/starch
11 serving portions of fruit and vegetable

Protein
14.5 serving portions fish or plant protein

Fat
4 serving portions anti-inflammatory fat

Breakfast
6, one-inch corn tortilla
½ cup egg substitute
1 ½ oz. fat-free cheese
¼ cup tomato salsa cream (½ serving)
½ cup melon
Fluids: water and blueberry white tea
Apo E high-quality multivitamin

Morning Snack
1 organic apple
½ tbsp. natural nut butter
Fluids: white mint tea*

Lunch
1 slice organic whole grain bread
4 oz. tofu
Onions, tomato, and lettuce
1 tbsp. fat-free mayonnaise
1 cup nonfat or soy milk
Fluids: iced lemon water (don't forget to
use a crystal glass)

Afternoon Snack
Trail mix: 1/8 cup nuts, ¼ cup cranberries/
raisins, and ½ cup low-fat granola
2/3 cup nonfat cottage cheese
Decaf matcha tea*

Evening Dinner
Vegetable spaghetti (¾ serving)
1 tbsp. parmesan cheese
1 serving mixed green salad*
1 slice whole grain bread
Fluids: sparkling lime juice water, hot
decaf peach green tea*

Supper or Evening Snack
1 cup blackberries
1 slice vanilla angel food cake (1/12 of a 10"
diam. tube)
1 cup nonfat milk

APO E GENE DIET
4/4 2000 KCAL DAY 4
Serving considerations per day
(Be mindful of serving sizes)

Carbohydrates
8.5 serving portions of grain/starch
10 serving portions of fruit and vegetable

Protein
13.5 serving portions fish or plant protein

Fat
3 serving portions anti-inflammatory fat

Breakfast
1 cup whole grain dry cereal
½ banana
1 cup soy milk or nonfat milk
Fluids: water and raspberry green tea
Apo E high-quality multivitamin

Morning Snack
1 snack break mix: ½ cup low-fat granola,
and 1/8 cup of your favorite dried fruit
such as dried apricots
½ cup nonfat cottage cheese

Lunch

3 oz. 1 serving Pam's baked potato
1 cup Cornish chili (1 serving)
1.5 oz. fat-free soy cheese, shredded
1 cup cooked broccoli
Lettuce, onions, and tomatoes
Fluids: iced hibiscus sparkling water

Afternoon Snack

Carrot, cucumber yogurt salad (1 serving)
Fluids: hot lemon ginger green tea*

Evening Dinner

4 oz. wild salmon with turmeric (4 oz.
  cooked salmon and 1 tsp. olive oil)
½ baked potato that is 2.5" X 4.5"
Wok-steamed kale (½ cup raw), garlic,
  onion (¼ cup) with
1 tomatoes and corn (¼ cup)
1 tbsp. parmesan cheese
Fluids: lemon sparkling water

Supper or Evening Snack

Apple blueberry crumble (½ serving)
Fluids: 1 cup nonfat, skim, or soy milk

APO E GENE DIET
4/4 2400 KCAL DAY 1

Serving considerations per day
(Be mindful of serving sizes)

Carbohydrates

6.5 serving portions of grain/starch
9.5 serving portions of fruit and vegetable

Protein

14.5 serving portions fish or plant protein

Fat

2.5 serving portions anti-inflammatory fat

Breakfast

Orange Shake to Go (½ serving)
½ whole grain bagel
½ tbsp. honey
$1/_8$ cup raisins/cranberries
1 cup nonfat milk or soy milk
Fluids: water, hot ginger green tea
Apo E high-quality multivitamin

Morning Snack

Granola mix: ¼ cup low-fat granola, $1/_8$ cup
  chopped walnuts, and $1/_8$ cup dried apricots
½ cup cottage cheese

Lunch

Vegetarian (meatless) tacos (1 serving) with
  tomato salsa cream (½ serving)
$1/_3$ cup black beans
½ medium apple
1 cup nonfat or soy milk
Fluids: fresh Cornish pixie green rose
  lemonade*

Afternoon Snack

Cornish chili (¾ serving)
4 whole grain crackers
Fluids: iced or hot apple spiced green tea*

Evening Dinner

5 oz. lime ginger halibut (5 oz. cooked
  halibut with 1 serving soy ginger sauce)
3 oz. Pam's baked potato with skin (1 serving)
1 ½ oz. nonfat cheese
1 tbsp. chives
½ cup grilled yellow squash and ½ cup
  asparagus
Fluids: iced water with lemon and fresh mint

Supper or Evening Snack

1 cup strawberries
1 slice angel food cake ($1/_{12}$ of a 10" diam.
  tube)
¾ cup nonfat warm vanilla yogurt
Fluids: iced water and chamomile peach
  herbal tea*

APO E 4/4 2400 KCAL

APO E GENE DIET
4/4 2400 KCAL DAY 2

Serving considerations per day
(Be mindful of serving sizes)

Carbohydrates

4.5 serving portions of grain/starch
15.5 serving portions of fruit and vegetable

Protein

12.5 serving portions fish or plant protein

Fat

3 serving portions anti-inflammatory fat

Breakfast

1 serving Scottish oats
1/8 cup raisins
1 cup nonfat milk
½ tbsp. honey
Fluids: water and black currant ginger tea*
Apo E high-quality multivitamin

Morning Snack

1 slice whole grain oat flax bread
1.5 tbsp. raisins
½ cup nonfat cottage cheese
Fluids: hot or cold peach green tea*

Lunch

½ slice whole grain bun or slice of bread
¾ serving tofu salad
½ medium apple
1 cup nonfat milk
Fluids: orange sparkling water*

Afternoon Snack

Carrot, cucumber and yogurt salad (1.5
    servings)
½ cup carrots/jicama slices
1 slice multi-grain bread
Fluids: sparkling orange ice water

Evening Dinner

Orange/rosemary mackerel (4 oz. cooked
    mackerel, 1 tsp. olive oil, juice of ½ orange)
Mixed greens*
½ baked potato that is 2.5" by 4.5"
Fluids: iced water and hot decaf raspberry
    green tea

Supper or Evening Snack

Kelly's Fore Street Dessert (½ serving)

APO E GENE DIET
4/4 2400 KCAL DAY 3

Serving considerations per day
(Be mindful of serving sizes)

Carbohydrates

8 serving portions of grain/starch
16.5 serving portions of fruit and vegetable

Protein

16.5 serving portions fish or plant protein

Fat

8.5 serving portions anti-inflammatory fat

Breakfast

2, six-inch corn tortillas
¾ cup egg white or substitute
3 oz. fat-free cheese
¼ cup tomato beans
1 oz. avocado
¼ cup salsa
½ cup melon
Fluids: water and hot white tea
Apo E high-quality multivitamin

Morning Snack

1 organic apple
½ tbsp. natural nut butter
½ cup nonfat cottage cheese
Fluids: white and mint tea*

Lunch

Fish salad (1 serving)

1 whole grain pita bread

1 cup nonfat milk

Fluids: iced lemon/lime sparkling ice water (don't forget a pretty glass)

Afternoon Snack

Fruit Shake to Go (¾ serving)

Evening Dinner

Vegetable spaghetti*

1 tbsp. parmesan cheese

1 green salad (1 serving)

1 slice whole grain bread

1 cup nonfat milk

Fluids: sparkling lime juice water and hot decaf peach green tea*

Supper or Evening Snack

½ cup frozen yogurt

Fruit pottage (2 servings)

Fluids: hot chamomile tea

APO E GENE DIET

4/4 2400 KCAL DAY 4

Serving considerations per day

(Be mindful of serving sizes)

Carbohydrates

9.5 serving portions of grain/starch

15 serving portions of fruit and vegetable

Protein

15 serving portions fish or plant protein

Fat

4.5 serving portions anti-inflammatory fat

Breakfast

Blueberry oat muffin (1 serving)

Baked apple with honey (½ serving)

Scrambled eggs (½–¾ cup egg whites or substitute)

1 cup nonfat milk

1 medium orange

Fluids: fresh water and hot jasmine green tea

Apo E high-quality multivitamin

Morning Snack

$1/3$ cup low-fat whole grain granola

¾ cup nonfat soy yogurt

1 cup fresh organic strawberries

Lunch

Rustic 1 serving Tuscany pizza

Green salad (1 serving)

Fluids: iced hibiscus tea, sparkling water*

Afternoon Snack

Carrot, cucumber and yogurt salad (1 serving)

¾ cup nonfat cottage cheese

Fluids: hot lemon ginger green tea*

Evening Dinner

Grilled tuna steak with teriyaki and shiitake mushrooms*

½ potato that is 2.5" by 4.5"

1 tsp. olive oil

Ratatouille from Cornwall (1 serving)

1 slice organic rustic whole grain bread

1 tbsp. parmesan cheese

1 tsp. avocado

Supper or Evening Snack

½ cup apple blueberry crumble*

¾ cup nonfat hot vanilla yogurt

APO E GENE DIET
4/3 1600 KCAL DAY 1
Serving considerations per day
(Be mindful of serving sizes)

Carbohydrates
6 serving portions of grain/starch
7 serving portions of fruit and vegetable

Protein
9 serving portions fish or plant protein

Fat
4.5 serving portions anti-inflammatory fat

Breakfast
1 slice whole grain toast
1 tbsp. organic nut butter
1 medium orange
1 cup nonfat milk
Fluids: water and hot matcha tea
Apo E high-quality multivitamin

Morning Snack
¼ cup whole grain granola
½ cup yogurt

Lunch
2 slices whole grain bread
1 tbsp. organic olive oil mayonnaise
3 oz. crabmeat
Lettuce and sliced tomato
1 oz. avocado
Lemon ice water*

Afternoon Snack
¼ cup nonfat cottage cheese
½ cup carrots
½ cup cherry tomatoes
Fluids: water and white tea

Evening Dinner
3 oz. wild organic black cod
3 oz. Pam's baked potato with skin (1 serving)
2 tbsp. tomato salsa cream (¼ serving)
1 tbsp. chives
1 cup steamed broccoli
1 whole grain bread
$1/_8$ avocado
Fluids: water with lemon and fresh mint

Supper or Evening Snack
Chilled strawberry pottage (1 serving)
½ cup nonfat frozen yogurt
Fluids: water and chamomile herbal tea

APO E GENE DIET
4/3 1600 KCAL DAY 2
Serving considerations per day
(Be mindful of serving sizes)

Carbohydrates
5 serving portions of grain/starch
8.5 serving portions of fruit and vegetable

Protein
7 serving portions fish or plant protein

Fat
2 serving portions anti-inflammatory fat

Breakfast
½ cup nonfat cottage cheese
½ banana
½ organic whole grain bagel
½ tbsp. local organic honey
Fluids: water and hot lemon mint green tea
Apo E high-quality multivitamin

Morning Snack
½ medium apple
½ tbsp. nut butter

Lunch

1 whole grain pita bread
Shredded lettuce and sliced tomato
2 oz. fresh crab
1 oz. low-fat soy cheese, shredded
2 tbsp. nonfat Caesar dressing
Fluids: orange sparkling water*

Afternoon Snack

1 serving carrot and cucumber yogurt salad
4 whole grain crackers
Fluids: 1 cup green lavender mint tea

Evening Dinner

Shiitake mushroom and spinach lasagna
(¾ serving)
1 tbsp. parmesan cheese
1 slice rustic whole grain bread
1 cup steamed spinach
Fluids: chamomile tea with essence of
rosehips and lemon

Supper or Evening Snack

3 diet raspberry ginger biscuits (cookies) (1
serving)
1 cup nonfat milk

APO E GENE DIET
4/3 1600 KCAL DAY 3

Serving considerations per day
(Be mindful of serving sizes)

Carbohydrates

9.5 serving portions of grain/starch
4 serving portions of fruit and vegetable

Protein

9.5 serving portions fish or plant protein

Fat

6 serving portions anti-inflammatory fat

Breakfast

Scrambled egg whites or ½ cup egg substitute
1 slice whole grain oat flax toast
$1/_8$ of an avocado
1 ½ oz. fat-free cheese
½ cup tomato salsa cream (1 serving)
Fluids: water and yerba tropical fruit green tea
Apo E high-quality multivitamin

Morning Snack

¼ cup nonfat cottage cheese
½ cup blueberries
Fluids: white and mint tea*

Lunch

¾ serving tofu salad
¾ cup grapes
¾ cup nonfat milk
Fluids: iced lemon water, hot green
raspberry ginger tea

Afternoon Snack

Trail mix: $1/_8$ cup almonds, $1/_8$ cup
Cranberries/raisins, and ½ cup low-fat granola
Fluids: Japanese matcha tea*

Evening Dinner

Grilled teriyaki sea bass (3 oz. raw sea bass
with 1 serving teriyaki sauce)
$1/_3$ cup black beans
Green salad (1 cup spinach, $1/_3$ cup cherry
tomatoes, $1/_3$ cup cabbage, $1/_3$ cup
shredded carrots)
Organic fat-free salad dressing, 1 tsp. olive oil
Sparkling lime juice water*
Fluids: hot decaf peach green tea

Supper or Evening Snack

¾ cup raspberries
1 serving angel food cake ($1/_{12}$ of a 10"
diam. tube)

APO E GENE DIET
4/3 1600 KCAL DAY 4

Serving considerations per day
(Be mindful of serving sizes)

Carbohydrates
6 serving portions of grain/starch
10.5 serving portions of fruit and vegetable

Protein
8 serving portions fish or plant protein

Fat
4 serving portions anti-inflammatory fat

Breakfast
1 serving Scottish oats
1 cup nonfat milk
Fluids: water and hot green tea
Apo E high-quality multivitamin

Morning Snack
¼ cup organic whole grain granola
1 cup nonfat soy yogurt (Nancy's brand-
www.nancysyogurt.com)

Lunch
1 whole grain pita bread
3 oz. water packet tuna
1 tbsp. fat-free ranch dressing
Lettuce, onions, and tomatoes
Fluids: hibiscus sparkling water

Afternoon Snack
1.5 oz. low-fat cheese
½ cup organic grapes
 Fluids: hot ginger green tea*

Evening Dinner
Vegetable spaghetti (¾ of a serving)
1 tbsp. grated soy cheese
1 serving organic green salad

Supper or Evening Snack
3 small lemon ginger biscuits (1 serving)

APO E GENE DIET
4/3 1800 KCAL DAY 1

Serving considerations per day
(Be mindful of serving sizes)

Carbohydrates
11.5 serving portions of grain/starch
5.5 serving portions of fruit and vegetable

Protein
10 serving portions fish or plant protein

Fat
2.5 serving portions anti-inflammatory fat

Breakfast
1 slice whole grain oat flax toast
½ tbsp. honey
½ cup blueberries
½ cup soy milk
Fluids: water and hot Japanese green tea
Apo E high-quality multivitamin

Morning Snack
½ cup cherries
¾ cup cottage cheese or yogurt

Lunch
1 serving vegetarian tacos
½ cup tomato salsa cream (1 serving)
Fluids: 1 cup low-fat soy milk and lemon
 ice green tea*

Afternoon Snack
1 serving sultana carrot ginger coleslaw (¾
 serving)
4 oz. whole wheat pretzels
½ cup cherry tomatoes
Fluids: apple spiced green tea

Evening Dinner
3 oz. wild grilled sea bass*
3 oz. Pam's baked potato with skin*
3 tbsp. plain yogurt
1 tbsp. chives

1 cup steamed broccoli
½ slice whole grain bread
¹/₈ of an avocado
Fluids: water with lemon and fresh mint

Supper or Evening Snack

Chilled strawberry pottage (1 serving)
½ cup frozen yogurt
Fluids: water and chamomile herbal tea

APO E GENE DIET
4/3 1800 KCAL DAY 2

Serving considerations per day
(Be mindful of serving sizes)

Carbohydrates
3.5 serving portions of grain/starch
12.5 serving portions of fruit and vegetable

Protein
11 serving portions fish or plant protein

Fat
2 serving portions anti-inflammatory fat

Breakfast

Scrambled eggs (½ cup egg substitute)
¼ cup tomato salsa cream (½ serving)
1 slice whole grain toast or whole wheat tortilla
½ tbsp. organic honey
Fluids: water and ginger green tea
Apo E high-quality multivitamin

Morning Snack

Sultana carrot ginger coleslaw (1 serving)
1.5 oz. soy cheese

Lunch

1 serving tofu salad
1 medium apple
1 cup nonfat milk
Orange sparkling water*

Afternoon Snack

1 serving carrot and cucumber yogurt salad
5 whole wheat crackers

Evening Dinner

Grilled lemon Pacific Rim ginger trout (3 oz.
  cooked trout with 1 serving soy ginger sauce)
3 oz. 1 serving Pam's baked potato
1 cup Mevagissey ratatouille (2 servings)

Supper or Evening Snack

Apple blueberry crumble (½ serving)
Vanilla custard (1 serving)

APO E GENE DIET
4/3 1800 KCAL DAY 3

Serving considerations per day
(Be mindful of serving sizes)

Carbohydrates
9.5 serving portions of grain/starch
10.5 serving portions of fruit and vegetable

Protein
12 serving portions fish or plant protein

Fat
4 serving portions anti-inflammatory fat

Breakfast

2, six-inch corn tortillas
¼ cup egg substitute
1 ½ oz. fat-free cheese
½ cup tomato salsa cream (½ serving)
Fluids: water and hot orange China green tea
Apo E high-quality multivitamin

Morning Snack

½ cup nonfat cottage cheese
1 cup blueberries
Fluids: white and mint tea*

Lunch

2 slices whole grain bread
3 oz. shrimp or crab
Onions, tomato, and lettuce
1 tbsp. organic fat-free mayonnaise
Fluids: sparkling iced lemon and fresh mint
water (don't forget to consider using a
crystal glass)

Afternoon Snack

Trail mix: ¼ cup almonds, ¼ cup cranberries/
raisins, and ½ cup low-fat granola
Fluids: decaf matcha tea*

Evening Dinner

1 slice multi-grain bread
Lime and tomato grilled sea bass (use 3 oz.
cooked sea bass and 1 serving or ½ cup
tomato salsa cream)
½ cup black beans
Organic mixed green salad (1 serving)
Fluids: sparkling lime juice water and hot
decaf peach green tea*

Supper or Evening Snack

1 cup raspberries
1 serving angel food cake ($^1/_{12}$ of a 10"
diam. tube)

APO E GENE DIET
4/3 1800 KCAL DAY 4

Serving considerations per day
(Be mindful of serving sizes)

Carbohydrates

7 serving portions of grain/starch
12 serving portions of fruit and vegetable

Protein

11 serving portions fish or plant protein

Fat

3 serving portions anti-inflammatory fat

Breakfast

1 serving Scottish oats
1 cup nonfat milk
Fluids: water and hot vanilla white tea
Apo E high-quality multivitamin

Morning Snack

¼ cup whole grain granola
1 cup nonfat yogurt with ½ cup berries

Lunch

1 whole grain pita bread
4 oz. water packed tuna
1 tbsp. fat free ranch
Lettuce (romaine), spring onions, and tomato
Fluids: hibiscus sparkling water

Afternoon Snack

1 oz. soy cheese
½ cup organic grapes
Fluids: hot ginger green tea*

Evening Dinner

Vegetable spaghetti dinner (1 serving)
1 tbsp. organic grated soy cheese
Green salad (1 serving)

Supper or Evening Snack

3 small ginger biscuits (1 serving)

APO E GENE DIET
4/3 2000 KCAL DAY 1
Serving considerations per day
(Be mindful of serving sizes)

Carbohydrates
5.5 serving portions of grain/starch
9 serving portions of fruit and vegetable

Protein
10 serving portions fish or plant protein

Fat
3 serving portions anti-inflammatory fat

Breakfast
Scottish oatmeal (1 serving)
$1/_8$ cup raisins/cranberries
1 cup nonfat milk or soy milk
Fluids: water and hot matcha green tea
Apo E high-quality multivitamin

Morning Snack
Granola mix: ¼ cup low-fat granola, 8
  chopped walnuts, and $1/_8$ cup dried apricots
¾ cup nonfat yogurt

Lunch
Vegetarian tacos (1.5 servings)
California tomato salsa cream (1 serving)
½ medium apple
Fluids: 1 cup nonfat or skim milk and
Lemon ice green tea*

Afternoon Snack
Black bean soup (½ serving)
¼ cup cherry tomatoes
Fluids: apple spiced green tea

Evening Dinner
4 oz. cooked baked roasting chicken
3 oz. Pam's baked potato with skin (1 serving)
1 ½ oz. nonfat cheese
1 tbsp. chives
Mevagissey ratatouilee (1 serving)
Fluids: water with cucumber, lemon and
  fresh mint

Supper or Evening Snack
½ cup low-fat chocolate frozen yogurt
Fluids: water and chamomile herbal tea

APO E GENE DIET
4/3 2000 KCAL DAY 2
Serving considerations per day
(Be mindful of serving sizes)

Carbohydrates
8.5 serving portions of grain/starch
7.5 serving portions of fruit and vegetable

Protein
13 serving portions fish or plant protein

Fat
2 serving portions anti-inflammatory fat

Breakfast
1 whole grain bagel
2 medium egg whites
½ banana
½ tbsp. honey
Fluids: water hot mint green tea
Apo E high-quality multivitamin

Morning Snack
½ cup cherries or cherry tomatoes
½ cup nonfat cottage cheese
8 whole grain crackers
1 cup hot green tea (don't forget to
  consider a bone china cup)

Lunch
1 slice whole grain bread
1 garden or veggie burger with lettuce and
  tomato
1 tbsp. organic fat-free mayonnaise
1 ½ oz. low-fat soy cheese
4 green or black olives
$1/_8$ of an avocado
1 cup nonfat milk
Fluids: orange sparkling water* (definitely
  consider a crystal glass)

Afternoon Snack

Fresh fruit Shake to Go (¾ serving)

Evening Dinner

Grilled Ahi tuna with black beans (4 oz. cooked ahi tuna with ½ cup black beans)
1 slice whole grain oat flax roll or bread
Mevagissey ratatouille (1 serving)
Fluids: iced or hot black currant China green tea

Supper or Evening Snack

3 small ginger cookies*
1 cup nonfat milk

**APO E GENE DIET
4/3 2000 KCAL DAY 3**
Serving considerations per day
(Be mindful of serving sizes)

Carbohydrates
7.5 serving portions of grain/starch
11 serving portions of fruit and vegetable

Protein
14.5 serving portions fish or plant protein

Fat
4 serving portions anti-inflammatory fat

Breakfast

1, six-inch corn tortilla
½ cup egg substitute
1 ½ oz. fat-free cheese
¼ cup tomato salsa cream (½ serving)
½ cup melon
Fluids: water and blueberry white tea
Apo E high-quality multivitamin

Morning Snack

1 organic apple
½ tbsp. natural nut butter
Fluids: white mint tea*

Lunch

1 slice organic whole grain bread
4 oz. tofu
Onions, tomato, and lettuce
1 tbsp. fat-free mayonnaise
1 cup nonfat or soy milk
Fluids: iced lemon water (don't forget to use a crystal glass)

Afternoon Snack

Trail mix: ¹/₈ cup nuts, ¼ cup cranberries/ raisins, and ½ cup low-fat granola
²/₃ cup nonfat cottage cheese
Decaf—matcha tea*

Evening Dinner

Vegetable spaghetti (¾ serving)
1 tbsp. parmesan cheese
1 serving mixed green salad*
1 slice whole grain bread
Fluids: sparkling lime juice water, hot decaf peach green tea*

Supper or Evening Snack

1 cup blackberries
1 slice vanilla angel food cake (¹/₁₂ cake 10" diam. tube)
1 cup nonfat milk

APO E 4/3 2000 KCAL

APO E GENE DIET
4/3 2000 KCAL DAY 4

Serving considerations per day
(Be mindful of serving sizes)

Carbohydrates

8.5 serving portions of grain/starch
10 serving portions of fruit and vegetable

Protein

13.5 serving portions fish or plant protein

Fat

3 serving portions anti-inflammatory fat

Breakfast

1 cup whole grain dry cereal
½ banana
1 cup soy milk or nonfat milk
Fluids: water and Raspberry green tea
Apo E high-quality multivitamin

Morning Snack

1 Snack Break mix: ½ cup low-fat granola,
and $1/_8$ cup of your favorite dried fruit
such as dried apricots
½ cup nonfat cottage cheese

Lunch

3 oz. Pam's Baked Potato (1 serving)
1 cup Cornish Chili (1 serving)
1.5 oz. fat-free soy cheese, shredded
1 cup cooked broccoli
Lettuce, onions, and tomatoes
Fluids: Iced hibiscus sparkling water

Afternoon Snack

Carrot, cucumber yogurt salad (1 serving)
Fluids: Hot Lemon Ginger green tea*

Evening Dinner

4 oz. Wild Salmon with Turmeric (4 oz.
cooked salmon and 1 tsp. olive oil)
½ baked potato that is 2.5" by 4.5"
Wok-steamed kale (½ cup raw), garlic,
onion (¼ cup) with
1 tomatoes and corn (¼ cup)
1 tbsp. parmesan cheese
Fluids: Lemon Sparkling Water

Supper or Evening Snack

Apple Blueberry Crumble (½ serving)
Fluids: 1 cup nonfat, skim, or soy milk

APO E 4/3 2000 KCAL

APO E GENE DIET
4/3 2400 KCAL DAY 1

Serving considerations per day
(Be mindful of serving sizes)

Carbohydrates
6.5 serving portions of grain/starch
9.5 serving portions of fruit and vegetable

Protein
14.5 serving portions fish or plant protein

Fat
2.5 serving portions anti-inflammatory fat

Breakfast

Orange Shake to Go (½ serving)
½ whole grain bagel
½ tbsp. honey
1/8 cup raisins/cranberries
1 cup nonfat milk or soy milk
Fluids: water, hot ginger green tea
Apo E high-quality multivitamin

Morning Snack

Granola mix: ¼ cup low-fat granola, 1/8 cup
   chopped walnuts, and 1/8 cup dried apricots
½ cup cottage cheese

Lunch

Vegetarian (meatless) tacos (1 serving) with
   tomato salsa cream (½ serving)
1/3 cup black beans
½ Fresh apple, medium
1 cup nonfat or soy milk
Fluids: fresh Cornish pixie green rose
   lemonade*

Afternoon Snack

Cornish chili (¾ serving)
4 whole grain crackers
Fluids: iced or hot apple spiced green tea*

Evening Dinner

5 oz. lime ginger halibut (5 oz. cooked
   halibut with 1 serving soy ginger sauce)

3 oz. Pam's baked potato with skin (1 serving)
1 ½ oz. nonfat cheese
1 tbsp. chives
½ cup grilled yellow squash and ½ cup
   asparagus
Fluids: iced water with lemon and fresh mint

Supper or Evening Snack

1 cup blueberries
1 slice angel food cake (1/12 of a 10" diam.
   tube)
¾ cup nonfat warm vanilla yogurt
Fluids: iced water and chamomile peach
   herbal tea*

APO E GENE DIET
4/3 2400 KCAL DAY 2

Serving considerations per day
(Be mindful of serving sizes)

Carbohydrates
4.5 serving portions of grain/starch
15.5 serving portions of fruit and vegetable

Protein
12.5 serving portions fish or plant protein

Fat
3 serving portions anti-inflammatory fat

Breakfast

1 serving Scottish oats
1/8 cup raisins
1 cup nonfat milk
½ tbsp. honey
Fluids: water and black currant, ginger tea*
Apo E high-quality multivitamin

Morning Snack

1 slice whole grain oat flax bread
1.5 tbsp. raisins
½ cup nonfat cottage cheese
Fluids: hot or cold peach green tea*

Lunch

½ slice whole grain bun or slice of bread
¾ serving tofu salad
½ Apple, medium
1 cup nonfat milk
Fluids: Orange sparkling water*

Afternoon Snack

Carrot, cucumber and yogurt salad (1.5 servings)
½ cup carrots/jicama slices
1 slice multi grain bread
Fluids: sparkling orange ice water

Evening Dinner

Flounder with oange/rosemary spice (4 oz. cooked flounder, 1 tsp.. olive oil, juice of ½ an orange)
Mixed greens*
½ baked potato that is 2.5" by 4.5"
Fluids: iced water and hot decaf raspberry green tea

Supper or Evening Snack

Kelly's Fore Street Dessert (½ serving)

APO E GENE DIET
4/3 2400 KCAL DAY 3

Serving considerations per day
(Be mindful of serving sizes)

Carbohydrates

8 serving portions of grain/starch
16.5 serving portions of fruit and vegetable

Protein

16.5 serving portions fish or plant protein

Fat

8.5 serving portions anti-inflammatory fat

Breakfast

2, six-inch corn tortillas
¾ cup egg white or substitute
3 oz. fat-free cheese
¼ cup tomato beans
1 oz. avocado
¼ cup salsa
½ cup melon
Fluids: water and hot white tea
Apo E high-quality multivitamin

Morning Snack

1 organic apple
½ tbsp. natural nut butter
½ cup nonfat cottage cheese
Fluids: white and mint tea*

Lunch

Fish salad (1 serving)
1 whole grain pita bread
1 cup nonfat milk
Fluids: iced lemon/lime sparkling water (don't forget a pretty glass)

Afternoon Snack

Fruit Shake to Go (¾ serving)

Evening Dinner

Vegetable spaghetti*
1 tbsp. parmesan cheese
1 green salad (1 serving)
1 slice whole grain bread
1 cup nonfat milk
Fluids: sparkling lime juice water and hot decaf peach green tea*

Supper or Evening Snack

½ cup orange frozen yogurt
Fruit pottage (2 servings)
Fluids: hot chamomile tea

APO E 4/3 2400 KCAL

APO E GENE DIET
4/3 2400 KCAL DAY 4

Serving considerations per day
(Be mindful of serving sizes)

Carbohydrates

9.5 serving portions of grain/starch
15 serving portions of fruit and vegetable

Protein

15 serving portions fish or plant protein

Fat

4.5 serving portions anti-inflammatory fat

Breakfast

Blueberry oat muffin (1 serving)
Baked apple with honey (½ serving)
Scrambled eggs (½ - ¾ cup egg whites or
   substitute)
1 cup nonfat milk
1 medium orange
Fluids: fresh water and hot jasmine green tea
Apo E high-quality multivitamin

Morning Snack

1/3 cup low-fat whole grain granola
¾ cup nonfat soy yogurt
1 cup fresh organic strawberries

Lunch

Rustic 1 serving Tuscany pizza
Green salad (1 serving)
Fluids: iced hibiscus tea, sparkling water*

Afternoon Snack

Carrot, cucumber and yogurt salad (1 serving)
¾ cup nonfat cottage cheese
Fluids: hot lemon ginger green tea*

Evening Dinner

Baked salmon with teriyaki and shiitake
   mushroom*
½ potato that is 2.5" by 4.5"
1 tsp. olive oil
Ratatouille from Cornwall (1 serving)
1 slice organic rustic whole grain bread
1 tbsp. parmesan cheese
1 tsp. avocado

Supper or Evening Snack

½ cup Apple Blueberry Crumble*
¾ cup nonfat hot vanilla yogurt

APO E 4/3 2400 KCAL

APO E GENE DIET
4/2 1600 KCAL DAY 1
Serving considerations per day
(Be mindful of serving sizes)

Carbohydrates
6 serving portions of grain/starch
13.5 serving portions of fruit and vegetable

Protein
7 serving portions protein

Fat
5 serving portions anti-inflammatory fat

Breakfast
1 slice whole grain toast
½ tbsp. organic nut butter
½ banana
1 tbsp. local organic honey
Fluids: water and hot silver needle white tea*
APO E high-quality multivitamin

Morning Snack
1 ½ cups jicama, radish and carrot sticks
2 tbsp. hummus

Lunch
2 slices whole grain bread
3 oz. sliced tuna Steak
Romaine lettuce, cucumber, red onion,
    and sliced tomato for sandwich
¹/₈ avocado
Fluids: lemon sparkling ice water*

Afternoon Snack
½ an apple, sliced
1 oz. soy cheese
Fluids: water and hot green lemon ginger tea*

Evening Dinner
Vegetable spaghetti (¾ serving)
1 tbsp. soy parmesan cheese
1 serving mixed green salad
Fluids: water with lemon and fresh mint

Supper:
1 cup nonfat milk
Black currant and rhubarb crumble (½
    serving)
Fluids: water and chamomile herbal tea

APO E GENE DIET
4/2 1600 KCAL DAY 2
Serving considerations per day
(Be mindful of serving sizes)

Carbohydrates
6.5 serving portions of grain/starch
10 serving portions of fruit and vegetable

Protein
8.5 serving portions protein

Fat
3 serving portions anti-inflammatory fat

Breakfast
Blueberry oat bread (¾ serving)
1 tbsp. local organic honey
Fluids: water and green tea
APO E high-quality multivitamin

Morning Snack
1 cup soy yogurt (1 serving)
¼ cup low-fat granola
1 cup grapes or cherries

Lunch
½ whole grain pita bread
1 serving organic lettuce, cucumber, onion,
    and tomato
2 oz. fresh crab
1 oz. avocado
1 tbsp. low-fat ranch dressing (olive or
    canola oil) and 1 oz. low-fat soy cheese
Fluids: orange sparkling water*

Afternoon Snack

1 serving carrot and cucumber yogurt salad
5 whole grain crackers
Fluids: 1 cup green lavender tea

Evening Dinner

4 oz. steamed cooked fish, such as salmon, with 1 tsp.. olive oil and lemon
1 serving mixed green salad
1 cup soy milk
1 slice rustic whole grain bread
½ cup steamed spinach
Fluids: chamomile tea with essence of rosehips and lemon

Supper:

1 slice orange angel food cake (¹/₁₂ of a 10" diam. tube)
1 cup nonfat milk and 1 cup hot green/ rosehip tea decaf*

APO E GENE DIET 4/2 1600 KCAL DAY 3

Serving considerations per day
(Be mindful of serving sizes)

Carbohydrates

5.5 serving portions of grain/starch
10 serving portions of fruit and vegetable

Protein

8 serving portions protein

Fat

8 serving portions anti-inflammatory fat

Breakfast

Breakfast omelet (¾ serving)
½ cup mixed berries
½ cup tomato salsa cream (2 serving)
Fluids: water and white tea with black currant*
APO E high-quality multivitamin

Morning Snack

1 sliced apple
½ tbsp. nut butter
Fluids: white and mint tea*

Lunch

1 slice whole grain bread
2 oz. herring or tuna
1 tbsp. olive/canola oil mayonnaise
1 cup chopped onions, cabbage, broccoli, and carrots
1 cup romaine lettuce
¹/₈ avocado
1 cup nonfat milk
Fluids: iced lemon water and 1 cup hot ginger green raspberry tea*

Afternoon Snack

Carrot, cucumber, and yogurt salad (1 serving)
¾ oz. pretzels
Fluids: Japanese matcha tea*

Evening Dinner

1½ cup salad (spinach, cherry tomatoes, cabbage, broccoli, carrots)*
2 oz. organic free-range cooked turkey
½ cup basmati rice
Simple salad dressing, (1 serving)
Fluids: sparkling lime juice water and hot decaf peach green tea*

Supper:

3 small ginger biscuits (cookies) (1 serving)
1 cup nonfat milk

APO E GENE DIET
4/2 1600 KCAL DAY 4
Serving considerations per day
(Be mindful of serving sizes)

Carbohydrates
4.75 serving portions of grain/starch
15 serving portions of fruit and vegetable

Protein
4.75 serving portions protein

Fat
5.5 serving portions anti-inflammatory fat

Breakfast
1 serving Scottish oats
½ cup nonfat milk
Water and green tea with orange slices
APO E high-quality multivitamin

Morning Snack
½ banana
½ serving snack mix
½ cup nonfat milk

Lunch
1 veggie burger*
2 slices toasted whole grain bread (cut in half)
1 serving lettuce and tomato
1 oz. low-fat soy cheese
¹/₈ of an avocado
Small salad of onions, tomatoes, and lettuce
1 tbsp. nonfat dressing
Fluids: hibiscus sparkling water*

Afternoon Snack
Carrot and cucumber yogurt salad (¾ serving)
Fluids: hot ginger green tea*

Evening Dinner
1 slice multi grain bread
½ serving shiitake mushroom and spinach lasagna
1 tbsp. grated low-fat cheese
1 ½ serving mixed green salad
Fluids: sparkling ice water with orange

Supper:
½ cup plain nonfat yogurt
½ cup fresh strawberries

APO E GENE DIET
4/2 1800 KCAL DAY 1
Serving considerations per day
(Be mindful of serving sizes)

Carbohydrates
7.5 serving portions of grain/starch
11.5 serving portions of fruit and vegetable

Protein
7 serving portions protein

Fat
5 serving portions anti-inflammatory fat

Breakfast
1 slice whole grain toast
½ tbsp. organic nut butter
1 banana
Fluids: water and hot China green tea with raspberry
APO E high-quality multivitamin

Morning Snack
1 cup nonfat yogurt
Snack mix (½ cup low-fat granola, and 1/8 cup apricots)

Lunch
2 slices whole grain bread
3 oz. fresh shrimp
Lettuce, cucumber, red onion, and sliced tomato
1/8 avocado
Fluids: lemon ice water*

Afternoon Snack
1 medium sliced apple
1 oz. whole organic soy cheese (not made from soy isolate)
Fluids: water and hot green lemon ginger tea*

Evening Dinner
Vegetable spaghetti (¾ serving)
1 tbsp. soy parmesan cheese
1 serving mixed green salad
1 slice whole grain bread
1/8 avocado
Fluids: water with lemon and fresh mint

Supper:
½ cup strawberry low-fat soy frozen yogurt
Fluids: water and chamomile herbal tea

APO E GENE DIET
4/2 1800 KCAL DAY 2
Serving considerations per day
(Be mindful of serving sizes)

Carbohydrates
8.5 serving portions of grain/starch
8 serving portions of fruit and vegetable

Protein
9.5 serving portions protein

Fat
4 serving portions anti-inflammatory fat

Breakfast
¾ serving blueberry oat bran bread
1 tbsp. organic local honey (honey from your local neighborhood)
Fluids: water and green tea with fresh squeezed lemon juice use ½ whole lemon
APO E high-quality multivitamin

Morning Snack
1 cup soy yogurt (2 servings)
¼ cup low-fat granola
½ cup grapes or cherries

Lunch
1 whole grain pita bread
1 serving romaine lettuce, cucumber, onion, and tomato

3 oz. organic sardines (Vitalchoice.com)
1 oz. avocado
8 olives
Orange sparkling water*

Afternoon Snack

1 serving carrot, cucumber and yogurt salad
4 whole grain crackers
Fluids: Japanese matcha tea*

Evening Dinner

3 oz. halibut with rosemary and lemon
½ cup steamed broccolini
½ cup steamed spinach
¾ cup wild rice
¼ cup white beans
2 tbsp. salsa cream*
1 tbsp. chives
Fluids: chamomile tea with essence of
Rosehips and lemon*

Supper:

½ cup red grapes
3 low-fat cookies made with
    monounsaturated fat (1 serving)
1 cup soy milk
1 cup hot green/rosehip tea decaf*

APO E GENE DIET
4/2 1800 KCAL DAY 3
Serving considerations per day
(Be mindful of serving sizes)

Carbohydrates
8 serving portions of grain/starch
6.5 serving portions of fruit and vegetable

Protein
10 serving portions protein

Fat
5.5 serving portions anti-inflammatory fat

Breakfast

1 cup organic bran cereal
1 cup soy milk
½ cup blueberries
1 tbsp. honey
Fluids: water and peach turmeric tea
APO E high-quality multivitamin

Morning Snack

¾ serving banana almond Shake to Go
Fluids: white mint tea*

Lunch

1 organic veggie burger*
2 slices whole grain bread
1/8 avocado
Onions, tomatoes, and lettuce
½ cup black beans
Fluids: iced lemon water—hot green
    raspberry ginger tea

Afternoon Snack

1 serving carrot and cucumber yogurt salad
Fluids: Japanese matcha tea*

Evening Dinner

12-inch corn tortilla or two 6-inch tortillas
3 oz. rosemary lime baked chicken (¾
    serving)
1 serving chopped romaine lettuce, vine-
    ripened tomatoes, and onions
1½ oz. organic low-fat soy cheese
1/8 avocado
2 tbsp. tomato salsa cream (¼ serving)
Fluids: sparkling lime juice water and hot
    decaf peach green tea

Supper:

½ cup Fresh sliced strawberries
5 Ginger biscuits (1.5 servings)
Fluids: hot green Rose Petal tea*

APO E GENE DIET
4/2 1800 KCAL DAY 4

Serving considerations per day
(Be mindful of serving sizes)

Carbohydrates

5.5 serving portions of grain/starch
11.5 serving portions of fruit and vegetable

Protein

7 serving portions protein

Fat

4 serving portions anti-inflammatory fat

Breakfast

1 serving Scottish oats
½ tbsp. honey
¹/₈ cup sultanas
1 cup nonfat milk
Fluids: water and 1 cup hot cinnamon
   white tea
APO E high-quality multivitamin

Morning Snack

¾ oz. whole wheat pretzels,
½ cup raspberry nonfat yogurt
   (carrageenan free)

Lunch

½ whole grain pita bread
1 serving chopped onions, celery, romaine
   lettuce, and tomato
¹/₈ avocado
3 oz. cooked black cod, also known as
   sablefish (vitalchoice.com)

Afternoon Snack

1 serving carrot and cucumber yogurt salad
4 whole grain crackers
Fluids: hot white tea with cranberry*

Evening Dinner

¾ serving shiitake mushroom and spinach
   lasagna
1 tbsp. organic parmesan cheese
1 serving mixed green salad with low-fat
   Italian salad dressing
½ slice rustic organic whole grain bread
4 steamed asparagus spears with lemon
Fluids: hot orange peel tea*

Supper:

3 small ginger biscuits
1 cup ice-cold nonfat milk
Fluids: hot chamomile rose petal tea*

APO E GENE DIET
4/2 2000 KCAL DAY 1
Serving considerations per day
(Be mindful of serving sizes)

Carbohydrates
6 serving portions of grain/starch
7 serving portions of fruit and vegetable

Protein
7 serving portions protein

Fat
5 serving portions anti-inflammatory fat

Breakfast

1 cup oatmeal
1 cup soy milk (organic and carrageenan free)
½ tbsp. honey
1 tbsp. flaxseed (organic and ground Spectrum brand)
$^1/_8$ cup sultanas
Fluids: water or hot white rosehip tea
APO E high-quality multivitamin

Morning Snack

1 apple
2 organic dates
½ tbsp. nut butter

Lunch

Mevagissey fish tacos (¾ serving)
2 tbsp. papaya salsa cream (¼ serving)
Fluids: lemon ice water*

Afternoon Snack

½ serving sultana, Carrot, Ginger Coleslaw
1 cup nonfat milk
Fluids: water and hot green lemon ginger tea*

Evening Dinner

3 oz. lime teriyaki grilled halibut (3 oz. cooked halibut with 1 serving teriyaki sauce)
6 steamed asparagus

½ potato (1.5" by 2.5")
½ slice whole grain bread with $^1/_8$ avocado
Fluids: water with lemon and fresh mint

Supper:

Peach blackberry crumble (¾ serving)
½ cup frozen yogurt
Fluids: water and chamomile herbal tea

APO E GENE DIET
4/2 2000 KCAL DAY 2
Serving considerations per day
(Be mindful of serving sizes)

Carbohydrates
10 serving portions of grain/starch
11 serving portions of fruit and vegetable

Protein
9 serving portions protein

Fat
5 serving portions anti-inflammatory fat

Breakfast

2 slices whole grain bread
1 tbsp. organic nut butter
1 banana
½ tbsp. local organic honey
Fluids: water and matcha green tea
APO E high-quality multivitamin

Morning Snack

½ cup low-fat granola
1 cup nonfat soy yogurt

Lunch

2 slices whole grain bread
1 veggie burger*
1 leaf romaine lettuce and ¼ of a vine-ripened tomato
1 tbsp. vegetarian fat-free mayonnaise
Fluids: orange sparkling water*

APO E 4/2 2000 KCAL

Afternoon Snack

½ serving sultana, carrot, ginger coleslaw
1 slice multi-grain bread
Fluids: Japanese green tea

Evening Dinner

4 oz. grilled tuna steak in teriyaki ginger
   sauce (4 oz. cooked tuna with 1 serving
   teriyaki sauce)
½ cup broccoli/broccolini
¼ cup cooked white beans
1 serving green salad
½ cup steamed spinach
1 cup nonfat milk
½ slice organic rustic whole grain bread
Fluids: chamomile tea with essence of
   rosehips and lemon*

Supper:

Mixed Berry Pottage (1 serving)
½ cup low-fat frozen soy yogurt
1 cup hot green/Rosehip tea decaf

APO E GENE DIET
4/2 2000 KCAL DAY 3

Serving considerations per day
(Be mindful of serving sizes)

Carbohydrates

10.5 serving portions of grain/starch
10 serving portions of fruit and vegetable

Protein

12 serving portions protein

Fat

5 serving portions anti-inflammatory fat

Breakfast

½ cup scrambled eggs*
½ cup vegetarian tomato beans (Amy's foods)
¼ cup fresh salsa*
$1/_8$ avocado
½ whole grain bagel toasted
½ cup fresh cut melon
Fluids: water and hot green tea
APO E high-quality multivitamin

Morning Snack

1 serving snack mix
1 serving fresh organic peach
Fluids: white and mint tea*

Lunch

1 whole wheat pita bread
Prawn salad (3 oz. grilled prawns, chopped
   onions, lettuce, tomato and 1 tbsp.
   vegetarian fat-free mayonnaise)
4 organic Mediterranean olives
1 cup nonfat milk
Fluids: iced lemon water and hot green
   raspberry ginger tea

Afternoon Snack

1 cup fresh vegetable soup*
7 whole grain crackers
Fluids: Japanese matcha tea*

Evening Dinner

3 oz. organic roasted rosemary chicken (¾
   serving)
1 serving Pam's baked potato
1 serving mixed green salad
1 small slice rustic whole grain bread
Fluids: sparkling lime juice water and hot
   decaf peach green tea*

Supper:

3 ginger biscuits (1 serving)
1 cup nonfat milk

APO E GENE DIET
4/2 2000 KCAL DAY 4
Serving considerations per day
(Be mindful of serving sizes)

Carbohydrates
10 serving portions of grain/starch
9 serving portions of fruit and vegetable

Protein
10.5 serving portions protein

Fat
4.5 serving portions anti-inflammatory fat

Breakfast
1 orange
¾ serving blueberry oat bread
½ cup scrambled eggs or egg substitute*
1 tbsp. honey
Water and hot white tea
APO E high-quality multivitamin

Morning Snack
1 apple
1 cup soy yogurt
$1/3$ cup low-fat granola

Lunch
1 whole grain pita breads
1 tbsp. fat-free ranch
1 serving chopped onions, celery, romaine
   lettuce, and tomato
$1/8$ avocado
3 oz. grilled sea bass cooked
Fluids: fresh iced water with black currant*

Afternoon Snack
$1/3$ cup fresh low-fat hummus
7 whole grain crackers
Fluids: hot white tea with cranberry*

Evening Dinner
3 oz. rosemary wild salmon (3 oz. cooked
   salmon and 1 tsp. olive oil)
1 tbsp. organic almonds
1 serving mixed green salad
1 cup nonfat milk
2 slices rustic organic whole grain bread
6 steamed asparagus spears with lemon
Fluids: hot orange peel tea*

Supper:
¾ cup sliced strawberries and blueberries
1 slice chocolate angel food cake ($1/12$ of a
   10" diam. tube)
Fluids: hot chamomile rose petal tea*

APO E 4/2 2000 KCAL

APO E GENE DIET
4/2 2400 KCAL DAY 1
Serving considerations per day
(Be mindful of serving sizes)

Carbohydrates
10 serving portions of grain/starch
11.5 serving portions of fruit and vegetable

Protein
12.5 serving portions protein

Fat
6 serving portions anti-inflammatory fat

Breakfast
½ cup scrambled egg whites
2 slices toasted oat bran bread*
1 tbsp. organic nut butter
½ cup fresh mixed berries
Fluids: water and 1 cup hot Japanese green tea
APO E high-quality multivitamin

Morning Snack
1 serving snack mix
½ cup nonfat soy cottage cheese
Fluids: hot green tea with Lemon

Lunch
1 whole grain pita bread
Shredded lettuce and chopped onions
2 oz. grilled mackerel cooked
⅛ avocado
1 cup fresh papaya slices
Fluids: lemon ice water*

Afternoon Snack
2 tbsp. almonds
1 serving vegetable soup
2 mandarin oranges
Fluids: water and hot green lemon ginger tea*

Evening Dinner
1 cup whole wheat spaghetti
3 oz. grilled Cornish game hen breast
1 tbsp. organic parmesan cheese
1 cup steamed broccoli
½ cup streamed carrots
1 cup nonfat milk
Fluids: water with lemon and fresh mint

Supper:
¾ serving peach blackberry crumble
½ cup low-fat vanilla soy ice cream
Fluids: water and chamomile herbal tea*

APO E GENE DIET
4/2 2400 KCAL DAY 2
Serving considerations per day
(Be mindful of serving sizes)

Carbohydrates
11 serving portions of grain/starch
8.5 serving portions of fruit and vegetable

Protein
14 serving portions protein

Fat
8 serving portions anti-inflammatory fat

Breakfast
2, six-inch corn tortillas
¼ cup egg substitute
¼ avocado
1 ½ oz. low-fat soy cheese
¼ cup salsa
½ cup melon
Fluids: water hot white tea with lemon
APO E high-quality multivitamin

Morning Snack
1 toasted organic whole grain bagel
1 tbsp. nut butter
1 cup soy milk
Fluid: hot spiced green tea

Lunch
1 serving blueberry sultana oat bread

1 veggie burger
1 serving romaine lettuce and vine-ripened
  tomatoes
1 tbsp. fat-free mayonnaise
$1/_8$ avocado
Fluids: orange sparkling water*

Afternoon Snack

½ serving sultana, carrot, ginger coleslaw
4 whole grain crackers
Fluids: Japanese matcha tea*

Evening Dinner

6 oz. grilled teriyaki shrimp (6 oz. cooked
  shrimp with 1 serving teriyaki sauce)
9 steamed asparagus
½ cup basmati rice
Sliced tomato with balsamic vinegar
1 serving Pam's baked potato
2 tbsp. low-fat salsa cream (¼ serving)
1 tbsp. fresh chopped chives
Fluids: chamomile tea with essence of
  rosehips and lemon*

Supper:

1 cup Mixed Berry Crumble*
½ cup low-fat frozen soy yogurt
1 cup hot green/Rosehip tea decaf*

APO E GENE DIET
4/2 2400 KCAL DAY 3

Serving considerations per day
(Be mindful of serving sizes)

Carbohydrates

9 serving portions of grain/starch
12.5 serving portions of fruit and vegetable

Protein

11 serving portions protein

Fat

5.5 serving portions anti-inflammatory fat

Breakfast

1 cup oat bran flakes
¼ cup sultanas
½ banana
1 cup soy milk
Fluids: water and ginger peach green tea*
APO E high-quality multivitamin

Morning Snack

1 tbsp. nut butter
1 slice toasted rustic whole grain bread
1 sliced apple
Fluids: white and mint tea*

Lunch

1 serving Tuscany pizza
1 serving mixed green salad
Fluids: iced lemon water and hot green
  raspberry ginger tea

Afternoon Snack

½ serving sultana, carrot, ginger coleslaw
8 whole grain crackers
Fluids: Japanese matcha tea*

Evening Dinner

5 oz. grilled halibut with mango salsa
  (5 oz. cooked halibut with ½ serving
  mango salsa, and 1 tsp. olive oil)
6 steamed asparagus
1 serving rustic whole grain bread
1 cup soy milk
Fluids: sparkling lime juice water and
hot decaf peach green tea*

Supper:

1 cup skim milk
½ serving Kelly's Fore Street Dessert
Fluids: hot decaf green tea*

APO E GENE DIET
4/2 2400 KCAL DAY 4

Serving considerations per day
(Be mindful of serving sizes)

Carbohydrates

9.5 serving portions of grain/starch
7.5 serving portions of fruit and vegetable

Protein

11 serving portions protein

Fat

6 serving portions anti-inflammatory fat

Breakfast

1 serving blueberry oat bread
1 cup nonfat strawberry yogurt
Fluids: water and hot green tea with mint*
APO E high-quality multivitamin

Morning Snack

¾ serving banana Shake to Go

Lunch

2 slices rustic organic whole grain bread
1 veggie burger*
Lettuce, sliced tomato, and onions
1 tbsp. low-fat canola or olive oil mayonnaise
1 ½ oz. slice organic low-fat soy cheese
Fluids: organic green tea and a touch of
  organic lemonade*

Afternoon Snack

2 organic fresh dates
1 serving fresh fruit such as an orange
Fluids: hot ginger green tea*

Evening Dinner

4 oz. roasted lime rosemary chicken (1
  serving)
1 medium baked red potato (2.5" by 4.5")
1 serving Mevagissey ratatouille
1 slice rustic organic whole grain bread
Fluids: iced water and hot decaf green
orange spiced tea

Supper:

1 serving peach and blackberry crumble
½ cup low-fat soy ice cream
Fluids: Hot Lemon Ginger Spiced tea

APO E GENE DIET
3/3 1600 KCAL DAY 1
Serving considerations per day
(Be mindful of serving sizes)

Carbohydrates
6 serving portions of grain/starch
13.5 serving portions of fruit and vegetable

Protein
7 serving portions protein

Fat
5 serving portions anti-inflammatory fat

Breakfast
1 slice whole grain toast
½ tbsp. organic nut butter
½ banana
1 tbsp. local organic honey
Fluids: water and hot silver needle white tea*
APO E high-quality multivitamin

Morning Snack
1½ cups jicama, radish and carrot sticks
2 tbsp. hummus

Lunch
2 slices whole grain bread
3 oz. sliced cooked chicken breast
Romaine lettuce, cucumber, red onion,
and sliced tomato for sandwich
$^1/_8$ avocado
Fluids: lemon sparkling ice water*

Afternoon Snack
½ sliced apple
1 oz. soy cheese
Fluids: water and hot green lemon ginger tea*

Evening Dinner
¾ serving vegetable spaghetti
1 tbsp. soy parmesan cheese
1 serving mixed green salad
Fluids: water with lemon and fresh mint

Supper:
1 cup nonfat milk
½ serving black currant and rhubarb crumble
Fluids: water and chamomile herbal tea

APO E GENE DIET
3/3 1600 KCAL DAY 2
Serving considerations per day
(Be mindful of serving sizes)

Carbohydrates
6.5 serving portions of grain/starch
10 serving portions of fruit and vegetable

Protein
8.5 serving portions protein

Fat
3 serving portions anti-inflammatory fat

Breakfast
¾ serving blueberry oat bread
1 tbsp. local organic honey
Fluids: water and green tea
APO E high-quality multivitamin

Morning Snack
1 cup soy yogurt (1 serving)
¼ cup low-fat granola
1 cup grapes or cherries

Lunch
½ whole grain pita bread
1 serving organic lettuce, cucumber, onion,
and tomato
2 oz. sliced chicken
1 oz. avocado
1 tbsp. low-fat ranch dressing (olive or
canola oil) and 1 oz. low-fat soy cheese
Fluids: orange sparkling water*

Afternoon Snack

1 serving carrot and cucumber yogurt salad
5 whole grain crackers
Fluids: 1 cup green lavender tea

Evening Dinner

4 oz. steamed cooked fish such as salmon
    with 1 tsp.. olive oil and lemon
1 serving mixed green salad
1 cup soy milk
1 slice rustic whole grain bread
½ cup steamed spinach
Fluids: chamomile tea with essence of
    rosehips and lemon

Supper:

1 slice orange angel food cake ($1/12$ of a 10"
    diam. tube)
1 cup nonfat milk and 1 cup hot green
    rosehip tea decaf*

APO E GENE DIET
3/3 1600 KCAL DAY 3

Serving considerations per day
(Be mindful of serving sizes)

Carbohydrates

5.5 serving portions of grain/starch
10 serving portions of fruit and vegetable

Protein

8 serving portions protein

Fat

8 serving portions anti-inflammatory fat

Breakfast

¾ serving breakfast omelet
½ cup mixed berries
½ cup tomato salsa cream (2 serving)
Fluids: water and white tea with black
    currant*
APO E high-quality multivitamin

Morning Snack

1 sliced apple
½ tbsp. nut butter
Fluids: white and mint tea*

Lunch

1 slice whole grain bread
2 oz. herring or tuna
1 tbsp. olive/canola oil mayonnaise
1 cup chopped onions, cabbage, broccoli,
    and carrots
1 cup romaine lettuce
$1/8$ avocado
1 cup nonfat milk
Fluids: iced lemon water and 1 cup hot
    ginger green raspberry tea*

Afternoon Snack

1 serving carrot, cucumber, and yogurt salad
¾ oz. pretzels
Fluids: Japanese matcha tea*

Evening Dinner

1½ cup salad (spinach, cherry tomatoes,
    cabbage, broccoli, carrots)*
2 oz. organic free-range cooked turkey
½ cup basmati rice
1 serving simple salad dressing
Fluids: sparkling lime juice water and hot
    decaf peach green tea*

Supper:

3 small ginger biscuits (cookies) (1 serving)
1 cup nonfat milk

APO E GENE DIET
3/3 1600 KCAL DAY 4

Serving considerations per day
(Be mindful of serving sizes)

Carbohydrates

4.75 serving portions of grain/starch
15 serving portions of fruit and vegetable

Protein

4.75 serving portions protein

Fat

5.5 serving portions anti-inflammatory fat

Breakfast

1 serving Scottish oats
½ cup nonfat milk
Water and green tea with orange slices
APO E high-quality multivitamin

Morning Snack

½ banana
½ serving snack mix
½ cup nonfat milk

Lunch

1 veggie burger*
2 slice toasted whole grain bread (cut in half)
1 serving lettuce and tomato
1 oz. low-fat soy cheese
¹/₈ of an avocado
1 small salad of onions, tomatoes, and lettuce
1 tbsp. nonfat dressing
Fluids: hibiscus sparkling water*

Afternoon Snack

¾ serving carrot and cucumber yogurt salad
Fluids: hot ginger green tea*

Evening Dinner

1 slice multi-grain bread
½ serving shiitake mushroom and spinach lasagna
1 tbsp. grated low-fat cheese
1½ serving mixed green salad
Fluids: sparkling ice water with orange

Supper:

½ cup plain nonfat yogurt
½ cup fresh strawberries

APO E GENE DIET
3/3 1800 KCAL DAY 1
Serving considerations per day
(Be mindful of serving sizes)

Carbohydrates
7.5 serving portions of grain/starch
11.5 serving portions of fruit and vegetable

Protein
7 serving portions protein

Fat
5 serving portions anti-inflammatory fat

Breakfast
1 slice whole grain toast
½ tbsp. organic nut butter
1 banana
Fluids: water and hot China green tea with
   raspberry
APO E high-quality multivitamin

Morning Snack
1 cup nonfat yogurt
Snack mix (½ cup low-fat granola, and 1/8
   cup apricots)

Lunch
2 slices whole grain bread
3 oz. organic sliced chicken breast
Lettuce, cucumber, red onion, and sliced
   tomato
1/8 avocado
Fluids: lemon ice water*

Afternoon Snack
1 medium sliced apple
1 oz. whole organic soy cheese (not made
   from soy isolate)
Fluids: water and hot green lemon ginger tea*

Evening Dinner
¾ serving vegetable spaghetti
1 tbsp. soy parmesan cheese
1 serving mixed green salad

1 slice whole grain bread
1/8 avocado
Fluids: water with lemon and fresh mint

Supper:
½ cup strawberry low-fat soy frozen yogurt
Fluids: water and chamomile herbal tea

APO E GENE DIET
3/3 1800 KCAL DAY 2
Serving considerations per day
(Be mindful of serving sizes)

Carbohydrates
8.5 serving portions of grain/starch
8 serving portions of fruit and vegetable

Protein
9.5 serving portions protein

Fat
4 serving portions anti-inflammatory fat

Breakfast
¾ serving blueberry oat bran bread
1 tbsp. organic local honey (honey from
   your local neighborhood)
Fluids: water and green tea with fresh
   squeezed lemon juice use ½ whole lemon
APO E high-quality multivitamin

Morning Snack
1 cup soy yogurt (2 servings)
¼ cup low-fat granola
½ cup grapes or cherries

Lunch
1 whole grain pita bread
1 serving romaine lettuce, cucumber,
   onion, and tomato
3 oz. organic sardines (Vitalchoice.com)
1 oz. avocado
1 serving 8 olives
Orange sparkling water*

Afternoon Snack

1 serving carrot, cucumber and yogurt salad
4 whole grain crackers
Fluids: Japanese matcha tea*

Evening Dinner

3 oz. halibut with rosemary and lemon
½ cup steamed broccolini
½ cup steamed spinach
¾ cup wild rice
¼ cup white beans
2 tbsp. salsa cream*
1 tbsp. chives
Fluids: chamomile tea with essence of
  rosehips and lemon*

Supper:

½ cup red grapes
3 low-fat cookies made with
  monounsaturated fat (1 serving)
1 cup soy milk
1 cup hot green/Rosehip tea decaf*

APO E GENE DIET
3/3 1800 KCAL DAY 3

Serving considerations per day
(Be mindful of serving sizes)

Carbohydrates

8 serving portions of grain/starch
6.5 serving portions of fruit and vegetable

Protein

10 serving portions protein

Fat

5.5 serving portions anti-inflammatory fat

Breakfast

1 cup organic bran cereal
1 cup soy milk
½ cup blueberries
1 tbsp. honey
Fluids: water and peach turmeric tea
APO E high-quality multivitamin

Morning Snack

¾ serving banana almond Shake to Go
Fluids: white mint tea*

Lunch

1 organic veggie burger*
2 slices whole grain bread
1/8 avocado
Onions, tomatoes, and lettuce
½ cup black beans
Fluids: iced lemon water and hot green
  raspberry ginger tea

Afternoon Snack

1 serving carrot and cucumber yogurt salad
Fluids: Japanese matcha tea*

Evening Dinner

12-inch corn tortilla or two 6-inch tortillas
3 oz. rosemary lime baked chicken (¾ serving)
1 serving chopped romaine lettuce, vine-
  ripened tomatoes, and onions
1½ oz. organic low-fat soy cheese
1/8 avocado
2 tbsp. tomato salsa cam (¼ serving)
Fluids: sparkling lime juice water and
Hot decaf peach green teas

Supper:

½ cup fresh sliced strawberries
5 ginger biscuits (1.5 servings)
Fluids: hot green rose petal tea*

APO E 3/3 1800 KCAL

APO E GENE DIET
3/3 1800 KCAL DAY 4

Serving considerations per day
(Be mindful of serving sizes)

Carbohydrates

5.5 serving portions of grain/starch
11.5 serving portions of fruit and vegetable

Protein

7 serving portions protein

Fat

4 serving portions anti-inflammatory fat

Breakfast

1 serving Scottish oats
½ tbsp. honey
¹/₈ cup sultanas
1 cup nonfat milk
Fluids: water and 1 cup hot cinnamon
  white tea
APO E high-quality multivitamin

Morning Snack

¾ oz. whole wheat pretzels,
½ cup raspberry nonfat yogurt
  (carrageenan free)

Lunch

½ whole grain pita bread
1 serving chopped onions, celery, romaine
lettuce, and tomato
¹/₈ avocado
3 oz. cooked black cod, also known as
  sablefish (vitalchoice.com)

Afternoon Snack

1 serving carrot and cucumber yogurt salad
4 whole grain crackers
Fluids: hot white tea with cranberry*

Evening Dinner

¾ serving shiitake mushroom and spinach
lasagna
1 tbsp. organic parmesan cheese
1 serving mixed green salad with low-fat
  Italian salad dressing
½ slice rustic organic whole grain bread
4 steamed asparagus spears with lemon
Fluids: hot orange peel tea*

Supper:

3 small ginger biscuits
1 cup ice-cold nonfat milk
Fluids: hot chamomile rose petal tea*

APO E GENE DIET
3/3 2000 KCAL DAY 1
Serving considerations per day
(Be mindful of serving sizes)

Carbohydrates
6 serving portions of grain/starch
7 serving portions of fruit and vegetable

Protein
7 serving portions protein

Fat
5 serving portions anti-inflammatory fat

Breakfast
1 cup oatmeal
1 cup soy milk (organic and carrageenan free)
½ tbsp. honey
1 tbsp. flaxseed (organic and ground
  Spectrum brand)
1/8 cup sultanas
Fluids: water or hot white rosehip tea
APO E high-quality multivitamin

Morning Snack
1 apple
2 organic dates
½ tbsp. nut butter

Lunch
Mevagissey fish tacos (¾ serving)
2 tbsp. papaya salsa cream (¼ serving)
Fluids: lemon ice water*

Afternoon Snack
½ serving sultana, carrot, ginger coleslaw
1 cup nonfat milk
Fluids: water and hot green lemon ginger tea*

Evening Dinner
3 oz. lime teriyaki grilled halibut (3 oz. cooked
  halibut with 1 serving teriyaki sauce)
6 steamed asparagus
½ potato (1.5" by 2.5")

½ slice whole grain bread with 1/8 avocado
Fluids: water with lemon and fresh mint

Supper:
¾ serving peach blackberry crumble
½ cup frozen yogurt
Fluids: water and chamomile herbal tea

APO E GENE DIET
3/3 2000 KCAL DAY 2
Serving considerations per day
(Be mindful of serving sizes)

Carbohydrates
10 serving portions of grain/starch
11 serving portions of fruit and vegetable

Protein
9 serving portions protein

Fat
5 serving portions anti-inflammatory fat

Breakfast
2 slices whole grain bread
1 tbsp. organic nut butter
1 banana
½ tbsp. local organic honey
Fluids: water and matcha green tea
APO E high-quality multivitamin

Morning Snack
½ cup low-fat granola
1 cup nonfat soy yogurt

Lunch
2 slices whole grain bread
1 veggie burger*
1 leaf romaine lettuce and ¼ of a vine-
  ripened tomato
1 tbsp. vegetarian fat-free mayonnaise
Fluids: Orange sparkling water*

APO E 3/3 2000 KCAL

Afternoon Snack

½ serving sultana, carrot, ginger coleslaw
1 slice multi-grain bread
Fluids: Japanese green tea

Evening Dinner

4 oz. grilled tuna steak in teriyaki ginger
   sauce (4 oz. cooked tuna with 1 serving
   teriyaki sauce)
½ cup broccoli/broccolini
¼ cup cooked white beans
1 serving green salad
½ cup steamed spinach
1 cup nonfat milk
½ slice organic rustic whole grain bread
Fluids: chamomile tea with essence of
   rosehips and lemon*

Supper:

1 serving mixed berry pottage
½ cup low-fat frozen soy yogurt
1 cup hot green, rosehip, decaf tea

APO E GENE DIET
3/3 2000 KCAL DAY 3

Serving considerations per day
(Be mindful of serving sizes)

Carbohydrates

10.5 serving portions of grain/starch
10 serving portions of fruit and vegetable

Protein

12 serving portions protein

Fat

5 serving portions anti-inflammatory fat

Breakfast

½ cup scrambled eggs*
½ cup vegetarian tomato beans (Amy's foods)
¼ cup fresh salsa*
1/8 avocado
½ whole grain bagel toasted
½ cup fresh cut melon
Fluids: water and hot green tea
APO E high-quality multivitamin

Morning Snack

1 serving snack mix
1 serving fresh organic peach
Fluids: white and mint tea*

Lunch

1 whole wheat pita bread
Prawn salad (3 oz. grilled prawns, chopped
   onions, lettuce, tomato and 1 tbsp.
   vegetarian fat-free mayonnaise)
4 organic Mediterranean olives
1 cup nonfat milk
Fluids: iced lemon water—hot green
   raspberry ginger tea

Afternoon Snack

1 cup fresh vegetable soup*
7 whole grain crackers
Fluids: Japanese matcha tea*

Evening Dinner

3 oz. organic roasted rosemary chicken (¾
   serving)
1 serving Pam's baked potato
1 serving mixed green salad
1 small slice rustic whole grain bread
Fluids: sparkling lime juice water and hot
   decaf peach green tea*

Supper:

3 ginger biscuits (1 serving)
1 cup nonfat milk

APO E GENE DIET
3/3 2000 KCAL DAY 4
Serving considerations per day
(Be mindful of serving sizes)

Carbohydrates
10 serving portions of grain/starch
9 serving portions of fruit and vegetable

Protein
10.5 serving portions protein

Fat
4.5 serving portions anti-inflammatory fat

Breakfast

1 orange
¾ serving blueberry oat bread
½ cup scrambled eggs or egg substitute*
1 tbsp. honey
Water and hot white tea
APO E high-quality multivitamin

Morning Snack

1 apple
1 cup soy yogurt
$^1/_3$ cup low-fat granola

Lunch

1 whole grain pita breads
1 tbsp. fat-free ranch
1 serving chopped onions, celery, romaine
    lettuce, and tomato
$^1/_8$ avocado
3 oz. grilled sea bass cooked
Fluids: fresh iced water with black currant*

Afternoon Snack

$^1/_3$ cup fresh low-fat hummus
7 whole grain crackers
Fluids: hot white tea withcranberry*

Evening Dinner

3 oz. rosemary wild salmon (3 oz. cooked
    salmon and 1 tsp. olive oil)
1 tbsp. organic almonds
1 serving mixed green salad
1 cup nonfat milk
2 slices rustic organic whole grain bread
6 steamed asparagus spears with lemon
Fluids: hot orange peel tea*

Supper:

¾ cup sliced strawberries and blueberries
1 slice chocolate angel food cake ($^1/_{12}$ of a
10" diam. tube)
Fluids: hot chamomile rose petal tea*

APO E 3/3 2000 KCAL

APO E GENE DIET
3/3 2400 KCAL DAY 1
Serving considerations per day
(Be mindful of serving sizes)

Carbohydrates
10 serving portions of grain/starch
11.5 serving portions of fruit and vegetable

Protein
12.5 serving portions protein

Fat
6 serving portions anti-inflammatory fat

Breakfast
½ cup scrambled egg whites
2 slices toasted oat bran bread*
1 tbsp. organic nut butter
½ cup fresh mixed berries
Fluids: water and 1 cup hot Japanese green tea
APO E high-quality multivitamin

Morning Snack
1 serving snack mix
½ cup nonfat soy cottage cheese
Fluids: hot green tea with lemon

Lunch
1 whole grain pita bread
Shredded lettuce and chopped onions
2 oz. grilled mackerel cooked
¹/₈ avocado
1 cup fresh papaya slices
Fluids: lemon ice water*

Afternoon Snack
2 tbsp. almonds
1 serving vegetable soup
2 mandarin oranges
Fluids: water and hot green lemon ginger tea*

Evening Dinner
1 cup whole wheat spaghetti
3 oz. grilled chicken breast

1 tbsp. organic parmesan cheese
1 cup steamed broccoli
½ cup steamed carrots
1 cup nonfat milk
Fluids: water with lemon and fresh mint

Supper:
¾ serving peach blackberry crumble
½ cup low-fat vanilla soy ice cream
Fluids: water and chamomile herbal tea*

APO E GENE DIET
3/3 2400 KCAL DAY 2
Serving considerations per day
(Be mindful of serving sizes)

Carbohydrates
11 serving portions of grain/starch
8.5 serving portions of fruit and vegetable

Protein
14 serving portions protein

Fat
8 serving portions anti-inflammatory fat

Breakfast
2, six-inch corn tortillas
¼ cup egg substitute
¼ avocado
1 ½ oz. low-fat soy cheese
¼ cup salsa
½ cup melon
Fluids: water hot white tea with lemon
APO E high-quality multivitamin

Morning Snack
1 toasted organic whole grain bagel
1 tbsp. nut butter
1 cup soy milk
Fluid: hot spiced green tea

Lunch
1 serving blueberry sultana oat bread

1 veggie burger
1 serving romaine lettuce and vine-ripened
   tomatoes
1 tbsp. fat-free mayonnaise
1/8 avocado
Fluids: orange sparkling water*

Afternoon Snack

½ serving sultana, carrot, ginger coleslaw
4 whole grain crackers
Fluids: Japanese matcha tea*

Evening Dinner

6 oz. grilled teriyaki shrimp (6 oz. cooked
   shrimp with 1 serving teriyaki sauce)
9 steamed asparagus
½ cup basmati rice
Sliced tomato with balsamic vinegar
1 serving Pam's baked potato
2 tbsp. low-fat salsa cream (¼ serving)
1 tbsp. fresh chopped chives
Fluids: chamomile tea with essence of
   rosehips and lemon*

Supper:

1 cup mixed berry crumble*
½ cup low-fat frozen soy yogurt
1 cup hot green/Rosehip tea decaf*

**APO E GENE DIET
3/3 2400 KCAL DAY 3**
Serving considerations per day
(Be mindful of serving sizes)

Carbohydrates
9 serving portions of grain/starch
12.5 serving portions of fruit and vegetable

Protein
11 serving portions protein

Fat
5.5 serving portions anti-inflammatory fat

Breakfast

1 cup oat bran flakes
¼ cup sultanas
½ banana
1 cup soy milk
Fluids: water and ginger peach green tea*
APO E high-quality multivitamin

Morning Snack

1 tbsp. nut butter
1 slice toasted rustic whole grain bread
1 sliced apple
Fluids: white and mint tea*

Lunch

1 serving Tuscany pizza
1 serving mixed green salad
Fluids: iced lemon water and hot green
   raspberry ginger tea

Afternoon Snack

½ serving sultana, carrot, ginger coleslaw
8 whole grain crackers
Fluids: Japanese matcha tea*

Evening Dinner

5 oz. grilled halibut with mango salsa
   (5 oz. cooked halibut with ½ serving
   mango salsa, and 1 tsp.. olive oil)
6 steamed asparagus
1 serving rustic whole grain bread
1 cup soy milk
Fluids: sparkling lime juice water and
hot decaf peach green tea*

Supper:

1 cup skim milk
½ serving Kelly's Fore Street Dessert
Fluids: hot decaf green tea*

APO E 3/3 2400 KCAL

APO E GENE DIET
3/3 2400 KCAL DAY 4

Serving considerations per day
(Be mindful of serving sizes)

Carbohydrates
9.5 serving portions of grain/starch
7.5 serving portions of fruit and vegetable

Protein
11 serving portions protein

Fat
6 serving portions anti-inflammatory fat

Breakfast
1 serving blueberry oat bread
1 cup nonfat strawberry yogurt
Fluids: water and hot green tea with mint*
APO E high-quality multivitamin

Morning Snack
¾ serving banana Shake to Go

Lunch
2 slices rustic organic whole grain bread
1 veggie burger*
Lettuce, sliced tomato, and onions
1 tbsp. low-fat canola or olive oil mayonnaise
1 ½ oz. slice organic low-fat soy cheese
Fluids: organic green tea and a touch of
   organic lemonade*

Afternoon Snack
2 organic fresh dates
1 serving fresh fruit such as an orange
Fluids: hot ginger green tea*

Evening Dinner
4 oz. roasted lime rosemary chicken (1
   serving)
1 medium baked red potatoe (2.5" by 4.5")
1 serving Mevagissey ratatouille
1 slice rustic organic whole grain bread
Fluids: iced water and hot decaf green
orange spiced tea

Supper:
1 serving peach and blackberry crumble
½ cup low-fat soy ice cream
Fluids: hot lemon ginger spiced tea

APO E GENE DIET
2/3 1600 KCAL DAY 1
Serving considerations per day
(Be mindful of serving sizes)

Carbohydrate
4 serving portions of grain/starch
9.5 serving portions of fruit and vegetable

Protein
8.5 serving portions protein

Fat
4.5 serving portions anti-inflammatory fat

Breakfast
¾ serving Shake to Go
Water and hot Japanese green tea
APO E high-quality multivitamin

Morning Snack
1 cup soy yogurt
¼ cup dried apricots
Water and hot Japanese green tea*

Lunch
1 slice whole grain bread
2 oz. sliced chicken breast
1 tbsp. low-fat olive oil or canola oil mayonnaise
Lettuce, cucumber, red onion, and sliced tomato
$^1/_8$ avocado
1 cup nonfat milk
Fluids: sparkling lemon ice water

Afternoon Snack
½ serving sultana carrot ginger coleslaw
7 whole grain crackers
Fluids: water and hot green, lemon ginger tea

Evening Dinner
3 oz. sockeye salmon
¼ cup organic white beans
2 tbsp. mango salsa cream (¼ serving)
1 serving green salad
Fluids: water with lemon and fresh mint

Supper:
3 nonfat ginger biscuits (1 serving)
Fluids: water and hot chamomile herbal tea

APO E GENE DIET
2/3 1600 KCAL DAY 2
Serving considerations per day
(Be mindful of serving sizes)

Carbohydrates
4.5 serving portions of grain/starch
7.5 serving portions of fruit and vegetable

Protein
8.5 serving portions protein

Fat
6 serving portions anti-inflammatory fat

Breakfast
1 slice whole grain bread
1 tbsp. nut butter
½ banana
1 tsp.. local organic honey
Fluids: water and hot Peach green tea*
APO E high-quality multivitamin

Morning Snack
Snack Mix (½ serving)
1 oz. soy cheese
½ cup grapes or cherries
Fluids: Sparkling Cranberry Water

Lunch
1 whole grain pita bread
Organic lettuce, cucumber, onion, and tomato
3 oz. sliced chicken
1 oz. avocado
1 tbsp. low-fat ranch dressing (olive or canola oil) and 1 oz. soy cheese
Fluids: Orange sparkling water*

Afternoon Snack

½ serving sultana, carrot, ginger coleslaw
1 cup soy milk
Fluids: 1 cup Green Lavender mint tea

Evening Dinner

1 cup organic whole wheat pasta
½ cup shiitake mushrooms
1 tsp. olive oil
$1/_8$ avocado
½ cup fresh marinara sauce
½ cup steamed spinach
1 oz. soy cheese
Fluids: chamomile tea with essence of
Rosehips and lemon*

Supper:

½ cup low-fat frozen yogurt or soy ice
cream
1 cup hot green/Rosehip tea decaf*

APO E GENE DIET
2/3 1600 KCAL DAY 3

Serving considerations per day
(Be mindful of serving sizes)

Carbohydrates

5.5 serving portions of grain/starch
7.5 serving portions of fruit and vegetable

Protein

4.5 serving portions protein

Fat

10 serving portions anti-inflammatory fat

Breakfast

Blueberry Sultana Oat Bread (1 serving)
Fluids: water and hot Orange Ginger green tea
APO E high-quality multivitamin

Morning Snack

1 apples, sliced
1 tbsp. nut butter
Fluids: white tea with lemon

Lunch

1 slice whole grain bread
3 oz. Grilled Teriyaki Tuna Steak (3 oz.
cooked tuna with 1 serving teriyaki
sauce)
1 tbsp. olive/canola oil mayonnaise
1 serving chopped onions, celery, and
romaine lettuce
$1/_8$ avocado
Fluids: iced lemon water—hot green
raspberry ginger tea*

Afternoon Snack

Snack Mix (½ serving)
1 cup nonfat yogurt
Fluids: Japanese matcha tea*

Evening Dinner

¾ serving shiitake mushroom and spinach
lasagna
1 slice whole grain bread with
$1/_8$ serving avocado
Mixed salad (5 ingredients—1 cup spinach
and ½ cup of veggies such as cherry
tomatoes, cucumber or carrots
Salad dressing with 1 tsp. olive oil
Fluids: Sparkling lime juice water and
hot decaf peach green tea*

Supper:

½ cup fresh mixed berries such as
blueberries
1 slice lemon angel food cake ($1/_{12}$ of 10"
diam. tube)

APO E GENE DIET
2/3 1600 KCAL DAY 4

Serving considerations per day
(Be mindful of serving sizes)

Carbohydrates

5 serving portions of grain/starch
5 serving portions of fruit and vegetable

Protein

9 serving portions protein

Fat

7 serving portions anti-inflammatory fat

Breakfast

1 serving Scottish oats 2
1 cup nonfat milk
Fluids: water and hot white tea
APO E high-quality multivitamin

Morning Snack

$^1/_8$ cup plain organic almonds
1 oz. soy cheese

Lunch

1 veggie burger*
1 slice whole grain bread
1 ½ oz. low-fat soy cheese
2 tbsp. soy salsa cream (¼ serving)
Salad with 1 cup lettuce, ½ cup veggies
   such as onions or tomatoes
Fluids: hibiscus sparkling water

Afternoon Snack

1 tbsp. nut butter
½ cup carrot slices
Fluids: hot ginger green tea*

Evening Dinner

1, six-inch tortilla
Diced tomato and shredded lettuce
1 ½ oz. low-fat soy cheese
¼ cup black beans
2 tbsp. soy salsa cream (¼ serving)
$^1/_8$ avocado
Fluids: peach and ginger green tea*

Supper:

Apple blueberry fruit crumble (¾ serving)
1 serving hot nonfat vanilla Custard

APO E GENE DIET
2/3 1800 KCAL DAY 1
Serving considerations per day
(Be mindful of serving sizes)

Carbohydrates
5.5 serving portions of grain/starch
9 serving portions of fruit and vegetable

Protein
9 serving portions protein

Fat
5 serving portions anti-inflammatory fat

Breakfast
¾ serving orange Shake to Go
Water and hot Japanese green tea
APO E high-quality multivitamin

Morning Snack
¾ serving blueberry sultana oat bread
1 cup soy milk
Fluids: water and hot Japanese green tea

Lunch
¾ serving Tuscany pizza
1 serving mixed salad
Fluids: lemon ice water*

Afternoon Snack
1 serving snack mix
Fluids: water and hot green lemon ginger tea*

Evening Dinner
4 oz. roasted chicken
1.5 oz. Pam's bked potato with skin (½ serving)
2 tbsp. salsa cream (¼ serving)
1 ½ oz. low-fat soy cheese
1 serving Mevagissey ratatouille
Fluids: water with lemon and fresh mint

Supper:
½ serving pear currant crumble
½ cup low-fat soy ice cream
Fluids: water and hot chamomile herbal tea

APO E GENE DIET
2/3 1800 KCAL DAY 2
Serving considerations per day
(Be mindful of serving sizes)

Carbohydrates
4.5 serving portions of grain/starch
12.5 serving portions of fruit and vegetable

Protein
7 serving portions protein

Fat
6 serving portions anti-inflammatory fat

Breakfast
½ cup scrambled egg white or egg
  substitute
2 slices whole grain oat flax toast
1 oz. avocado (for your toast—green toast)*
1 serving fresh orange slices
Fluids: tea: hot apricot green tea*
APO E high-quality multivitamin

Morning Snack
1 tbsp. nut butter
1 serving sliced apple
1 cup nonfat milk

Lunch
¾ serving tofu and bean tacos
2 tbsp. low-fat salsa cream (¼ serving)
Fluids: orange sparkling water*

Afternoon Snack
1 serving sultana, carrot, ginger coleslaw
4 whole grain crackers
Fluids: 1 cup green lavender mint tea*

Evening Dinner
¾ serving vegetable spaghetti or pasta
1 serving mixed green salad
½ cup steamed spinach
Fluids: chamomile tea with rosehips and
  lemon*

Supper:

3 small ginger biscuits (cookies) (1 serving)
1 cup nonfat milk
Fluids: 1 cup hot green tea decaf

APO E GENE DIET
2/3 1800 KCAL DAY 3

Serving considerations per day
(Be mindful of serving sizes)

Carbohydrates

7.5 serving portions of grain/starch
3 serving portions of fruit and vegetable

Protein

10 serving portions protein

Fat

6.5 serving portions anti-inflammatory fat

Breakfast

1 tbsp. almond butter
1 slice multi grain toast
1 cup soy milk
Fluids: lemon water and hot white tea
APO E high-quality multivitamin

Morning Snack

1 cup nonfat yogurt
¼ cup low-fat granola
Fluids: white tea with lemon*

Lunch

1 Garden Burger*
2 slices whole grain bread
1 serving romaine lettuce, red onion and
   organic vine-ripened tomatoes
1 ½ oz. low-fat soy cheese
1 tbsp. light canola mayonnaise
$1/_8$ avocado
Fluids: iced lemon water and hot creen
   raspberry ginger tea*

Afternoon Snack

½ serving wheat pasta salad
10 ripe, green olives
Fluids: Japanese matcha tea*

Evening Dinner

3 oz. salmon with Pacific Rim Sauce (3
   oz. cooked salmon with 1 serving thai
   hazelnut sauce)
1 serving basmati rice
8 steamed asparagus
Fluids: sparkling lime juice water and hot
   decaf peach green tea*

Supper:

¾ serving peach blackberry crumble
1 cup hot soy custard (½ serving)
Fluids: hot decaf orange green tea

APO E GENE DIET
2/3 1800 KCAL DAY 4

Serving considerations per day
(Be mindful of serving sizes)

Carbohydrates

5 serving portions of grain/starch
12.5 serving portions of fruit and vegetable

Protein

2.5 serving portions protein

Fat

8 serving portions anti-inflammatory fat

Breakfast

1 serving Scottish oats with dates
Fluids: water and hot Japanese apricot tea*
APO E high-quality multivitamin

Morning Snack

Organic trail mix: ½ cup oat bran cereal,
   $1/_8$ cup nuts, ¼ cup currants
$2/_3$ cup nonfat cottage cheese

Lunch

1 serving vegetarian taco
2 tbsp. low-fat soy yogurt
½ cup salsa
Fluids: sparkling hibiscus water hot green
   tea with lemon*

Afternoon Snack

1 slice whole grain bread
1 tbsp. nut butter
Fluids: hot ginger green tea*

Evening Dinner

¾ serving shiitake mushroom and spinach
   lasagna
1 tbsp. parmesan cheese
1 serving mixed green salad
1 tbsp. fat free salad dressing

Supper:

1 slice lemon angel food cake ($1/_{12}$ cake 10"
   diam. tube)
¾ cup fresh sliced organic strawberries
Fluids: hot chamomile, lavender tea*

APO E GENE DIET
2/3 2000 KCAL DAY 1

Serving considerations per day
(Be mindful of serving sizes)

Carbohydrates

8 serving portions of grain/starch
6.5 serving portions of fruit and vegetable

Protein

10 serving portions protein

Fat

7.5 serving portions anti-inflammatory fat

Breakfast

Scrambled eggs*
1 slice whole grain toast
1 serving fresh orange
1 tbsp. honey
Fluids: water and hot Japanese green tea
APO E high-quality multivitamin

Morning Snack

¾ serving blueberry sultana oat bread
Water and hot Japanese green tea

Lunch

1 serving Tuscany pizza
1 serving mixed green salad
1 serving cilantro soy ginger dressing
½ oz. kalamata olives
Fluids: lemon ice water*

Afternoon Snack

1 serving fresh sliced apples
1 tbsp. nut butter
1 serving soy cheese
Fluids: water and hot green, lemon ginger tea*

Evening Dinner

4 oz. lime rosemary baked bhicken (1
   serving)
3 oz. Pam's baked potato with skin (1
   serving)
2 tbsp. salsa cream (¼ serving)
1 serving fresh chives
1 cup cooked broccoli
1 cup nonfat milk
Fluids: water with lemon, hot green tea

Supper:

½ serving pear currant crumble
½ cup low-fat soy ice cream
Fluids: water and hot chamomile herbal tea

APO E GENE DIET
2/3 2000 KCAL DAY 2

Serving considerations per day
(Be mindful of serving sizes)

Carbohydrates

5.5 serving portions of grain/starch
5.5 serving portions of fruit and vegetable

Protein

8 serving portions protein

Fat

6 serving portions anti-inflammatory fat

Breakfast

1 serving Scottish oats
¼ cup black currants
1 cup soy milk
Fluids: water and hot Japanese green tea
APO E high-quality multivitamin

Morning Snack

1 tbsp. nut butter
1 serving whole grain bread
Fluids: white tea with lemon*

Lunch

¾ serving vegetarian black bean soup
1 slice whole grain bread
1 serving romaine lettuce and organic vine-
   ripened tomatoes
1½ oz. low-fat soy cheese
1 tbsp.* vegetarian light canola mayonnaise
1/8 avocado
Fluids: iced lemon water and hot green
   raspberry ginger tea*

Afternoon Snack

½ serving snack mix
Fluids: Japanese matcha tea*

Evening Dinner

¾ serving fish tacos
2 tbsp. salsa cream (¼ serving)
½ cup black beans
Fluids: sparkling lime juice water and hot
   decaf peach green tea*

Supper:

1 cup organic hot chocolate with milk
Fluids: water

APO E GENE DIET
2/3 2000 KCAL DAY 3

Serving considerations per day
(Be mindful of serving sizes)

Carbohydrates

7 serving portions of grain/starch
9.5 serving portions of fruit and vegetable

Protein

7.5 serving portions protein

Fat

9 serving portions anti-inflammatory fat

Breakfast

1 serving omelet or burrito
1/8 avocado
½ cup olive oil grilled potatoes
2 tbsp. fresh diced tomato
Fluids: water and hot white tea*
APO E high-quality multivitamin

Morning Snack

1 tbsp. nut butter
1 slice whole grain toast

Lunch

1 Garden Burger*
2 slices whole grain bread
1 serving romaine lettuce with sliced red onion and vine-ripened tomatoes
1½ oz. low-fat soy cheese
1 tbsp. canola oil mayonnaise
¹/₈ avocado
Fluids: orange sparkling water*

Afternoon Snack

1 blueberry oat muffin (1 serving)
Fluids: 1 cup hot green lavender tea*

Evening Dinner

1 serving shiitake mushroom and spinach lasagna*
1 cup romaine salad with 1 tbsp. fat free Caesar dressing
Mevagissey ratatouille (1 serving)
Fluids: chamomile tea with rosehips and lemon

Supper:

½ cup soy ice cream
1 serving mixed berry pottage
1 cup hot green/rosehip tea decaf*

APO E GENE DIET
2/3 2000 KCAL DAY 4

Serving considerations per day
(Be mindful of serving sizes)

Carbohydrates

7 serving portions of grain/starch
9.5 serving portions of fruit and vegetable

Protein

8.5 serving portions protein

Fat

8 serving portions anti-inflammatory fat

Breakfast

¾ serving orange Shake to Go
Fluids: water and green tea
APO E high-quality multivitamin

Morning Snack

1 fresh organic peach
8 almonds

Lunch

2 slices whole grain bread
3 oz. organic sliced chicken
¼ avocado
¼ cup sliced tomato
¼ cup sliced maui onion
½ cup baked sweet potato fries (www.alexiafoods.com) or ½ cup homemade sweet potato with 1 tsp. olive oil
Fluids: hibiscus sparkling water*

Afternoon Snack

1 cup carrots
¼ cup hummus
Fluids: hot ginger green tea*

Evening Dinner

3 oz. wild salmon
1 tbsp. chopped almonds
1 cup fresh romaine salad with 1 tbsp. olive oil based dressing
3 oz. Pam's baked potato (1 serving)

Supper:

½ serving apple peach crumble
1 cup nonfat milk
1 serving fresh sliced organic strawberries

APO E GENE DIET
2/3 2400 KCAL DAY 1
Serving considerations per day
(Be mindful of serving sizes)

Carbohydrates
8.5 serving portions of grain/starch
11.5 serving portions of fruit and vegetable

Protein
14 serving portions protein

Fat
5.5 serving portions anti-inflammatory fat

Breakfast
½ serving banana almond Shake to Go
½ whole grain bagel
1 tbsp. honey
Fluids: water and jasmine green tea*
APO E high-quality multivitamin

Morning Snack
¹/₈ cup raisins
1 tsp. flaxseed (ground)
1 peach sliced
1 cup nonfat soy yogurt
Fluids: water and Japanese green tea

Lunch
1 whole grain pita bread
1 serving romaine lettuce and vine-ripened
tomatoes
3 oz. grilled chicken breast, sliced
1 tbsp. organic cilantro ginger soy salad
dressing (¾ serving)
1½ oz. low-fat soy cheese
¹/₈ avocado
1 serving romaine lettuce
Fresh maui onion
Sliced red pepper
Fluids: lemon ice water*

Afternoon Snack
Black gean soup (¾ serving)
3 tbsp. chopped tomato
3 tbsp. chopped green onion
1 serving whole grain bread
Fluids: water and hot green ginger tea

Evening Dinner
5 oz. grilled black cod cooked
¼ cup salsa cream (½ serving)
½ cup pinto beans
1 cup broccoli
Fluids: water with lemon and fresh mint

Supper:
3 ginger biscuits (cookies) (1 serving)
1 cup organic soy milk
Fluids: water and hot chamomile herbal tea

APO E GENE DIET
2/3 2400 KCAL DAY 2
Serving considerations per day
(Be mindful of serving sizes)

Carbohydrates
7 serving portions of grain/starch
10.5 serving portions of fruit and vegetable

Protein
13.5 serving portions protein

Fat
9 serving portions anti-inflammatory fat

Breakfast
¾ cup egg scrambled substitute*
6" whole wheat tortilla
½ cup fresh salsa
¹/₈ avocado
½ cup mixed melon
1 cup soy milk
Fluids: water and green, red, black, or
white tea
APO E high-quality multivitamin

Morning Snack

1 serving organic sliced apple
1 cup peach yogurt
8 raw almonds
1 tbsp. organic ground flaxseed (Spectrum brand)
Fluids: white tea with lemon*

Lunch

1 Garden Burger
2 slices whole grain bread
1 serving romaine lettuce and organic vine-ripened tomatoes
1 tbsp. light canola mayonnaise
¼ avocado
Fluids: iced lemon water and hot green raspberry ginger tea*

Afternoon Snack

1 serving vegetarian black bean soup
Fluids: Japanese matcha tea*

Evening Dinner

1 slice multi-grain bread
5 oz. baked salmon cooked
1 cup Fresh steamed broccoli
½ cup cooked white beans
1½ cup mixed green salad
2 tbsp. organic salad dressing
Fluids: Sparkling lime juice water and hot decaf peach green tea*

Supper:

1 serving mixed fresh berry crumble
½ cup low-fat soy frozen yogurt
Fluids: hot decaf o range green tea*

APO E GENE DIET
2/3 2400 KCAL DAY 3

Serving considerations per day
(Be mindful of serving sizes)

Carbohydrates

6 serving portions of grain/starch
13.5 serving portions of fruit and vegetable

Protein

7.5 serving portions protein

Fat

9 serving portions anti-inflammatory fat

Breakfast

1 serving berry and oat muffin
1 pear sliced
1 tbsp. nut butter
½ cup nonfat cottage cheese
Fluids: raspberry green tea
APO E high-quality multivitamin

Morning Snack

¾ serving fresh fruit Shake to Go

Lunch

2 slices whole grain bread
1 serving chicken salad
¼ cup mixed melons
2 cups romaine mixed salad
Fluids: orange sparkling water*

Afternoon Snack

½ serving sultana, carrot, ginger coleslaw
1/8 cup almonds
Fluids: 1 cup green lavender mint tea*

Evening Dinner

¾ serving shiitake mushroom and spinach
lasagna
1 tbsp. parmesan cheese
1½ spinach salad
2 tbsp. organic fat free salad dressing
1 rustic whole grain bread
Fluids: chamomile tea with essence of
Rosehips and lemon*

Supper:

¾ cup blackberries and ½ cup low fat
frozen yogurt
1 cup hot green/Rosehip tea decaf*

**APO E GENE DIET
2/3 2400 KCAL DAY 4**
Serving considerations per day
(Be mindful of serving sizes)

Carbohydrates
7.5 serving portions of grain/starch
12.5 serving portions of fruit and vegetable

Protein
13.5 serving portions protein

Fat
4.5 serving portions anti-inflammatory fat

Breakfast

1 apple
1 serving red pepper tofu scramble
½ cup grilled wax red potato
Fluids: white earl grey tea
APO E high-quality multivitamin

Morning Snack

Snack mix: ½ cup oat bran squares, and ¼
cup dried cranberries/raisins
2 oz. soy cheese
Fluids: lemon green tea*

Lunch

2 slices whole grain bread
4 oz. sliced organic chicken with no skin
1 serving romaine lettuce, fresh tomato,
and onions
1 tbsp. canola mayonnaise
Organic sliced peaches
Fluids: hibiscus sparkling water*

Afternoon Snack

1 serving vegetarian tacos
1 oz. soy cheese
$^1/_8$ avocado
Fluids: hot ginger green tea*

Evening Dinner

5 oz. black cod
Spinach, red pepper, fresh tomatoes, and corn
1 medium red skin potato
$^1/_8$ avocado
1 cup steamed broccoli
½ cup cooked carrots

Supper or Evening Snack

½ cup low-fat soy ice cream or frozen yogurt
1 serving fresh sliced strawberries

APO E 2/3 2400 KCAL

APO E GENE DIET
2/2 1600 KCAL DAY 1

Serving considerations per day
(Be mindful of serving sizes)

Carbohydrates
4.5 serving portions of grain/starch
14 serving portions of fruit and vegetable

Protein
4.5 serving portions protein

Fat
7 serving portions anti-inflammatory fat

Breakfast
¾ serving fresh fruit Shake to Go
Water and hot Japanese green tea
APO E high-quality multivitamin

Morning Snack
1 cup soy yogurt
¼ cup dried apricots
Water and hot Japanese green tea*

Lunch
1 slice whole grain bread
2 oz. sliced chicken breast
1 tbsp. low-fat olive oil or canola oil
mayonnaise
Lettuce, cucumber, red onion, and sliced
   tomato
¼ avocado
1 cup nonfat milk
Fluids: sparkling lemon ice water*

Afternoon Snack
1 apple
7 whole grain crackers
Fluids: water and hot green, lemon ginger tea

Evening Dinner
1 slice whole grain bread
¹/₈ cup almonds
2 oz. sockeye salmon

2 tbsp. mango salsa cream (¼ serving)
1 serving mixed green salad
Fluids: water with lemon and fresh mint

Supper:
3 nonfat ginger biscuits (1 serving)
Fluids: water and hot chamomile herbal tea

APO E GENE DIET
2/2 1600 KCAL DAY 2

Serving considerations per day
(Be mindful of serving sizes)

Carbohydrates
5 serving portions of grain/starch
8.5 serving portions of fruit and vegetable

Protein
7 serving portions protein

Fat
8 serving portions anti-inflammatory fat

Breakfast
2 slices whole grain bread
2 tbsp. nut butter
½ banana
Fluids: water and hot peach green tea*
APO E high-quality multivitamin

Morning Snack
½ serving snack mix
1 oz. soy cheese
½ cup grapes or cherries
Fluids: sparkling cranberry water*

Lunch
½ whole grain pita bread
Organic lettuce, cucumber, onion, and
   tomato
2 oz. sliced chicken
1 oz. avocado
1 tbsp. fat-free ranch dressing
1 oz. soy cheese
Fluids: Orange sparkling water*

Afternoon Snack

½ serving sultana, carrot, ginger coleslaw
1 cup soy milk
Fluids: 1 cup green lavender mint tea*

Evening Dinner

1 cup organic whole wheat pasta
½ cup shiitake mushrooms
1 tsp. olive oil
¹/₈ serving avocado
½ cup fresh marinara sauce
½ cup steamed spinach
½ oz. soy cheese
Fluids: chamomile tea with essence of
    rosehips and lemon*

Supper:

½ cup low-fat frozen yogurt or soy ice cream
1 cup hot green/rosehip tea decaf*

**APO E GENE DIET
2/2 1600 KCAL DAY 3**

Serving considerations per day
(Be mindful of serving sizes)

Carbohydrates

5.5 serving portions of grain/starch
9.5 serving portions of fruit and vegetable

Protein

4 serving portions protein

Fat

9 serving portions anti-inflammatory fat

Breakfast

¾ serving blueberry sultana oat bread
Fluids: water and hot orange ginger green tea
APO E high-quality multivitamin

Morning Snack

1 serving sliced apples
1 tbsp. nut butter
Fluids: white tea with lemon

Lunch

2 slices whole grain bread
2 oz. grilled teriyaki tuna steak (2 oz.
    cooked tuna with 1 serving teriyaki sauce)
1 tbsp. olive/canola oil mayonnaise
1 serving chopped onions, celery, and
    romaine lettuce
¼ avocado
Fluids: iced lemon water and hot green
    raspberry ginger tea

Afternoon Snack

1 sliced carrot with 1 cup nonfat yogurt
Fluids: Japanese matcha tea*

Evening Dinner

½ serving shiitake mushroom and spinach
    lasagna
¹/₈ avocado
Mixed salad (5 ingredients—spinach,
    cherry tomatoes, cucumber, carrots, salad
    dressing with 1 tbsp. olive oil
Fluids: sparkling lime juice water and hot
    decaf peach green tea*

Supper:

½ cup fresh mixed berries
1 serving lemon angel food cake

APO E GENE DIET
2/2 1600 KCAL DAY 4

Serving considerations per day
(Be mindful of serving sizes)

Carbohydrates

4 serving portions of grain/starch
6.5 serving portions of fruit and vegetable

Protein

6 serving portions protein

Fat

10 serving portions anti-inflammatory fat

Breakfast

½ serving Scottish oats with dates
1 cup nonfat milk
Fluids: water and hot white tea
APO E high-quality multivitamin

Morning Snack

¹/₈ cup plain organic almonds
1 oz. soy cheese

Lunch

1 veggie burger
1 slice whole grain bread
2 tbsp. soy salsa cream (¼ serving)
¹/₈ avocado
Onions, tomatoes, and lettuce—medium
   salad
Fluids: hibiscus sparkling water*

Afternoon Snack

2 tbsp. nut butter
10 carrot slices
Fluids: hot ginger green tea*

Evening Dinner

6-inch tortilla
Diced tomato and shredded lettuce
1 ½ oz. low-fat soy cheese
¼ cup black beans
2 tbsp. soy salsa cream*
¹/₈ avocado
Fluids: Peaches and Ginger green tea*

Supper:

Apple peach Fruit Crumble (½ serving)
Nonfat Vanilla Custard (½ serving)

APO E GENE DIET
2/2 1800 KCAL DAY 1

Serving considerations per day
(Be mindful of serving sizes)

Carbohydrates

6.5 serving portions of grain/starch
9.5 serving portions of fruit and vegetable

Protein

6.5 serving portions protein

Fat

6 serving portions anti-inflammatory fat

Breakfast

¾ serving orange Shake to Go
Water and hot Japanese green tea
APO E high-quality multivitamin

Morning Snack

¾ serving blueberry sultana oat bread
1 cup soy milk
Fluids: water and hot Japanese green tea

Lunch

¾ serving Tuscany pizza
1 serving mixed green salad
8 olives, green
Fluids: lemon ice water*

Afternoon Snack

1 serving snack mix
Fluids: water and hot green lemon ginger tea*

Evening Dinner

2 oz. roasted chicken
1.5 oz. Pam's baked potato with skin (½ serving)
2 tbsp. salsa cream (¼ serving)
1 oz. low-fat soy cheese
Mevagissey ratatouille (1 serving)
Fluids: water with lemon and fresh mint

Supper:

½ cup pear currant crumble*
½ cup low-fat soy ice cream
Fluids: water and hot chamomile herbal tea

APO E GENE DIET
2/2 1800 KCAL DAY 2

Serving considerations per day
(Be mindful of serving sizes)

Carbohydrates

5.5 serving portions of grain/starch
12.5 serving portions of fruit and vegetable

Protein

7 serving portions protein

Fat

6.5 serving portions anti-inflammatory fat

Breakfast

Scrambled egg substitute*
1 slice whole grain oat flax toast
1 oz. avocado (for your toast—green toast)*
1 serving fresh orange
Fluids: tea: hot cpricot green tea*
APO E high-quality multivitamin

Morning Snack

1 tbsp. nut butter
½ sliced apple
½ cup nonfat milk

Lunch

1 serving tofu tacos
2 tbsp. low-fat salsa cream (¼ serving)
Fluids: Orange sparkling water*

Afternoon Snack

½ serving sultana, carrot, ginger coleslaw
6 whole grain crackers
Fluids: 1 cup green lavender mint tea*

APO E 2/2 1800 KCAL

Evening Dinner

¾ serving vegetable spaghetti or pasta
1 serving mixed green salad
½ cup steamed spinach
Fluids: chamomile tea with rosehips and lemon

Supper:

3 small ginger biscuits (1 serving)
1 cup soy yogurt
Fluids: 1 cup hot green tea decaf

**APO E GENE DIET
2/2 1800 KCAL DAY 3**
Serving considerations per day
(Be mindful of serving sizes)

Carbohydrates
8 serving portions of grain/starch
5 serving portions of fruit and vegetable

Protein
6.5 serving portions protein

Fat
7 serving portions anti-inflammatory fat

Breakfast

²/₃ cup low fat granola
¾ cup soy milk
Fluids: lemon water and hot white tea
APO E high-quality multivitamin

Morning Snack

1 banana
2 tbsp. almond butter
Fluids: white tea with lemon*

Lunch

½ Garden Burger patty
1 slice whole grain bread
1 serving romaine lettuce, red onion and
    organic vine-ripened tomatoes
1 tbsp. light canola mayonnaise
¼ avocado

Fluids: iced lemon water and hot green
    raspberry ginger tea*

Afternoon Snack

½ serving wheat pasta salad
8 ripe, green olives
Fluids: Japanese matcha tea*

Evening Dinner

2 oz. salmon with pacific rim Sauce (2
    oz. cooked salmon with 1 serving thai
    hazelnut sauce)
½ cup basmati rice
8 steamed asparagus
Fluids: sparkling lime juice water and
    hot decaf peach green tea*

Supper:

1 serving peach blackberry crumble
½ serving hot soy custard
Fluids: hot decaf orange green tea

**APO E GENE DIET
2/2 1800 KCAL DAY 4**
Serving considerations per day
(Be mindful of serving sizes)

Carbohydrates
6.5 serving portions of grain/starch
13.5 serving portions of fruit and vegetable

Protein
2.5 serving portions protein

Fat
8.5 serving portions anti-inflammatory fat

Breakfast

1 cup Scottish oats*
¾ cup fresh blackberries
Fluids: water and hot Japanese apricot tea
APO E high-quality multivitamin

Morning Snack

Organic trail mix: ½ cup oat bran cereal,
 ¹/₈ cup almonds, ¼ cup currants*
¼ cup nonfat cottage cheese

Lunch

1 serving vegetarian tacos
2 tbsp. low-fat soy yogurt
½ cup salsa
1 serving fresh organic olives
Fluids: sparkling hibiscus water and hot
 green tea with lemon

Afternoon Snack

1 slice whole grain bread
1 tbsp. nut butter
Fluids: hot ginger green tea*

Evening Dinner

¾ serving shiitake mushroom and spinach
 lasagna
1 cup mixed green salad*
1 tbsp. fat-free salad dressing

Supper:

1 slice lemon angel food cake (¹/₁₂ of a 10"
 diam. tube)
¾ cup fresh sliced organic strawberries
Fluids: hot chamomile, lavender tea

APO E GENE DIET
2/2 2000 KCAL DAY 1
Serving considerations per day
(Be mindful of serving sizes)

Carbohydrates
8 serving portions of grain/starch
10.5 serving portions of fruit and vegetable

Protein
9 serving portions protein

Fat
7.5 serving portions anti-inflammatory fat

Breakfast
½ cup scrambled egg whites
1 slice whole grain toast
1 serving fresh orange
1 tbsp. almond butter
Fluids: water and hot Japanese green tea
APO E high-quality multivitamin

Morning Snack
¾ serving blueberry sultana oat bread
Water and hot Japanese green tea

Lunch
1 serving Tuscany pizza
1 serving mixed green salad
¼ serving cilantro soy ginger dressing
½ oz. kalamata olives
Fluids: lemon ice water*

Afternoon Snack
1 serving fresh sliced apples
2 tbsp. nut butter
1 serving soy cheese
Fluids: water and hot green lemon ginger tea*

Evening Dinner
3 oz. rosemary thyme roasted chicken (¾ serving)
3 oz. Pam's baked potato with skin (1 serving)

2 tbsp. salsa cream (¼ serving)
1 serving fresh chives
1 cup cooked broccoli
1 cup nonfat milk
Fluids: water with lemon, hot green tea

Supper:
½ serving pear currant crumble
½ cup low-fat soy ice cream
Fluids: water and hot chamomile herbal tea

APO E GENE DIET
2/2 2000 KCAL DAY 2
Serving considerations per day
(Be mindful of serving sizes)

Carbohydrates
5 serving portions of grain/starch
5 serving portions of fruit and vegetable

Protein
5 serving portions protein

Fat
8 serving portions anti-inflammatory fat

Breakfast
1 serving Scottish oats
½ cup black currants
Fluids: water and hot Japanese green tea
APO E high-quality multivitamin

Morning Snack
1 tbsp. nut butter
1 serving whole grain bread
Fluids: white tea with lemon*

Lunch
1 serving vegetarian black bean soup
1 slice whole grain bread
1 serving romaine lettuce and organic vine-ripened tomatoes
1½ oz. low-fat soy cheese
1 tbsp. vegetarian light canola mayonnaise

¼ avocado
Fluids: iced lemon water and hot green raspberry ginger tea*

Afternoon Snack

Snack Mix (¾ serving)
Fluids: Japanese matcha tea*

Evening Dinner

10 olives
Fish Tacos (¾ serving)
2 tbsp. salsa cream (¼ serving)
1 cup black beans
Fluids: sparkling lime juice water and hot decaf peach green tea*

Supper:

1 cup organic hot chocolate with nonfat milk
Fluids: water

**APO E GENE DIET
2/2 2000 KCAL DAY 3**
Serving considerations per day
(Be mindful of serving sizes)

Carbohydrates

6.5 serving portions of grain/starch
10 serving portions of fruit and vegetable

Protein

6 serving portions protein

Fat

10.5 serving portions anti-inflammatory fat

Breakfast

1 serving omelet or burrito
1/8 avocado
2 tbsp. fresh diced tomato
1 serving fresh orange slices
Fluids: water and hot white tea
APO E high-quality multivitamin

Morning Snack

1 tbsp. nut butter
1 slice whole grain toast

Lunch

1 Garden Burger*
2 slices whole grain bread
1 serving romaine lettuce with sliced red onion and vine-ripened tomatoes
1½ oz. low-fat soy cheese
1 tbsp. canola oil mayonnaise
¼ avocado
Fluids: orange sparkling water*

Afternoon Snack

1 blueberry oat muffin (1 serving)
Fluids: 1 cup hot green lavender tea

Evening Dinner

¾ serving shiitake mushroom and spinach lasagna
1 cup romaine lettuce with 1 tbsp. reduced-fat olive oil dressing
1 serving Mevagissey ratatouille
Fluids: chamomile tea with rosehips and lemon

Supper:

½ cup soy ice cream
1 serving mixed berry pottage
1 cup hot green/rosehip tea decaf

APO E 2/2 2000 KCAL

APO E GENE DIET
2/2 2000 KCAL DAY 4

Serving considerations per day
(Be mindful of serving sizes)

Carbohydrates

6 serving portions of grain/starch
8 serving portions of fruit and vegetable

Protein

6 serving portions protein

Fat

9.5 serving portions anti-inflammatory fat

Breakfast

¾ serving orange Shake to Go
Fluids: water and green tea
APO E high-quality multivitamin

Morning Snack

1 fresh organic peach
8 almonds

Lunch

2 slices whole grain bread
2 oz. cooked organic sliced chicken
¼ avocado
Sliced tomato
Sliced Maui onion
½ cup baked sweet potato fries
    (www.alexiafoods.com) or homemade
    with 1 tsp. olive oil
Fluids: hibiscus sparkling water*

Afternoon Snack

1 cup carrots
¼ cup hummus
Fluids: hot ginger green tea*

Evening Dinner

3 oz. wild salmon
1 tbsp. chopped almonds
1 cup fresh romaine salad with olive oil
    based dressing
1 medium Pam's baked potato*

Supper:

Apple pear crumble (½ serving)
1 cup nonfat milk
¾ cup fresh sliced organic strawberries

APO E GENE DIET
2/2 2400 KCAL DAY 1

Serving considerations per day
(Be mindful of serving sizes)

Carbohydrates

9 serving portions of grain/starch
12 serving portions of fruit and vegetable

Protein

9.5 serving portions protein

Fat

8.5 serving portions anti-inflammatory fat

Breakfast

¾ serving fresh fruit Shake to Go
1 slice whole grain toasted
1 tbsp. honey
Fluids: water and jasmine green tea*
APO E high-quality multivitamin

Morning Snack

1 tbsp. ground flaxseed
1 peach sliced
1 cup nonfat soy yogurt
Fluids: water and Japanese green tea

Lunch

1 whole grain pita bread
1 serving romaine lettuce and vine-ripened
    tomatoes
2 oz. grilled chicken breast sliced
1 tbsp. organic ginger soy salad dressing (½
    serving)
¼ avocado
1 serving romaine lettuce
Fresh Maui onion
Sliced red pepper
Fluids: lemon ice water

Afternoon Snack

½ serving black bean soup
3 tbsp. chopped tomato
3 tbsp. chopped green onion
1.5 slices whole grain bread
Fluids: water and hot green ginger tea

Evening Dinner

3 oz. grilled black cod (3 oz. cod cooked
  with 1 tsp. olive oil)
¼ cup salsa cream (½ serving)
¼ avocado
½ cup pinto beans
1 cup broccoli
Fluids: water with lemon and fresh mint

Supper:

3 ginger biscuits (cookies) (1 serving)
1 cup organic soy milk
Fluids: water and hot chamomile herbal tea

**APO E GENE DIET
2/2 2400 KCAL DAY 2**

Serving considerations per day
(Be mindful of serving sizes)

Carbohydrates

6.5 serving portions of grain/starch
8.5 serving portions of fruit and vegetable

Protein

10 serving portions protein

Fat

10 serving portions anti-inflammatory fat

Breakfast

½ cup egg sramble substitute*
6" whole wheat tortilla
½ cup fresh salsa
¼ avocado
½ cup mixed melon
1 cup soy milk
Fluids: water and green, red, black, or
  white tea
APO E high-quality multivitamin

Morning Snack

1 serving organic sliced apple
1 cup peach yogurt
8 raw almonds
1 tbsp. organic ground flaxseed (Spectrum
  brand)
Fluids: white tea with lemon*

Lunch

Garden Burger
1 slice whole grain bread
1 serving romaine lettuce and organic
vine-ripened tomatoes
1 tbsp. light canola mayonnaise
½ avocado
Fluids: iced lemon water and hot Green
raspberry ginger tea*

Afternoon Snack

Vegetarian black bean soup (½ serving)
1 cup basmati rice
Fluids: Japanese matcha tea*

Evening Dinner

3 oz. baked salmon (3 oz. cooked salmon
  with 1 tsp. olive oil)
½ cup Fresh steamed broccoli
1 cup cooked white beans
1 ½ cup mixed green salad
2 tbsp. fat free organic salad dressing
Fluids: Sparkling lime juice water and
hot decaf peach green tea*

Supper:
¾ serving black currant/rhubarb crumble
½ cup low-fat soy frozen yogurt
Fluids: hot decaf orange green tea

APO E GENE DIET
2/2 2400 KCAL DAY 3
Serving considerations per day
(Be mindful of serving sizes)

Carbohydrates
4 serving portions of grain/starch
15.5 serving portions of fruit and vegetable

Protein
6 serving portions protein

Fat
13 serving portions anti-inflammatory fat

Breakfast
1 serving blueberry and oat muffin
1 pear sliced
1 tbsp. organic fruit preserves
1 tbsp. nut butter
1 cup soy milk
Fluids: raspberry green tea*
APO E high-quality multivitamin

Morning Snack
1 serving fresh fruit Shake to Go

Lunch
1 slice whole grain bread
½ serving chicken salad*
¼ cup mixed melons
2 cups romaine mixed salad
Fluids: orange sparkling water*

Afternoon Snack
½ serving sultana, carrot, ginger coleslaw
¼ cup almonds
Fluids: 1 cup green lavender mint tea*

Evening Dinner
¾ serving shiitake mushroom and spinach lasagna
1 tbsp. parmesan cheese
1½ spinach salad
2 tbsp. organic fat free salad dressing
Fluids: chamomile tea with essence of rosehips and lemon*

Supper:
¾ cup blackberries and 1 cup nonfat ice cream
1 cup hot green/Rosehip tea decaf*

APO E GENE DIET
2/2 2400 KCAL DAY 4
Serving considerations per day
(Be mindful of serving sizes)

Carbohydrates
8 serving portions of grain/starch
11 serving portions of fruit and vegetable

Protein
9.5 serving portions protein

Fat
8 serving portions anti-inflammatory fat

Breakfast
1 serving red pepper scramble
½ cup grilled wax red potato
Fluids: white earl grey tea
APO E high-quality multivitamin

Morning Snack
Snack Mix: ½ cup oat bran squares, ¼ cup almonds, and ¼ cup dried cranberries*
1 oz. soy cheese
Fluids: lemon green tea

Lunch

2 slices whole grain bread

3 oz. sliced organic chicken with no skin

1 serving romaine lettuce, fresh tomato,
   and onions

1 tbsp. canola mayonnaise

Organic sliced peaches

Fluids: hibiscus sparkling water

Afternoon Snack

½ serving vegetarian tacos

1/8 avocado

Fluids: hot ginger green tea*

Evening Dinner

4 oz. black cod (4 oz. cooked black cod
   with 1 tsp. olive oil)

Spinach, red pepper, fresh tomatoes, and corn

½ cup red skin potato

1 cup steamed broccoli

½ cup cooked carrots

Supper or Evening Snack

1 cup low-fat soy ice cream

¾ cup fresh sliced strawberries

APO E 2/2 2400 KCAL

Chapter Twenty

THE APO E GENE DIET RECIPES

Here I offer a wide variety of recipes to make your Apo E Gene Diet experience more fun and enjoyable.

For the recipes in this book, use truly organic ingredients whenever possible. When it's not possible, use ingredients free of pesticides, antibiotics, preservatives and genetically-modified organisms (GMO).

Breakfast Food Choices

Have you every wondered what the word "breakfast" means? Very simply, it means "breaking" the "fast." What this means is that you must refuel your body with the energy that was used while you were sleeping; and also providing new energy for the coming day.

Here are some recipes my patients have enjoyed.

History of Scottish Oatmeal

Oatmeal comes from a grain (Avena sativa), and it is actually the seed of the plant. Also known as porridge, oatmeal has been eaten in Scotland and England for centuries, although in England, oats were mainly fed to horses. Oats is truly a native food in the British Isles, directly related to the climate being better suited to growing oats more effectively than wheat.

In Scotland, oatmeal is used in a variety of recipes ranging from the delicious, simple morning oatmeal with fruit, to the outright yucky in my book—although some people love these cultural foods. One example is "Marag geal" from the Outer Hebrides. This is a white pudding made with oatmeal and vegetables that are boiled in a sheep's bladder. Another recipe is the traditional Scottish Highland Black Pudding—far from a pudding in my book—that includes oatmeal mixed with sheep's blood and an assortment of varying spices, and sometimes meat and fat are added to make an old traditional Scottish highland sausage. Personally, I prefer the traditional Scottish Oatmeal in its simplest form. Unprocessed Scottish Oats offers a highly nutritional heart healthy food.

APO E GENE DIET APO E SCOTTISH OATS[29]

Ingredients

¼ cup organic Scottish oats[30]   4 oz. soy milk[31] or nonfat milk
½ banana   1 tsp. chopped walnuts
1 tsp. freshly ground flaxseed

Directions

Cook oats in a pan with milk or soy milk. After completely cooking–'til the oats are soft and creamy–add a yummy topping, in this case banana topped with organic honey and nuts. Serve in your favorite cereal bowl.

1 serving.

Nutritional serving information: carbohydrate—grain 1
protein ½
fat 1

APO E GENE DIET SCOTTISH OATS 2

Ingredients

¼ cup organic Scottish oatmeal   1 tsp. ground flaxseed
4 oz. vanilla soy milk or skim milk   ½ tsp. organic honey
Try flavoring with organic ginger and cinnamon, if you like.

Directions

Combine all ingredients in a pan. Bring to boil, and cook for 4-6 minutes. Serve in a favorite breakfast cereal bowl.

1 serving.

Nutritional serving information: carbohydrate—grain 1
protein ½
fat 1

APO E GENE DIET SCOTTISH OATMEAL WITH DATES

Ingredients

¼ cup organic Scottish oatmeal   1 tsp. ground flaxseed
4 oz. organic soy or skim milk   1 small cooked apple
1 tbsp. currants   2 dates[32], chopped
½ tsp. organic honey

---

29 From the children's book Cornish Pixie-Fairy Conference, see resources.
30 See The Apo E Gene Diet Organic Scottish Oatmeal at www.bobsredmill.com, or use organic quick oats
31 A note about soy milk, soy dairy products, and carageenan: Certain soy milk makers add a substance called carrageenan to their products. Carrageenan has been connected to cancer and gastrointestinal disorders. I recommend avoiding this additive
32 Dates are known for a high tannin level and are used to help with intestinal conditions. Dates have also been known to help with fever, sore throat, colds and bronchila conditions.

Directions

Combine all ingredients in a pan. Bring to boil and simmer for 4-6 minutes.

Add dates and honey. Serve in favorite breakfast cereal bowl.

1 serving.

Nutritional serving information: carbohydrate—fruit 1
carbohydrate—grain 1
protein ½
fat 1

APO E GENE DIET SCOTTISH FRUIT OATMEAL

Ingredients

½ cup Scottish oatmeal
8 oz. vanilla soy or skim milk
1 tbsp. sultanas
½ tsp. honey

2 tsp. ground flaxseed
1 small diced and cooked apple
1 tbsp. cranberries
cinnamon to flavor, if desired

Directions

Combine all ingredients in a pan. Bring to boil and simmer for 4–6 minutes.
Serve in favorite breakfast cereal bowl.

1 serving.

Nutritional serving information: carbohydrate—fruit 2
carbohydrate—grain 2
protein 1
fat 2

THE APO E GENE DIET SCOTTISH SPICED PEAR OATMEAL

Ingredients

½ cup Scottish oatmeal
8 oz. soy or skim milk
Sprinkle of clove spice to taste
1 tsp. ginger spice
Ground cinnamon to taste

2 tsp. ground flaxseed
1 small baked pear
½ tsp. honey
1 tsp. currants and/or 1 tsp. sultanas

Directions

Heat on stove top: ½ cup oats, 1 cup soy milk. Add clove and honey. If you like, you can also add cinnamon and ginger. Bring all ingredients to a low boil and simmer for 2–3 minutes. Add 2 tbsp. currants or sultanas, pear, and some flaxseed. Serve in your favorite English bone china bowl.

1 serving.

Nutritional serving information: carbohydrate—fruit 1
carbohydrate—grain 2
protein 1
fat 2

BREAKFAST BREAD[33]

Ingredients

2 cups whole grain wheat flour

1 tsp. baking soda

2 egg whites or egg substitute

¼ cup honey

¹/₈ cup canola oil and

2 cups oat bran

2 cup blueberries

2 cups low-fat soy milk

¼ cup hazelnuts or walnuts

¹/₈ cup peanut oil (double canola oil if you don't wish to use peanut oil)

Directions

Preheat oven to 375° F. Use a nonstick tin or pan. In medium bowl, combine all dry ingredients (do not add blueberries yet). In a large bowl, mix all liquid ingredients. Add dry ingredients to liquid mixture and mix well. Carefully fold in blueberries. Pour batter in cake pan. Bake for about 30 minutes. Test with a toothpick to see if fully baked. Remove from pan and allow to cool before slicing.

8 servings.

Nutritional serving information: carbohydrate—fruit ½
carbohydrate—grain 2
protein ½
fat 2

THE APO E RASPBERRY OAT BREAD

Ingredients

1¾ cups whole grain flour

1 tsp. baking powder

¼ cup canola oil

1 tsp. orange rind

2 cups soy honey

2 ¼ cups oat bran

2 egg whites

2 tsp. freshly squeezed orange juice

¼ cup honey

2 cups fresh or frozen raspberries

Directions

Preheat to 350° F. In a mixing bowl, mix all dry ingredients. In a separate bowl, combine all wet ingredients—egg whites, canola oil, honey, and soy milk. When the wet ingredients are completely blended, slowly add dry ingredients to your blended mixture and stir well. Gently add in the berries. Pour mixture into nonstick bread pan. Bake for 40–50 minutes or until cooked.

8 servings.

Nutritional serving information: carbohydrate—fruit ½
carbohydrate—grain 2
protein 1
fat 1

33   From the children's book *Cornish Fairy-Pixie Conference,* see resources.

THE APO E BLUEBERRY SULTANA OAT BREAD

Ingredients

1 ¾ cups whole grain flour

1 tsp. baking powder

¼ cup canola oil

1 tsp. orange rind

2 cups soy honey

1 ½ cup fresh or frozen blueberries

2 ¼ cups oat bran

2 egg whites

2 tsp. freshly squeezed orange juice

¼ cup honey

¼ cup sultanas

Directions

Set oven to 350° F. In a mixing bowl, combine all dry ingredients. In a separate bowl, combine all wet ingredients: egg whites, canola oil, honey, and soy milk. After the wet ingredients are completely blended, slowly add dry ingredients to your blended wet mixture and stir well. Gently add in berries and sultanas. Pour mixture into nonstick bread pan. Bake for 40-50 minutes or until bread is brown on top.

8 servings.

Nutritional serving information: carbohydrate—fruit ½
carbohydrate—grain 2
protein 1
fat 1

THE APO E GENE DIET BLACK CURRANT OAT BREAD

Ingredients

1 ¾ cups whole grain flour

1 tsp. baking powder

¼ cup canola oil

1 tsp. orange rind

2 cups soy honey

2 ¼ cups oat bran

2 egg whites

2 tsp. freshly squeezed orange juice

¼ cup honey

2 cups fresh or frozen black currants

Directions

Preheat oven to 350° F. In a mixing bowl, combine all dry ingredients. In a separate bowl, combine all wet ingredients and blend together—egg whites, canola oil, honey, and soy milk. When the wet ingredients are completely blended, slowly add dry ingredients to your blended mixture and stir well. Gently add the berries to this mixture. Pour mixture into nonstick bread pan. Bake for 40–50 minutes or until cooked.

8 servings.

Nutritional serving information: carbohydrate—fruit ½
carbohydrate—grain 2
protein 1
fat 1

THE APO E GENE DIET BANANA BERRY MUFFINS (JEN'S)

Ingredients

2 very ripe bananas, mashed

2 tbsp. canola oil

½ cup unsweetened applesauce

½ cup whole grain flour

¼ tsp. salt

3 tbsp. honey

1 tsp. vanilla

1 cup whole wheat pastry flour

1 ½ tsp. baking soda

¾ cup chopped walnuts

2 cups coarsely chopped mixed berries (blackberries, blueberries, raspberries or black currants)

Directions

Preheat oven to 350° F. Mix bananas, honey, oil, vanilla, and applesauce. In a separate bowl, stir together flours, baking soda, salt, and walnuts. Add dry ingredients to liquid mixture and blend together until just combined. Add berries and stir gently. Spoon batter into nonstick muffin pan or paper-lined cups in pan. Bake for 16 minutes and check to see if fully baked. Remove from pan and allow to cool completely on rack.

12 servings.

Nutritional serving information: carbohydrate—fruit ½
carbohydrate—grain 2
protein ½
fat 1

THE APO E GENE DIET BLUEBERRY MUFFINS (JEN'S)

Ingredients

1 cup whole wheat pastry flour

1 ½ tsp. baking soda

2 tbsp. canola oil

½ cup unsweetened applesauce

¾ cup chopped walnuts

½ cup whole grain flour

3 tbsp. honey

1 tsp. vanilla

¼ tsp. salt

2 cups coarsely chopped mixed berries (blackberries, blueberries, raspberries or black currants)

Directions

Preheat oven to 350° F. Mix honey, oil, vanilla, and applesauce. In a separate bowl, stir together flours, baking soda, salt, and walnuts. Add dry ingredients to liquid mixture and blend together until just combined. Add berries and stir gently. Spoon batter into nonstick pan or paper-lined cups in pan. Bake for 16 minutes for muffins or 25 minutes for bread. Check to see if fully baked. Remove from pan and allow to cool completely on rack.

12 servings.

Nutritional serving information: carbohydrate—fruit ½
carbohydrate—grain 2
protein ½
fat 1

THE APO E GENE DIET BLUEBERRY OAT MUFFINS

Ingredients

1 cup whole wheat pastry flour

½ cup organic oats

3 tbsp. honey

1 tsp. vanilla

¼ tsp. salt

½ cup whole grain flour

1 ½ tsp. baking soda

2 tbsp. canola oil

½ cup unsweetened applesauce

¾ cup chopped walnuts

2 cups coarsely chopped mixed berries (blackberries, blueberries, raspberries or black currants)

Directions

Preheat oven to 350° F. Mix honey, oil, vanilla, and applesauce. In a separate bowl, stir together flours, ¼ cup oats, baking soda, salt, and walnuts. Add dry ingredients to liquid mixture and blend together until just combined. Add berries and stir gently. Spoon batter into nonstick bread pan or paper-lined cups in muffin pan. Sprinkle remaining oats on top of muffins. Bake for 16 minutes for muffins or 25 minutes for bread. Check to see if fully baked. Remove from pan and allow to cool completely on rack.

12 servings.

Nutritional serving information: carbohydrate—grain 2
protein ½
fat 1

THE APO E GENE DIET "GREEN" TOAST

Pam's "Green Toast" is a fun breakfast for children. Try it!

Ingredients

1 slice of oat bran flax bread or a whole grain rustic bread.[34]

1 serving of avocado–spread over the freshly toasted bread. Umm, Good!

Directions

Toast one slice of organic bread to your liking. Top with a serving of avocado (the green stuff). Cut into to green fingers and enjoy.

1 serving.

Nutritional serving information: carbohydrate—grain 1
fat 1

34   See http://www.vitalvittles.com

THE APO E GENE DIET OMELET OR BURRITO

Ingredients

2 egg whites (free-range, hormone-free, antibiotic-free) or ½ cup egg substitute

Extra-virgin olive oil in a pump spray bottle

$^1/_8$ avocado   1 small chopped shallot

2 tbsp. diced red bell pepper   1 tomato, sliced

½ tsp. curry mix with turmeric or turmeric powder

1 whole wheat tortilla or corn (purchase or make either fat-free tortilla or
    tortillas made with olive oil). Note: when purchasing tortillas make sure they
    do not contain trans fat, a common ingredient in commercial tortillas.

Directions

When making your eggs, follow the directions for your individual serving
recommendation. You may wish to add some low-fat soy cheese if included in
your recommended dietary plan.

In your favorite frying pan, spray some olive oil so your omelet doesn't stick.
Turn on the heat to medium. Mix your eggs, shallots, and bell pepper, and curry
mix with turmeric in a bowl and cook in the pan. For omelets place ingredients
into the pan and stir eggs. After the eggs have cooked place all the topping in
the center of the omelet and fold the omelet in half. Cook for additional minute
and place on your plate.

For the burrito version:

Heat the tortilla. Place cooked eggs and all your toppings on top of it. Roll up
and enjoy. I have to say this is one of my personal favorite breakfasts!

1 serving.

Nutritional serving information: carbohydrate—vegetable 1
                                         carbohydrate—grain 1
                                         protein 2
                                         fat 1

THE APO E GENE DIET RED PEPPER TOFU SCRAMBLE

Ingredients

4 oz. firm tofu or egg whites

2 tbsp. diced red bell pepper

1 vine-ripened fresh tomato

1/8 of an avocado

1 small whole wheat tortilla or oat flax toast (optional)

1 small chopped shallot

Extra-virgin olive oil in spray pump bottle

1/4-1/2 tsp. curry mix with turmeric (optional)

You may wish to add some low-fat soy cheese if this is included in your recommended dietary plan.

Directions

In a bowl, break tofu into small pieces. Brown the garlic, mushrooms, and chopped pepper with the olive oil in a pan until lightly browned. Add the tofu, then the curry/turmeric mixture, salt, and pepper. Cook for 2-3 more minutes, stirring constantly. Serve with salsa, sliced avocado, and warm whole wheat tortillas or toast.

1 serving.

Nutritional serving information: carbohydrate—vegetable 1/2
carbohydrate—grain 1
protein 1
fat 1

THE APO E GENE DIET BANANA ALMOND SHAKE TO GO

A shake is an excellent way to include fresh fruit in to your diet. Here are four shakes to go. This can also be a snack selection.

Ingredients

1/2 banana

1 1/3 tbsp. natural almond butter

1 tbsp. honey to taste

1/4 cup fresh or frozen mixed berries

2 tbsp. Scottish oatmeal

8 oz. vanilla Vita soy milk (carrageenan-free)

1 tbsp. ground flaxseed, fresh ground, or Spectrum brand organic pre-ground (Note: refrigerate if pre-ground)

Directions

Put all ingredients in food processor. Liquidize until you have a smooth consistency.

1 serving.

Nutritional serving information: carbohydrate—fruit 1 1/2
carbohydrate—grain 1/2
protein 2
fat 2

THE APO E GENE DIET QUICK FRESH FRUIT SHAKE TO GO

This can also be a snack selection.

Ingredients

4 medium strawberries

1 tbsp. raspberries

1 cup fresh pineapple, crushed or sliced

2 tbsp. Scottish oatmeal

1 cup soy plain or vanilla nonfat yogurt (carrageenan-free)

1 tbsp. blueberries

½ tbsp. ground flaxseed

1 medium fresh banana

4 ice cubes

Directions

Place all ingredients in a blender and liquidize until smooth. Serve in a cup to go. Or if serving at home, serve in a glass dessert dish.

1 serving.

Nutritional serving information: carbohydrate—fruit 5
carbohydrate—grain ½
protein 1
fat ½

THE APO E GENE DIET LEMON SHAKE TO GO

Ingredients

1 small peach

½ medium size fresh banana

Juice of 1 lemon

1 cup plain soy yogurt (carrageenan-free)

2 tbsp. Scottish oatmeal

1 tsp. vanilla extract

4 ice cubes

Directions

Place all ingredients in a blender and liquidize until smooth. Serve in a cup to go. Or if staying home, serve in a glass dessert dish.

1 serving.

Nutritional serving information: carbohydrate—fruit 2
carbohydrate—grain ¼
protein 1

THE APO E GENE DIET ORANGE SHAKE TO GO

Ingredients

1 medium orange

2 tbsp. Scottish oatmeal

½ medium size fresh banana

4 ice cubes

1 small peach

1 tbsp. ground flaxseed

1 tsp. vanilla extract

1 cup soy plain yogurt (carrageenan-free)

Directions
Place all ingredients in a blender and liquidize until smooth. Serve in a cup to go. Or if staying home, serve in a glass dessert dish.

1 serving.

Nutritional serving information: carbohydrate—fruit 2
carbohydrate—grain ½
protein 1
fat 1

THE APO E GOLF SNACK MIX

A lot of my patients are avid golfers. The big question was, "Pam, you don't want me to have a hot dog on the course. So what do I do for my morning snack?" Yep, you guessed it! The Apo E Gene Diet Golf Snack Mix slips, oh so nicely, into that golf bag. The serving amount is based on your individual diet. By the way, this can be a great for kids, too morning or afternoon. It slips nicely into a backpack.

Tip for moms and dads—this is a great fun activity to do with your children. Get them measuring and mixing all the ingredients in a big bag, then dance around the kitchen with a big baggie of The Apo E Gene Diet Golf Snack Mix. See who can do the best shake dance. Dads usually do the silliest dances, and children think this is really funny. Then use a measuring cup to measure out serving sizes into individual baggies.

Mix ½ cup of any of the following nuts or seeds: pumpkin seeds, almonds, walnuts, along with ½ cup of any of the following: dried blueberries, diced dried apricots, sultanas, currants, or dried cranberries.

Add 1 cup oat bran cereal flakes or whole oat bran biscuit pieces. Mix all ingredients in a bowl and pop into paper or wax snack bag for a morning or afternoon snack. Do the big shake. Make a big batch of this snack mix on Sunday evenings to last (maybe) through the whole week.

4 servings.

Nutritional serving information: carbohydrate—fruit 1
carbohydrate—grain ½
protein ½
fat 1

Apo E Gene Diet Soups

SIMPLE VEGETABLE BROTH (4 SERVINGS)

Ingredients

3 cups carrots, sliced

8 cups water

1 cup chopped turnip

2 crushed garlic cloves

1 cup celery, chopped

1 bay leaf

Salt to taste

2 tbsp. extra-virgin olive oil

1 cup shallots, chopped

1 cup chopped onion

1 cup fresh parsley

½ cup fresh thyme

1 tsp. white pepper

3 sticks astragalus root
(available at health food stores)

Directions

Combine all ingredients in a large saucepan. Cover the vegetables with water. Bring to a boil and then reduce heat and simmer for 45 minutes. Liquidize in blender and strain for broth.

4 servings.

Nutritional serving information: carbohydrate—vegetables 1 ½
                                          fat 1

CREAMED SPINACH CARROT SOUP

Ingredients

2 tbsp. extra-virgin olive oil

4 crushed cloves of garlic

3 cups chopped carrots

2 tbsp. whole wheat flour

1 ½ cup organic lentils

1 tsp. flaxseed

2 cups soy milk

4 cups vegetable stock

1 cup chopped leeks

2 shallots, chopped

1 large potato

4 cups fresh spinach

2 sticks astragalus root

1 sprig cilantro or parsley

¼ tsp. ginger

White pepper to taste

Add additional ½ cup broth or water if needed

Directions

Heat olive oil in medium size skillet. Add shallots, leek, and garlic. Add lentils, potato, and carrots and cook for 5–7 minutes until they begin to soften. Gradually add in the wheat flour and flaxseed, and stir well. Slowly add in 1 cup of vegetable broth. Transfer all ingredients to a larger sauce pan for further cooking. Allow to cook for another 5 minutes. Add the remaining 3 cups of broth. Then add the spinach. Bring soup to a boil, then lower heat to a simmer for 20 to 30 minutes. After 20 to 30 minutes, add the soy milk, and any additional water (if needed). Simmer for another

7–10 minutes. Liquidize in a food processor or blender for 1 minute. Serve hot in a china bowl. Top with cilantro or parsley.

8 servings.

Nutritional serving information: carbohydrate—vegetables 1 ½
protein 1
fat 1

MISO PASTA SOUP

Ingredients

2 tbsp. extra-virgin olive oil
2 cups shallots
2 cups celery
2 cups spinach
2 tbsp. fresh miso

6 cups water
4 cups carrots
1 cup chopped shiitake mushrooms
1 cup whole wheat noodles

Directions

In a medium skillet, heat olive oil. Add chopped shiitake mushrooms, shallots, carrots, and celery, and stir until brown 2–3 minutes. Then add the boiling water, vegetables, and pasta. Simmer for 7–10 minutes. Add the spinach. Dissolve miso in a bowl of warm water. Add this to the pasta and vegetables. Serve in a Japanese-type bowl. Top with chopped green onion if desired.

8 servings.

Nutritional serving information: carbohydrate—vegetables 2
carbohydrate—grain 1
fat 1

THE APO E GENE DIET TOMATO, CARROT AND BUTTERNUT SQUASH SOUP

Ingredients

1 tbsp. extra-virgin olive oil
4 garlic cloves, crushed
2 cups organic tomato soup
3 cups chopped carrots
½ cup soy milk
¼ tsp. cumin
Salt and white pepper to taste

1 cup chopped shallots
2 sticks astragalus root
2 cups butternut squash
1 cups cooked white navy beans
¼ tsp. ground ginger
2 cups vegetable broth

Directions

Heat olive oil in a skillet. Add shallots and garlic. Then add beans, carrots, astragalus, and squash. Stir well. Add vegetable broth and bring to a boil. Simmer and cook for about 20–30 minutes until the beans and carrots are soft. Add salt and white pepper liquidized with ½ cup soy milk. Serve in a china bowl. Add parsley to garnish.

8 servings.

Nutritional serving information: carbohydrate—vegetables 2
protein ½
fat 1

BUTTERNUT LEMON SOUP

Ingredients

2 tbsp. extra-virgin olive oil

Juice from ½ a lemon

¼ tsp. cinnamon

½ cup soy milk

Salt and white pepper to taste
   or liquidized fresh butternut squash

1 cup chopped shallots

¼ tsp. nutmeg (if desired)

4 cloves crushed garlic

4 cups vegetable broth

2 cups organic butternut squash, soup

Directions

Heat olive oil in a skillet. Add shallots and garlic. Brown lightly. Add squash, vegetable broth, and lemon juice and bring to a boil. Turn down to a simmer and cook for about 20–25 minutes. Add ½ cup of soy milk. Add seasonings, and liquidize. Serve in a china bowl. Top with avocado chunks and some grated lemon rind.

4 servings.

Nutritional serving information: carbohydrate—vegetables 1 ½
                                        fat 1

SUNFLOWER SPLIT PEA SOUP

Ingredients

2 cups yellow split peas

2 tsp. extra-virgin olive oil

2 cloves crushed garlic

1 cup chopped celery

½ tsp. toasted sunflower seeds

Salt and pepper to taste

8 cups vegetable broth

1 cup chopped shallots

4 cups chopped carrots

½ cup soy milk

1 cup chopped potato

Directions

If you can, soak yellow split peas overnight (this helps with cooking). In a medium saucepan, warm olive oil. Add shallots, garlic, carrots, celery, and potato—cook for 3-5 minutes. Add vegetable broth, then bring to a boil. Reduce heat and simmer for 45-50 minutes or until the peas are cooked. Add white pepper and soy milk. Liquidize. Serve in a white china bowl. Top with toasted sunflower seeds.

8 servings.

Nutritional serving information: carbohydrate—vegetables 1 ½
                                        carbohydrate—grain ½
                                        protein 1
                                        fat 1

CORNISH PEA SOUP

Ingredients

1 cup split peas	1 tbsp. olive oil
¼ cup fresh thyme	¼ cup shallots
4 cups cold water	1 medium leek, chopped
¼ cup fresh parsley	1 cup carrots
1 cup celery	1 cup chopped potato
2 cups soy milk	Salt and pepper

Directions

Soak peas in warm water for 4 hours—if possible. Rinse and place peas in a large saucepan with 4 cups of cold water. Add remaining ingredients—leaving out the soy milk. Bring soup to a boil, then turn down to low and simmer for 2 hours. When soup is cooked, add soy milk and bring back to the boil. Simmer for another 10 minutes. Serve in your English china soup bowl. Add the croutons and chopped mint as a garnish.

6 servings.

Nutritional serving information: carbohydrate—vegetables 1
carbohydrate—grain 1
protein 1
fat 1

SIMPLE VEGETARIAN BLACK BEAN SOUP

Ingredients

1 tbsp. organic olive oil	3 cups vegetable broth
1 can organic black beans[35]	1 tsp. cumin
1 tsp. turmeric	2 stalks of astragalus root
2 shallots, chopped	1 cup peeled carrots coarsely chopped
1 cup red pepper	1 cup tomato puree
1 cup organic chopped tomatoes	Add ground pepper to taste
¼ cup fresh ginger root slices	¼ cup fresh parsley

Directions

In a heavy pot add olive oil and heat for 30 seconds. Add shallots, carrots, and red pepper. Cook for 3–5 minutes. Then add in vegetable stock, spices, astragalus root, tomato puree, beans, and tomatoes. Cook for about 25 minutes. Serve in your favorite bowl. Add parsley and sliced fresh ginger root to the top.

4 servings.

Nutritional serving information: carbohydrate—vegetables 2
carbohydrate—grain 1
protein 1
fat ½

35 Amy's brand–www.amys.com

GARBAGE CAN VEGETABLE SOUP

Ingredients

8 cups vegetable broth

1 cup lentils

1 cup whole wheat pasta shells

2 cups black beans

2 cloves crushed garlic

8 cups chopped potato

2 cups chopped zucchini

2 cups chopped shallots

White pepper and salt

4 cups additional broth if needed

2 sticks astragalus root

2 cups fresh tomatoes

1 cup pearl barley

3 tbsp. extra-virgin olive oil

4 cups chopped carrots

2 cups chopped yellow squash

2 cups fresh spinach

Directions

In a very large saucepan, heat olive oil. Add shallots and garlic, and cook for 2–3 minutes then add carrots, celery, and potato. Cook for additional 5 minutes. Then add in all other ingredients. Bring to a boil, boil slowly for 5 minutes. Reduce heat to a simmer. Simmer for 45–60 minutes or until done. Serve in a rustic bowl, topped with chunks of avocado. Serve with whole grain crusty bread.

18 servings.

Nutritional serving information: carbohydrate—vegetables 2
protein ½
fat ½

CREAM POTATO CORN SOUP

Ingredients

1 cup chopped onion

2 cloves crushed garlic

3 cups vegetable broth

2 cups fresh cut white corn

4 cups chopped celery

2 cups white beans

1 cup chopped shallots

2 tbsp. extra-virgin olive oil

8 cups chopped potatoes

4 cups chopped carrots

1 cup soy milk

White pepper and salt to season

Directions

Heat olive oil in a saucepan. Add shallots and garlic. Cook for 2–3 minutes then add carrots, celery, and potato. Cook for additional 5 minutes. Then add remaining ingredients. Bring to a boil, boil for 5 minutes and then turn down to a simmer. Simmer for 45–50 minutes or until done. Mash soup with a potato masher immediately after cooking. Serve in a china bowl, topped with a spoonful of white corn. Serve with whole grain, old-fashioned, crusty bread.

10 servings.

Nutritional serving information: carbohydrate—vegetables 2
carbohydrate—grain 1
protein 1
fat 1

SPRING AND FALL TIME NETTLE SOUP

Yes, this is the stinging nettle that may have stung you as a young child. However, nettles have been found to be helpful with prostate disorders, joint disorders, allergies, and certain respiratory disorders. Now I am sure you are wondering whether the nettles keep their sting—well, they don't. When you cook stinging nettle, the sting goes away.

6 servings.

Ingredients

2 tbsp. extra-virgin olive oil

2 tbsp. whole wheat flour

2 cup shallots

2 cloves crushed garlic

Juice of quarter of a lemon

2 sticks astragalus root

4 cups small leaf stinging nettles—Caution with fresh nettle handling!

1 cup soy milk

2 cups vegetable stock

Salt and pepper to taste

Directions

Heat olive oil in a saucepan, then add shallots, and garlic. Cook for 2–3 minutes, then add nettle. Cook for an additional 5 minutes. Add whole wheat flour, stir through, then gradually add vegetable stock. Bring to a boil, boil slowly for 5 minutes, and then turn down to simmer. Simmer for 30 minutes or until done. Liquidize immediately after cooking. Serve in a china bowl, topped with a mint leaf and grated lemon rind.

Nutritional serving information: carbohydrate—vegetables 1 ½
fat 1

Entrees and Side Dishes

THE APO E HEATHER'S LIME ROSEMARY BAKED CHICKEN

My sister Heather made this chicken dish while I was visiting her in England. The herbs and juices from the chicken roasting made her English Tudor kitchen smell divine. As she made the chicken, we reviewed her recipe and together came up with ingredients to add even further flavor and healthy benefits to it. Here you have it all!

Ingredients

1 large chicken (6–7 lbs), free range, certified 100% organic, antibiotic- and hormone-free
4 whole garlic cloves, crushed
1 fresh lime cut and squeezed over chicken, and then inside the chicken
2 sprigs fresh sage, lavender, and rosemary, 1 each for inside chicken and 1 each for outside
1 tbsp. extra-virgin olive oil to coat chicken
¼ tsp. fresh ground pepper

Directions

Preheat oven to 350° F. Prepare chicken with herbs, oils, and garlic in a large roasting pan. Cook for 60-90 minutes—basting occasionally. Cut breast meat off the bone. Serve in 3-5 oz. portions.

15 servings.   Exchanges per serving = 4 protein.

FREE-RANGE ROASTED ROSEMARY TURKEY

Ingredients

1 large turkey, free-range, certified 100% organic, antibiotic- and hormone-free
1 fresh lime cut and squeezed over turkey and then placed inside the turkey
2 sprigs each fresh thyme and rosemary, 1 each for inside and 1 for outside the turkey
1 tbsp. extra-virgin olive oil to coat turkey
1 pinch fresh ground pepper

Directions

Preheat oven to 350° F. Prepare turkey with herbs, oil, and garlic in a large roasting pan. Cooking time based on size of turkey, approximately 15–20 minutes per pound. Baste occasionally. Cut breast meat off the bone. Serve in 3–5 oz. portions.

1 serving.   Exchanges per serving = 3 protein.

APO E LIME AND THYME ROASTED TURKEY

Ingredients

1 large turkey, free-range, certified 100% organic, antibiotic- and hormone-
  free
4 whole garlic cloves, crushed
1 fresh lime cut and squeezed over turkey and then placed inside the turkey
2 sprigs each fresh thyme and rosemary, 1 each for inside and 1 for outside the
  turkey
1 pinch fresh ground pepper

Directions

Preheat oven to 350° F. Prepare turkey with herbs, oils, and garlic in a large
roasting pan. Cooking time based on size of turkey, approximately 15–20
minutes per pound. Baste occasionally. Cut breast meat off the bone. Serve in
3–5 oz portions.

1 serving.   Exchanges per serving = 3 protein

THE APO E GENE DIET CORNISH CHILI

Ingredients

16 oz. chili beans (black)   ½ cup water
8 oz. tomatoes   1 tbsp. chopped scallions
2 medium sweet onions (Maui if   8 oz. firm tofu
  available), coarsely chopped
1 chopped red bell pepper   1 tsp. extra-virgin olive oil
2 tbsp. jalapeño peppers—if desired   1 tsp. turmeric and chili spices (to taste)

Directions

Combine all ingredients in medium saucepan. Bring to boil, cover and simmer
over a low heat for 20–30 minutes.

4 servings.

Nutritional serving information: carbohydrate—vegetables 1
                                       carbohydrate—grain 1
                                       protein 3

THE APO E GENE DIET VEGETABLE SPAGHETTI OR PASTA

Ingredients

2 tbsp. extra-virgin olive oil

2 garlic cloves, crushed

4 baby eggplants, quartered
sieved

2 tbsp. tomato paste

1 cup shiitake mushrooms

1 cup zucchini, chopped

½ cup kalamata olives

1 large shallots, chopped

1 tbsp. lemon juice

2 ½ cups coarsely cut vine-ripened tomatoes,

2 tsp. honey

1/8 cup fresh grated ginger

16 oz organic tofu

½ cup basil sprigs

16 oz. whole wheat dried spaghetti or any kind of whole wheat pasta

Directions

Heat 1 tbsp. of the oil in a large, heavy skillet. Add the tofu, shallots or onion, garlic, mushrooms, zucchini, lemon juice, and eggplant and cook over low heat, stirring occasionally, for 4–5 minutes or until lightly browned. Pour in the sieved tomatoes, season with salt and pepper to taste, and stir in the honey and tomato paste. Bring to a boil, reduce the heat, and simmer gently for 25 minutes. Meanwhile, bring a large pan of lightly salted water to the boil. Add the pasta, bring back to a boil, and cook for 8–10 minutes or until tender, but still firm to the bite. Drain, toss in the remaining oil. Serve with tomato veggie sauce. Sprinkle with olives and basil.

6 servings.

Nutritional serving information: carbohydrate—vegetables 4
carbohydrate—grain 2
protein 2
fat 1

THE APO E GENE DIET SHIITAKE MUSHROOM AND SPINACH LASAGNA

Ingredients

2 cups shiitake mushrooms, roughly cut

1 cup chopped shallots

1 tsp. crushed garlic

½ tsp. salt to taste

10 oz. fresh spinach, torn
preferred

1 cup high-quality tofu

1 tsp. extra-virgin olive oil

1 cup sliced zucchini

¼ cup fresh basil

½ lb. whole wheat lasagna

3 cups nonfat marinara sauce, fresh

2–4 oz. low-fat soy cheese (optional)

Directions

Preheat oven 450° F. In frying pan, heat 1 tbsp. olive oil, then add shallots, garlic, and shiitake mushrooms. Cook until all reach a soft consistency, about 5–7 minutes. Add spinach and cook slowly throughout, about 7 minutes. Do not drain. Move ingredients to a large bowl and mix in all other ingredients. Stir well. Boil lasagna in a large pot of boiling water until slightly soft. Do not cook completely. Drain. Alternate layers of noodles, sauce, tofu, and vegetables until the pan is filled, ending with noodles and cheese to cover the top of the lasagna. Bake covered for the first 20 minutes. Then uncover and cook for an additional 10–15 minutes or until cooked. End with a 2–3 minute broil to brown the cheese on top of the dish. Let 10 minutes before serving.

6 servings.

Nutritional serving information: carbohydrate—vegetables 3
carbohydrate—grain 1
protein 1
fat 1

THE APO E GENE DIET GRILLED OR BAKED FISH LUNCH OR DINNER PLATE

A tip I learned from my Nana, Bertha McDonald, as a young girl: "You want to know the secret of good eating, my love? Eat the best fish you can find and eat it often."

The fisherman of Cornwall are on their fishing boats, catching fish for your dinner tonight. For centuries the Cornish fishing industry has made Cornwall what it is today. An abundance of fresh fish, including pilchards, mackerel, and cod, was hauled into the famous harbors of Polperro, Mevagissey, Fowey, and Charlestown. The Cornish pilchards were so fresh and delicious, they were shipped far and wide, even to Italy as far back as the mid-1700s.

Make sure your fish is fresh, wild fish, not farm-raised. Farm-raised fish has been shown to contain food color, environmental toxins, PCBs, heavy metals such as mercury and lead, and other toxic contaminants, as well as residues of antibiotics and other drugs. Wild salmon is only available between April and October. Two reliable sources of wild fish I have found are Whole Foods markets and an Internet site called Vital Choice Seafood (www. vitalchoice.com).

Ingredients
You can use these types of fish: mackerel, shrimp, scallops, black cod, sea bass, herring, salmon, halibut, tuna, sardines, pilchards.

Consider herbs and flavors for fish: lemons, limes, garlic, shallots, lavender, thyme, rosemary, cilantro, parsley, teriyaki, Thai peanut, and soy ginger.

Directions
Preheat oven to 350° F. Place raw fish on your favorite baking sheet that has been brushed with a little olive oil. Brush fish with a little olive oil. Squeeze fresh lime over the fish. Add fresh herbs: rosemary, cilantro, thyme, lavender, etc. Bake for 12–15 minutes. As an alternative, you can use your grill.

Fish serving size—average 3 to 5 oz.—as per your individual dietary recommendation. Consume the recommended amount of fish per your suggested protein allowance.

1 serving.   Exchanges per serving = 3 protein.

GRILLED OR BAKED SALMON WITH TERIYAKI SHIITAKE MUSHROOM SAUCE

Ingredients

5 oz. fresh wild salmon

Sliced shiitake mushrooms

1 clove fresh garlic

Teriyaki sauce (see sauce section)

1 shallot, chopped finely

Juice of half a lime

Directions

Marinate the fish in the sauce for about 20–30 minutes. Then bake or grill with shallot, mushroom, garlic, and lime until done to your liking.

1 serving.   Exchanges per serving = 3 protein.

FRESH GRILLED WILD HALIBUT WITH RASPBERRY HONEY GINGER GLAZE

Ingredients

5 oz. fresh wild halibut

¼ cup fresh raspberries

1 clove fresh garlic

¼ cup soy ginger sauce (see sauce recipes)

1 shallot, chopped finely

Juice of half a lime

Directions

Marinate by covering the fish with all the ingredients and juice/sauce for about 30–40 minutes. Then grill or bake until cooked to your liking.

1 serving.   Exchanges per serving = 4 protein.

THE APO E GENE DIET FISH SALAD

Ingredients

1 tsp. lemon

1 tsp. mustard—optional

2 tsp. chopped avocado

1 tbsp. diced tomato

1 tsp. vinegar

4 finely chopped almonds

2 tsp. chopped sweet onions

2 tbsp. chopped red pepper

3-5 oz. shrimp, black cod, or tuna, cooked

1 tsp. olive oil mayonnaise (e.g., Spectrum brand)

Directions

Mix together in bowl. Serve.

1 serving.

Nutritional serving information: carbohydrate—vegetables 1
protein 3
fat 3

THE APO E GENE DIET GREEN SALAD

Ingredients

2 cups torn romaine lettuce

½ cup cilantro
   cucumber

3 vine-ripened chopped tomatoes

¼ cup Apo E vinaigrette dressing

¼ tsp. white pepper

2 cups spinach leaves

½ cup peeled and chopped English

½ cup red pepper

1 tbsp. broken soy cheese

Directions

Combine lettuce, spinach, cilantro, cucumbers, tomatoes, red pepper and ¼ cup vinaigrette. Toss. Sprinkle each serving with soy cheese. Add fresh ground pepper.

4 servings.

Nutritional serving information: carbohydrate—vegetables 3
                                         fat 2

THE APO E GENE DIET CHICKEN SALAD

Ingredients

3-5 oz. chicken, cooked
   brand)

1 tsp. lemon

2 tsp. cilantro

2 tbsp. chopped sweet onions

1 tsp. olive oil mayonnaise (e.g., Spectrum

1 tsp. vinegar

1 tsp. chardonnay mustard

2 tbsp. chopped red pepper

Directions

Mix all ingredients together in bowl. Serve.

1 serving.

Nutritional serving information: carbohydrate—vegetables 4
                                         protein 1
                                         fat 1

THE APO E GENE DIET TUNA OR TOFU SALAD

Ingredients:

4 oz. tuna or tofu

2 cups fresh spinach

1 cup broccoli tips

1 cup shiitake mushrooms

1 cup sweet onion

1 cup vine-ripened tomatoes

3 tsp. extra-virgin olive oil

1 tsp. turmeric

1 cup grated carrot

1 cup cabbage

1 cup red bell pepper

1 cup asparagus

2 tbsp. chopped walnuts

1 tbsp. balsamic vinegar

Directions

Mix all ingredients in salad bowl. Serve.

4 servings.

Nutritional serving information: carbohydrate—vegetables 4
protein 1
fat 1

THE APO E GENE DIET VEGETARIAN (MEATLESS) TACOS

Ingredients

2 corn tortillas

½ cup diced red pepper

½ cup grilled vegetables (red onion, red peppers, zucchini)

¼ cup fresh vine-ripened tomatoes, chopped cilantro

¼ cup romaine lettuce

½ cup pinto beans

2 tsp. extra-virgin olive oil

1/8 avocado

¼ cup low-fat soy cheese

¼ cup fresh salsa with garlic and

Directions

In the center of each corn tortilla place half of each ingredient: lettuce black beans, avocado, grilled or chopped vegetables, tomato, low-fat soy cheese, and top with salsa.

2 servings.

Nutritional serving information: carbohydrate—vegetables 1 ½
carbohydrate—grain 1 ½
fat 1 ½

THE APO E GENE DIET MEVAGISSEY FISH TACOS

Ingredients

5 oz. fresh wild white fish, cooked
¼ cup romaine lettuce
½ cup grilled vegetables (red onion, red peppers, zucchini)
¼ cup diced tomato
¼ cup fresh mango or tomato, cilantro salsa

2 corn tortillas
1 oz. of ground turmeric or to your flavor
2 tsp. extra-virgin olive oil
¹/₈ avocado
¼ cup nonfat soy cheese

A little fresh sliced ginger for garnish adds a sparkle to your taco and a tingle to your tongue

Directions

In the center of each tortilla place half of each ingredient: lettuce, fish, avocado, grilled or chopped vegetables, tomato, soy or fat-free cheese, and top with mango or tomato salsa and ginger.

2 servings.

Nutritional serving information: carbohydrate—vegetables 1
carbohydrate—grains 1
protein 2 ½
fat 1 ½

THAI HAZELNUTS CURRANT TOFU

Ingredients

3 oz. tofu per person or per recommendation in suggested menu table
½ cup chopped red pepper
Extra-virgin olive oil in a pump spray bottle
Thai hazelnut sauce (see sauce section) to taste

honey
¹/₃ cup currants
½ cup mango
1 cup young English pea pods

Directions

Brown tofu using olive oil spray. Add chopped red pepper, currants, mango. Add sauce and honey then cook for 7–12 minutes. Add pea pods and simmer for an additional 5–7 minutes.

1 serving.

Nutritional serving information: carbohydrate—vegetables 5
protein 1
fat ½

THE APO E GENE DIET TOFU AND BEAN TACOS - VEGETARIAN

Ingredients

1 serving of cooked pinto or black beans
¼ cup fresh chopped romaine lettuce
⅛ cup finely chopped red cabbage
½ cup sweet white onion, chopped (mild Maui onion, if available)

1 serving firm tofu	¼ cup vine-ripened tomatoes
1 serving fresh avocado	1 serving white corn tortillas
½ tsp. extra-virgin olive oil	2 cloves garlic, if you desire garlic flavor

Directions

Chop tofu into bite-size pieces, grate cheese, finely chop garlic. Combine these three ingredients and mix well. Brown tofu mixture in a lightly seasoned skillet over medium heat until golden brown. Heat beans in a saucepan over medium heat. Mix beans and tofu together. Set aside. Cut up onions, tomatoes, and avocado. Warm tortillas in lightly seasoned pan with olive oil, fold in half, and fill tortillas with tofu and beans. Add all desired toppings: lettuce, cabbage, onions, tomatoes, and avocado.

1 serving

Nutritional serving information: carbohydrate—vegetables 1 ½
carbohydrate—grain 1
protein 2
fat 1 ½

THE APO E GENE DIET SHRIMP CURRY

Ingredients

4 oz. cooked, peeled, de-veined shrimp	1 tsp. cumin powder
⅛ tsp. cayenne	⅛ tsp. paprika
2 small cooked and diced potatoes	¼ tsp red pepper
1 tsp. tomato paste	¼ tsp. whole wheat flour—very little
½ tsp. honey mustard	¼ tsp. dried lavender
1 tbsp. lime juice	2 tbsp. low-fat soy yogurt

Directions

Mix all ingredients in bowl; chill for at least 1–2 hours before serving.

1 serving.

Nutritional serving information: carbohydrate—grains 2
protein 4

THE APO E GENE DIET VEGETABLE AND GARBANZO BEAN CURRY

Ingredients

1 tbsp. extra-virgin olive oil
1 tbsp. whole grain flour
2 garlic cloves, crushed
3 tsp. freshly grated ginger
1 cup coarsely cut carrots
1 large red potato
1 ½ cups garbanzo beans
2 tsp. lemon juice

1 tbsp. tomato paste
½ cup stock
2 shallots, chopped
1 tbsp. ground curry powder, pre-made,
   or freshly ground.
1 cup organic green peas
1 cup low-fat soy milk

Optional herbs and seasonings. You may include any or all of these: Freshly ground coriander seeds, turmeric, fenugreek, ginger, black pepper, dried chilies, cardamoms, cinnamon.

Directions

Cut all vegetables into bite size pieces. Heat oil in a nonstick pan. Add shallots, tomato paste, potato, carrots, whole grain flour, garlic, and ginger. Add in stock slowly, and cook for a few minutes. Add curry spices. Cook, stirring, for 1–2 minutes. Add remaining vegetables, and soy milk. Cook until vegetables are soft. Stir in lemon juice.

4 servings.

Nutritional serving information: carbohydrate—vegetables 2
carbohydrate—grain ½
protein 1
fat 1

THE APO E GENE DIET WHEAT PASTA SALAD

Ingredients

1 lb whole wheat noodles
1 cup asparagus
1 tsp. extra-virgin olive oil
1 small tomato, chopped
¼ cup sweet potato, chopped
¹/₈ cup fresh grated ginger

1 cup garbanzo beans
10 kalamata olives
1 red bell pepper
4 oz. soy cheese
¼ cup shiitake balsamic vinegar
¼ cup fresh basil

Directions

Cook pasta and asparagus in separate saucepans. When pasta and asparagus are cooked, combine with all other ingredients. Serve.

6 servings.

Nutritional serving information: carbohydrate—vegetables 1
carbohydrate—grains 2
protein 2
fat 1

THE APO E GENE DIET PAM'S BAKED POTATO

Ingredients

1 medium baked potato   ½ tsp. extra-virgin olive oil
A pinch of salt on the potato and a pinch of salt over your shoulder for good
    luck

Directions

Preheat oven to 350° F. Wash potato well under warm water and pat dry. Cover the potato with the olive oil and sprinkle a little sea salt for perfection of taste and flavor. Bake your potato in the preheated oven 45–60 minutes.

1 serving.

Nutritional serving information: carbohydrate—grain 1

THE APO E GENE DIET RUSTIC TUSCANY PIZZA

Ingredients

1 packet yeast   1 cup white flour
½ cup whole wheat flour   1 ¼ cups lukewarm water
1 tbsp. honey   ½ cup red onion, chopped
½ cup fresh tomato sauce   1 thinly sliced tomato
1 tsp. extra-virgin olive oil   ¼ cup shiitake mushrooms
1 small roasted garlic clove   4 oz. soy cheese
¼ cup kalamata olives   1 cup chopped red bell pepper

Herbs:

1 tbsp. chopped fresh sweet basil   Chopped fresh parsley
1 tbsp. fresh cilantro   1 tbsp. fresh marjoram
1 tsp. fresh sage   1 tsp. rosemary

Directions

Step One: Make pizza dough. Prepare yeast. Make yeast mixture in a bowl with lukewarm water, yeast, and honey. Allow to stand and rise. In a bowl add the yeast to the whole wheat and white flours. Mix all ingredients until the dough forms a ball. Place freshly made dough in a large bowl with inside of bowl rubbed with olive oil. Cover dough with a clean damp cloth and let it rise in a warm place for approximately 30 minutes or until it has doubled in size.

After dough has risen, knead again and roll out on a clean, dry, floured surface. Divide into equal portions and roll each piece into a ball. Place the dough, covered, in the refrigerator to rest for 1 hour. Bring the dough to room temperature before preparing to use.

Preheat oven to 450° F.

Step Two: Now that you have made your whole wheat crust, coat pizza pan with a little olive oil. Add pizza crust to the pan. Combine tomato sauce and herbs, spread over the dough, and add soy cheese evenly over the surface. Top with vegetables, spreading them evenly over the dough. Bake for 10–14 minutes or until crust is cooked to a light brown.

4 servings.

Nutritional serving information: carbohydrate—grains 3
carbohydrate—vegetables ½
protein 1
fat ¼

THE APO E GENE DIET OLIVE OIL POTATO WEDGEWOOD FRIES

I call these "Wedgewood" fries because they are big wedges and look like wood.

Ingredients

3 russet potatoes

1 tbsp. extra-virgin olive oil (in pump spray bottle)

Salt and ground pepper

Directions

Preheat oven to 450° F.

Cut fresh potatoes into thick wedges. Place cut potatoes into boiling water. Boil for 5 minutes. Drain and place on a cookie sheet which has been lightly sprayed with olive oil. Lightly spray potato wedges with olive oil. Bake for 25 minutes or until golden brown.

6 servings

Nutritional serving information: carbohydrate—grain 1
fat 1

THE APO E GENE DIET MEVAGISSEY RATATOUILLE

I first had this dish in a little bistro in Mevagissey, Cornwall, when I was about 15 or 16. It was so delicious. The flavors from this dish were extremely memorable. What a clever way to eat vegetables, I thought to myself, and to make them taste great!

Ingredients

2 tomatoes, roughly cut

1 small sweet red onion, roughly cut

4 small shallots, roughly chopped pieces

1 clove garlic, crushed

2 tsp. extra-virgin olive oil

1 small red bell pepper, roughly cut

1 small eggplant and zucchini, roughly cut

1 bunch of fresh spinach, rinsed and torn into

$^1/_8$ tsp. lavender

1 cup cooked corn

Directions
Preheat oven to 350° F. Heat olive oil in pan over a low to medium-high heat. Add onions, peppers, eggplant and zucchini, shallots, and garlic to the pan. When lightly browned, add spinach with ½ cup of water. When greens are wilted, add corn and tomatoes and cook for another 5–7 minutes. Pour all ingredients into an oval ceramic baking dish. Bake for 30–40 minutes. Garnish with lavender before serving.

12 servings.

Nutritional serving information: Carbohydrate—vegetables 2

APO E GENE DIET SULTANA, CARROT, GINGER COLESLAW

Ingredients

¹/₈ cup fresh grated ginger

½ cup sultanas

½ cup nonfat plain soy yogurt

1 ½ cups organic grated carrots, raw

¼ cup almonds

1 tsp. fresh squeezed lime juice

Directions
Combine all ingredients. Chill for at least 1 hour.

2 servings.

Nutritional serving information: Carbohydrate—vegetables 1
Carbohydrate—fruit 1
Protein–½
Fat 1

THE APO E GENE DIET GUACAMOLE

I just love the natural goodness of avocado. Until I moved to the United States in 1981, I had never eaten an avocado. Since I arrived I have eaten them often for the healthful qualities—and flavor! Don't forget, avocado contains large amounts of good fat and plant stanols. Plant stanols may reduce cholesterol and are a promising addition to interventions aimed at lowering heart disease risk. One serving of avocado has 137 mg of plant stanol and no partially hydrogenated fats. Compare this to the leading margarine butter substitute spread that has 2–7 mg of plant stanols per serving. Yep, I choose to put fresh avocado in my food.

Ingredients

1 medium soft avocado

½ cup mild sweet onion chopped

½ green pepper

2 medium garlic cloves, finely chopped

2 ripe tomatoes

1 jalapeno

2 tbsp. lime juice

Directions
Combine all ingredients in blender, and blend until smooth.

Or for a fun game your children will love, place all ingredients into a zip lock bag and squish to your heart's content until all the ingredients are blended. Cut off one corner of the zip lock bag and squeeze into a bowl.

4 servings.

Nutritional serving information: Carbohydrate—vegetables 1
                                         Fat 2

SOY YOGURT

Ingredients
1 package yogurt starter   Sea salt—to taste
1 quart soy milk, heated to boiling and cooled to lukewarm

Directions
Sprinkle sea salt over a bowl of moist soy yogurt and allow to set. Refrigerate, stirring occasionally when curds develop.

8 servings.

Nutritional serving information: Protein ½
                                         Fat 1

THE APO E GENE DIET CARROT AND CUCUMBER YOGURT SALAD

Ingredients
¹/₈ cup fresh ginger   2 peeled, grated carrots
1 ½ peeled, grated cucumbers   ¹/₈ tsp. lavender
½ tsp. freshly ground cumin seeds   1 tbsp. chardonnay vinegar
½ tsp. fresh cilantro   3 cups nonfat plain soy yogurt
1 tsp. fresh squeezed lemon juice

Directions
Mix together all ingredients. Chill for at least 1 hour.

4 servings.

Nutritional serving information: carbohydrate—vegetables ½
                                         carbohydrate—fruit ½
                                         protein ½

THE APO E GENE DIET CILANTRO SOY GINGER DRESSING

Ingredients

¼ cup of extra-virgin olive oil

¼ cup fresh chopped cilantro

1 tsp. low sodium soy sauce

¼ tsp. white pepper

1 crushed roasted garlic clove

¼ cup balsamic vinegar

1 tsp. fresh grated ginger

Directions

Make dressing ahead of time: Place all ingredients in a glass salad dressing container, mix well. For best results, let stand in the refrigerator for 8–24 hours.

4 servings.

Nutritional serving information: fats 3

THE APO E GENE DIET SIMPLE SALAD DRESSING

Ingredients

¼ cup extra-virgin olive oil

1 fresh lime—juice of 1 lime

1 tsp. fresh grated ginger

¼ cup chardonnay vinegar

1 tsp. low sodium soy sauce

¼ tsp. white pepper

Directions

Make dressing ahead of time: Place all ingredients in a glass salad dressing container, mix well. For best results, let stand in the refrigerator for 8–24 hours.

4 servings.

Nutritional serving information: fats 3

Food for Thought

At the second nutrition conference Dr. Andrew Weil held in Tucson, Arizona, a physician from Norway spoke about a group of older ladies who used to get together and have tea, sandwiches, and cake while they socialized and shared the traditional recipes of an afternoon tea. Eventually, two of these ladies were told by their doctors that they had to change their diet and stop eating the foods they loved. Soon after they quit attending the daily gatherings, they become much sicker, depressed, and lonely.

Based on this situation, the Norwegian physician learned that these daily gatherings served much more than a meal. They were also a cultural experience and welcome social occasion. What the women needed was a little recipe modification and nutritional help—not orders to disband a cherished get-together. It was this doctor's nurse who actually said, "No, all you need to do is make some changes, not break up the party."

Food has long been a big part of humans communicating love for their family and friends. Along with sustaining the physical body and satisfying basic physiological needs, food also fills emotional, mental, and spiritual needs. It is only recently that we began looking at food from a health-preserving and disease-preventing perspective in such detail.

Having begun to examine the benefits of good whole food, we need to look at some of the foods our families may have eaten in the past, which we may today call "comfort foods." While we don't necessarily need to remove these comforting foods from our diet, we may need to rework old family recipes. In order to maintain a healthy nutritional regimen, good food must include traditional, local, cultural, and high-quality ingredients. Take some time to look over some of your family recipes and see how you can modify the contents to make them healthier. And it can be fun to share with your family the memories you associate with these recipes.

I want to share with you some of my family traditions and recipes from Scotland and England. These are not foods I eat every day or even every week, yet they are traditional foods of my English-Scottish heritage that I prepare occasionally for my family and friends. While it is important to eat a healthy diet for your Apo E genotype most of the time, it is important not to leave behind you those wonderful foods that brought you so much joy. Keep such foods close to your heart and use them to generate good feelings whenever you need them in your life.

A Cornish Tradition—Pasties

Pasties are a cultural food for me and an example of how traditional foods can be enjoyed once in a while so as not to lose the traditional cultural aspect of one's upbringing. I include below the following recipe for Cornish pasties, one I have enjoyed since childhood, in memory of my Nana, Peggy Caine, who died just before this book was published, and my Uncle Brian. Nana Caine lived in Bodmin, Cornwall, all her life, and, believe me, she was a master Cornish pasty maker. I loved her very much. Her very presence emanated love, comfort, and joy. I was not able to share much time with her over the past few years, since she lived in the south of England and I live in California but she taught me the importance of the family dinner table in keeping the family together. Research today shows us that this is true, and I imagine she would be delighted to know that. So always make sure you and your children share at least one meal together each day, and if possible, make that meal dinner. It's such a good way to end the day. I assure you, the end result is a happy family.

Nana had a very specific way of making her pasties (pronounced "pass-tees"), and I am going to share the recipe she taught to me from about the age of 10. But first I would like to tell you a little history of the Cornish pasty. Pasties are said to be the original handheld convenience food, with a lineage that dates back to the Middle Ages, although no one knows for certain when they showed up on our ancestors' lunch plates—possibly as far back as the 1100s or 1300s, or maybe centuries afterward in the late 1700s or early 1800s. A common story told in Cornish inns, fishing villages, misty moorlands, and coastlines is that the history of the Cornish Pasty stretches back to the time of King Arthur—pasties may have come from Tintagel, his birthplace. Stories of King Arthur's Cornwall, with the legends of Camelot, are without question the best known and most fascinating of all Cornish folklore.

But no matter when they were first created, we have no doubt that Cornish pasties came from Cornwall. This dish grew out of a basic need to take hot, satisfying, high-calorie food into the cold Cornish tin mines. Served at lunchtime, pasties were meant to provide the miners with the fuel to get them through the rest of the day. The classic tin-mine pasty contained meat and root vegetables in one end and fruit such as apples, plums, or fruit preserves in the other end. It was also common to see a person's initials on one side of the pasty casing, in order to avoid mix-up at lunchtime. Nana carried on this time-bound tradition by putting our initials on the pasties so we didn't get someone else's, which was good because I would never want a pasty that was made for my sister. She never liked turnips, and turnips were my favorite part.

One very distinct feature of the Cornish pasty is the way it is put together. To close the pasty you need to perform a special seal technique called crimping, the wave-like seal that holds the pasty together. It is a little tricky to learn, but once you get the crimping down, it becomes a most enjoyable part of the whole pasty-making process. Essentially, to "crimp," you hold the two sides of the dough together and by making little twists and folds, you seal the dough on the top. A never-ending debate about the Cornish pasty is whether the sealing crimp should be on the side or on top. My vote is to crimp on the side because that makes the pasty easier to eat.

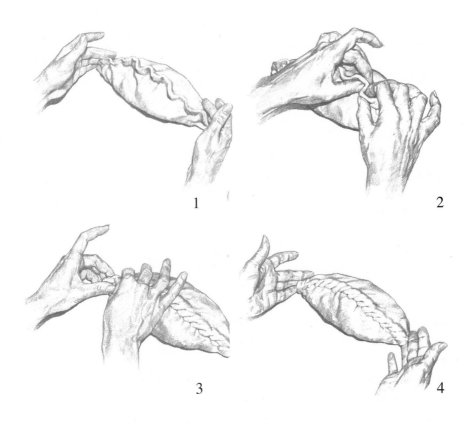

1

2

3

4

As you can see, there is a lot of history and debate surrounding the Cornish pasty, which nourishes the tummy as well as the heart and soul. Luckily, though, one thing that all true traditional pasty makers can definitely agree upon is the quality of the ingredients: The food should be the highest quality. If meat is used, it should be the leanest, best cuts available, and it should be cut into bite-size pieces, rendering true flavor. The vegetables should always be neatly sliced and diced, and the ingredients must never be cooked before they are wrapped inside the pasty. All of the ingredients are to be raw and cooked all at once inside the pasty in the oven.

Cornish pasty-making is an art, as my Uncle Brian would say. This is the "Culture of our Land," and if you want to experience a Cornish pasty you need to make it with the spirit of the past. As a child, when I delivered dairy products for Uncle Brian's dairy delivery company to authentic pasty shops and kitchens, I saw how the cooks followed the old rules of making pasties. A prime requirement was having the intention of delivering healthy food for good, hard-working people: Use garden-fresh, wholesome ingredients, such as turnips, onions, potatoes, and parsley, and this will feed your body and soul for hours. (Remember to cut parsley with scissors, not a knife).

The goodness and love wrapped neatly in this little packet we call a Cornish pasty helps me imagine the tin miners taking a break to enjoy theirs. Before you make your pasty, take a minute to set your own mind to good intention—to provide a tasty meal for today made with love and devotion to the delicious details of the Cornish tradition from hundreds of years ago.

Nana Caine's recipe for Cornish pasties has meat in it. If you do not eat meat, you can leave it out. You may want to substitute the traditional lean beef with chicken, fish, tofu, beans, lentils, salmon, lamprey eels, or carrots (even though some say putting carrot in a pasty is a sin, I love carrot in my pasty so I put it in, transgression or not). Even though these ingredients are not in the traditional recipe, I have tried them all, and they are all delicious. Tales from the past tell us that some miners actually ate only the filling and discarded the buttery crust. So if you wanted to do that, you could.

Slàinte mhòr agad! (SLAHN-tchuh VORR AH-kut!) Scottish for "Great health to you!"

NANA CAINE AND UNCLE BRIAN'S CORNISH PASTY
Pasty Crust
Ingredients
3 cups unbleached flour
Traditional recipe: 1 ½ sticks butter (never use margarine, as this is very bad fat)
Heart healthy version: 1 ½ cups canola oil
1 ½ tsp. salt
6 tbsp. water

Directions
In a large bowl, combine unbleached flour, butter or oil, and salt. Mix ingredients until well combined. Add water, one tablespoon at a time, to form a dough. Incorporate mixture well until it is a ball. Knead dough with heel of the hand to distribute butter evenly. Lightly dust the dough with a little flour, cover with wax paper. Place the dough, covered, in the refrigerator to rest for 30 minutes. Bring the dough to room temperature before preparing to use.

Pasty Filling

Ingredients

1 lb. round steak, very coarsely ground	2 large onions, chopped
2 potatoes, peeled and chopped	½ cup turnip or rutabaga, chopped
2 tsp. salt	1 egg, beaten
½ tsp. pepper	A tiny piece of butter on top with the salt and pepper

Directions

Preheat oven to 350° F. Combine all filling ingredients in a large bowl, then set aside. Next, divide the dough into 6 pieces and roll one of the pieces into a 10-inch round on a lightly floured surface. Put 1 ½ cups of filling in the middle of the pastry round, add salt and pepper to taste and your tiny piece of butter. Moisten the edges with a little water and fold the edges together to enclose the pasty. Pinch the edges together to seal them, and crimp (see directions above). Place pasty onto a lightly greased baking sheet and draw your initials in the top of your pasty. Also, use a knife to make 1 slit in the top. Brush the top of whole pasty with beaten egg to help seal the crimping and give it a beautiful glazed finish. Bake in preheated oven for 60 minutes. Remove from oven, cover with a tea towel, cool for 15 minutes. Humm humm—I can hear Nana tell me it is time for my pasty right now.

6 servings.   Exchanges per serving = 10 fat, 3 protein, 3 grains.

Nutritional serving information: carbohydrate—grains 3
protein 3
fat 10

The Magic Ingredient for Cornish Pasties

One winter afternoon around 4 o'clock, I was making Cornish Pasties in our kitchen when my daughter Paige, who was 5 years old, dragged her little wooden stool next to me so she could help me and also hear the stories of the Cornish pixies and fairies, Blue Bell Woods, the Cornish castles, and King Arthur. (Victoria and Alison, my older daughters, used to cook with me, too, but they are 11 and 20 years of age now, and while they don't quite believe in my fairy stories anymore, they believe in my pasties.)

Paige said, "So, Mum, do fairies and pixies from Blue Bell Woods like Cornish Pasties, too?"

"Of course they do," I replied. "Cornish fairies love vegetables and fruit, and Cornish pasties have lots of those. Cornish fairies are a big part of making pasties. Who do you think collects all those herbs for the green grocer to sell to all the mummies to bake our pasties? Parsley is the magic ingredient of pasties. That magic comes from the fairies."

"Oh, that's right, Mum, I forgot. How silly of me!" Then she pauses, thinking about the information I had just given her. "So, Mum, how do they carry so many herbs, when fairies are so small?"

"They have a magic herb pouch," I said, "just like the pixie and fairy dust pouch, that they carry with them wherever they fly."

"They do? Fairies must be very strong. No, I think they have help, mom."

Oh boy, these 5 year olds keep you thinking! However, at dinner time, Paige told the whole family about how the fairies collected the magic herbs for the green grocer so Mummy could make the pasties.

Keep your children dreaming and cooking with you. And always allow them to sprinkle the magical ingredients into the dish you are making.

PAM'S CORNISH PASTIES—THE HEART HEALTHY VERSION

Pasty short-crust ingredients

1 ½ cups whole wheat flour	¾ cup of olive oil
Pinch of salt	Water

Pasty filling ingredients

Note: all filling ingredients are to be kept separate. All kinds of vegetables and herbs can be placed inside a pasty, potatoes being one main ingredient. Additional possibilities include fish, spinach, shallots, leeks, carrots, parsnips, onion, parsley, turnip, watercress .

For this recipe, I am going to use: Fish, potatoes, carrots, onion, and the magic ingredient—parsley.

Directions

Make your short-crust and allow to cool in the refrigerator. Bring out your short-crust and roll it out, on a floured kitchen counter, to the size of a dinner plate. In the middle of the short-crust, ingredient by ingredient, layer the vegetables and fish filling, ending with the fish and a magic sprinkle of parsley. Dampen the edge of the pastry with water. Then take one edge of the circle of short-crust and fold it over to meet the other edge and press the edges of the dough together, to make a half-moon shape. Then crimp (see directions above) the edges of the pasty. Make a small hole with a knife to let out steam while cooking. Brush with an egg white and soy milk wash glaze. Place your pasty on a lightly greased metal baking sheet, bake for 1 hour at 450° F. Allow to cool and serve on your best English china plate with a fresh mixed garden salad.

The Apo E Pacific Rim Sauces

These sauces can be used on fish, beans, tofu, lentils, and chicken. If you don't have the time to make a sauce yourself, you may be able to locate a pre-made sauce similar to this recipe at a local store. Choose one that has the best possible ingredients in it. Look for a product made with natural flavorings and a monounsaturated or polyunsaturated oil, such as olive oil or canola oil. Choose a product that does not have artificial flavorings or preservatives. Stay with natural whole foods as much as possible.

The Ancient Chinese Wok

The wok has been used in Chinese cooking for approximately 2,000 years. Usually made out of metal, the wok has a distinct wide, deep bowl shape and can be used for either slow or rapid cooking. The versatility of this cooking tool is one of the main reasons why it has remained a major part of Asian cooking and is now used by cooks around the world. In addition, it requires little fuel, making it economical to use.

PACIFIC RIM FISH AND VEGETABLES IN A WOK

This recipe may include any of the Pacific Rim Sauces. When choosing your Pacific Rim Sauce, keep in mind your available daily servings of fat based on your individual Apo E genotype and calories allowed.

Ingredients

½ tsp. olive oil

¼ cup water chestnuts

¼ cup green onion

¹/₈ cup shallots

3 oz. organic tofu or fish

¼ cup vegetable stock

¼ cup red bell pepper

¼ cup grated carrots

¼ cup young English pea pods

Directions

Lightly spray the wok first with olive oil and then heat remaining olive oil. Cook the onion and shallots lightly. Add all other vegetables and cook for 2–3 minutes more. Then add tofu or fish and cook until lightly brown. Add Pacific Rim Sauce of your choosing after tofu has browned. Continue to warm for an additional 2–3 minutes or until the sauce is well heated. Serve over Basmati rice or Chinese noodles.

1 serving.   Exchanges per serving = 3 protein, ½ fat, 2 vegetables.

Nutritional serving information: carbohydrate—vegetables 2
protein 1
fat 1

THE APO E GENE DIET PEANUT SAUCE

This all-around delicious sauce can be stirred into rice, noodles, or cooked with vegetables, as well as on beans, fish, tofu etc.

Ingredients

1 tbsp. freshly ground peanut butter

¼ cup fresh cilantro

¼ cup water

2 tbsp. tamari sauce

1 tbsp. lime juice and lemon juice

¼ cup nonfat soy milk

1 tbsp. extra-virgin olive oil

1 tsp. fresh grated ginger

1 tsp. turmeric

1 tsp. ready-made tomato paste

1 tbsp. honey

3 tsp. fresh crushed garlic

1 small onion or scallion

Directions

Heat the olive oil in a pan over moderate heat. Brown the onion, garlic, and ginger until the onion is transparent. Add turmeric; cook for 1 minute until well mixed. Add the soy milk, peanut butter, cilantro, honey, lime and lemon juice, tomato paste, and water. Bring the sauce to a gentle boil, then reduce heat and simmer for 12–15 minutes.

4 servings.

Nutritional serving information: fat 2

THE APO E GENE DIET THAI HAZELNUT SAUCE

Ingredients

1 cup freshly ground hazelnut butter 2 ½ tsp. tamari
¼ cup honey   1 tsp. soy sauce
1 ½ tsp. vinegar   ¼ tsp. cayenne
¼ tsp. paprika   ½ cup miso soup
¼ cup sweet vinegar   2 chopped garlic cloves
2 tsp. fresh grated ginger—(grate with a medium-sized grater)

Directions

Combine all ingredients. Let sit for 1 hour in refrigerator to allow all the flavors to mingle together.

4 servings.

Nutritional serving information: fat 2

THE APO E GENE DIET TERIYAKI SAUCE

Ingredients

¼ cup low-sodium soy sauce   1 tsp. fresh grated ginger
1 tbsp. honey   ¼ cup of water
¼ cup apple cider   ¼ cup organic vinegar
1 tsp. sesame oil   1 tbsp. lime juice
2 tsp. shallots, finely chopped

Directions

Add oil to a low heat skillet. Then add garlic and cook for 2 minutes. Add all other ingredients slowly, stirring as you add ingredients. Once all ingredients have been added, cook for another 5–7 minutes on medium heat.

8 servings.

Nutritional serving information: fat 1

THE APO E GENE DIET SOY GINGER SAUCE

Ingredients

1 tsp. fresh ginger   ¼ cup low-sodium soy sauce
¼ tsp. turmeric   1 tbsp. honey
¼ cup of water   ¼ cup chardonnay vinegar
1 tbsp. lime juice and lemon juice   2 tsp. fresh crushed garlic
1 tbsp. extra-virgin olive oil

Directions
Heat oil in skillet on low heat. Add garlic and cook for 2 minutes. Add all other ingredients slowly stirring as you add each ingredient. Once all ingredients have been added, cook for another 5–7 minutes on medium heat.

4 servings.

Nutritional serving information: fat ½

THE APO E GENE DIET TOMATO SALSA CREAM

Ingredients
1 cup fresh tomato salsa   1 cup soy yogurt
1 tsp. lemon juice   1 tsp. fresh grated ginger

Directions
Combine all ingredients together. Chill for 1 hour before serving.

2 servings.

Nutritional serving information: carbohydrate–fruit 1
                                        protein ½
                                        fat ½

THE APO E GENE DIET MANGO SALSA CREAM

Ingredients
1 cup fresh mango salsa (see below)   1 cup soy yogurt
1 tsp. lemon   ¹/₃ cup chopped cilantro
1 tsp. fresh ginger

Directions
Mix ingredients together. Chill for 1 hour before serving.

2 servings.

Nutritional serving information: carbohydrate–fruit 1
                                        protein ½
                                        fat ½

THE APO E GENE DIET HAWAIIAN MANGO SALSA

Ingredients
½ cup of red pepper   1 finely diced Jalapeno pepper–mild
   type
1 cup English cucumber   ½ cup of cilantro chopped
Juice of two fresh limes   1 avocado–chopped if desired
1 ½ cups ripe mango fruit–chopped into small pieces
1 cup of Maui sweet onion–chopped into small pieces

Directions
Mix all ingredients in a bowl.

4 servings.

Nutritional serving information: carbohydrate–vegetable 1
carbohydrate–fruit 1
fat ½

THE APO E GENE DIET PAPAYA SALSA CREAM

This is one of my favorite salsa creams. When our family goes to Maui for a vacation, we often lease a home and invite our friends along. One great thing about staying in a home in Hawaii instead of a hotel is cooking your own meals. We love to prepare food and grill together—our friend Cleve Palmer is an excellent griller. Our favorite foods include fresh Hawaiian fish (heads removed), fresh vegetables, and salads. We love potatoes baked in olive oil and topped with this fresh Papaya Salsa cream. Life doesn't get any better—great place, great friends, and fantastic food. My dear friend Cleve inspired this recipe, since we share a real love for fresh ingredients, fresh vine-ripened tomatoes, basil, extra-virgin olive oil, and our Papaya Salsa Cream. (Cleve should have been a chef.)

Ingredients
1 cup fresh chopped papaya salsa   1 cup nonfat soy yogurt
1 tsp. lime   1 tsp. fresh grated ginger
½ cup sweet onion (Maui onion)   ⅓ cup chopped cilantro

Directions
Mix both ingredients together. Chill for 1 hour before serving.

4 servings.

Nutritional serving information: carbohydrate–fruit 1
protein ¼

THE APO E PAPAYA SALSA CREAM

Ingredients
1 cup fresh papaya salsa   1 cup soy yogurt
1 tsp. lemon   1 tsp. fresh grated ginger

Directions
Mix both ingredients together. Chill for 1 hour before serving.

4 servings.

Nutritional serving information: carbohydrate–fruit 1
protein ½
fat ½

Desserts

THE APO E GENE DIET CRUMBLES

Here are some examples of crumble recipes. Fresh fruit crumbles are a well-known English dessert, which I grew up eating at dinner. Our crumble usually consisted of apple, blackberry, raspberry, gooseberry, and rhubarb—the fruits my grandmother had in our garden. Of course, the crumbles I ate were made a little differently back then and usually were smothered with either Cornish clotted cream (a delicious decadent cream with 60 g of saturated fat per serving) or Kelly's Cornish Ice Cream. Very delicious memories! Today my focus is on modifying this delicious food to a healthy alternative. I hope you enjoy these recipes. The love from my grandmothers, Nana McDonald and Nana Caine, is in every one.

THE APO E GENE DIET VERY BERRY FRUIT SALAD

Ingredients

1 cup black currants

1 cup blackberries

1 cup blueberries

1 cup strawberries, cut in quarters

1 cup raspberries

Directions

Wash all fruit well. Cut fruit and place in a chilled bowl. Serve with your favorite frozen yogurt.

Alternative Directions

Freeze fresh berries in individual baggies in ¾ cup portions. When you are ready to serve a dessert, remove berries directly from the freezer, place on your favorite china dessert plates, and cover berries with warm Apo E Gene Diet English Vanilla Custard. This makes a delicious after-dinner or night-time snack.

10 servings.

Nutritional serving information: carbohydrate–fruit 1

Consider Black Currants

In World War II England, fresh citrus fruit was difficult to get from 1940 on, so black currant became a very popular fruit for its vitamin C, and the British government encouraged people to cultivate it. The taste became so popular, a black currant cordial was given out free to all British children, including me. Even Rowntrees, one of the largest candy makers in England, produced a candy called Fruit Gums, and the best flavor in my book is black currant. Ask any British Fruit Gum lover and they will tell you the black currant Fruit Gums are one of the best candies. Whether black currant is eaten fresh off the bushes in the garden or in popular candies, or whether it's turned into juice, the flavor is very good. Why should you consider eating black currant? In addition to vitamin C, black currants contain a very important source of essential fatty acid called gamma-linolenic acid (GLA).

THE APO E GENE DIET PEAR AND CURRANT CRUMBLE

Ingredients

2 pears, peeled, cored, and sliced
1 ½ cup organic Scottish rolled oats
¼ tsp. vanilla extract
²/₃ cup apple juice

1 cup currants
½ tsp. cinnamon
¹/₃ cup organic local honey
1 tsp. arrowroot

Directions

Preheat oven to 350° F. Layer sliced pears and currents in a nonstick baking dish. Mix the remaining ingredients in a bowl. Spread over fruit. Bake for 40 minutes. Delicious alone or serve with your recommended accompaniment such as nonfat ice cream or low-fat soy yogurt.

4 servings.

Nutritional serving information: Carbohydrate–fruit 1 ½
Carbohydrate–grain 2

THE APO E GENE DIET APPLE AND PEACH CRUMBLE

Ingredients

2 fresh peaches, peeled and sliced	1 Russet apple, peeled and sliced
1 cup sultanas	1 ½ cups organic Scottish rolled oats
½ tsp. cinnamon	1 sprinkle of lavender, if desired
1/8 tsp. vanilla extract	1/3 tsp. honey
2/3 cup apple juice	1 tsp. arrowroot

Directions

Preheat oven to 350° F. Layer sliced pears in a nonstick baking dish. Mix the remaining ingredients in a bowl. Spread over fruit. Bake for 40 minutes. Delicious alone or serve with your recommended accompaniment such as nonfat ice cream or soy yogurt, such as Nancy's brand soy yogurt, carrageenan-free.

4 servings.

Nutritional serving information: carbohydrate–fruit 1 ½
                                          carbohydrate–grain 2

THE APO E GENE DIET APPLE AND GRAPE CRUMBLE

Ingredients

2 fresh apples, peeled and sliced	1 cup concord red grapes
¾ cup organic Scottish rolled oats	¾ cup low-fat granola
½ tsp. cinnamon	1/8 tsp. vanilla extract
1/3 tsp. honey	2/3 cup red grape juice
1 tsp. arrowroot	

Directions

Preheat oven to 350° F. Layer apples and grapes in a nonstick baking dish. Mix the remaining ingredients in a bowl. Spread over fruit. Bake for 40 minutes. Delicious alone or serve with your favored accompaniment—nonfat ice cream or soy yogurt.

4 servings.   Exchanges per serving = 1 ½ fruit, 2 grain

Nutritional serving information: carbohydrate–fruit 1 ½
                                          carbohydrate–grain 2

THE APO E GENE DIET PEAR AND BLUEBERRY CRUMBLE

Ingredients

2 pears, peeled and sliced	1 cup fresh or frozen blueberries
1 ½ cup organic Scottish rolled oats	½ tsp. cinnamon
1/8 tsp. vanilla extract	1/3 honey
2/3 cup blueberry juice	1 tsp. arrowroot

Directions
Bake in a 350° F oven. Layer sliced pears and blueberries in a nonstick baking dish. Mix the remaining ingredients in a bowl. Spread over fruit. Bake for 40 minutes. Delicious alone or serve with your recommended accompaniment—nonfat soy ice cream or low-fat soy yogurt.

4 servings.

Nutritional serving information: carbohydrate–fruit 2
                                        carbohydrate–grain 1
                                        protein ½

THE APO E GENE DIET PEACH AND BLACKBERRY CRUMBLE

Ingredients
2 fresh peaches, peeled and sliced   1 cup fresh or frozen blackberries
1 ½ cup organic Scottish rolled oats   ¹/₈ tsp. vanilla extract
¹/₃ tsp. honey   ½ cup black currant or blackberry juice
1 tsp. arrowroot

Directions
Bake in a 350° F oven. Layer sliced peaches and add blackberries in a nonstick baking dish. Mix the remaining ingredients in a bowl. Spread over fruit. Bake for 40 minutes. Delicious alone or serve with your recommended accompaniment—nonfat soy ice cream or soy yogurt.

4 servings.   Exchanges per serving = 1 ½ fruit, 2 grain.

Nutritional serving information: carbohydrate–fruit 1 ½
                                        carbohydrate–grain 2

THE APO E BLACK CURRANT AND RHUBARB CRUMBLE

Ingredients
2 stalks fresh rhubarb, peeled and sliced 1 cup fresh or frozen black currants
1 ½ cups rolled oats   ¹/₈ tsp. vanilla extract
¹/₃ tsp. honey   ½ cup black currant juice
1 tsp. arrowroot

Directions
Preheat oven to 350° F. Layer sliced rhubarb in a nonstick baking dish, add black currants. Mix the remaining ingredients in a bowl. Spread over fruit. Bake for 40 minutes. Delicious alone, or serve with your recommended accompaniment—nonfat soy ice cream or soy yogurt.

4 servings.   Exchanges per serving = 1 ½ fruit, 2 grain.

Nutritional serving information: carbohydrate–fruit 1 ½
                                        carbohydrate–grain 2

THE APO E GENE DIET BAKED PEARS OR APPLES

Ingredients

4 medium organic pears or apples   1 ½ cups of water
¼ cup black currant juice   1 tsp. lemon juice
¼ cup organic honey   2 tsp. fresh whole cloves
¼ tsp. fresh ground cinnamon   ½ cup of sultanas
¼ cup slivered almonds   Fresh mint

Directions

Preheat oven to 350° F. Peel pears, leaving the stems on for decoration. Combine sultanas, black currant juice, honey, and lemon together in a saucepan. Bring sauce to a boil and remove to cool. Sprinkle cinnamon over pears. Place cinnamon, peeled pears, and water with cloves in a heavy dish and place in the oven. Bake on 350° F. until pears are tender, approximately 20–30 minutes. After pears are baked, remove them to individual decorative plates. Drizzle some of the warm sultana, honey, and black currant sauce over each pear. Top with slivered almonds and fresh mint. This recipe can also be made with an apple instead of a pear.

4 servings.

Nutritional serving information: carbohydrate–fruit 1 ½

THE APO E GENE DIET SCOTTISH FRUIT POTTAGE

Ingredients

2 ½ cups fresh mixed berries, mix and match: loganberry, gooseberry, blueberry, bilberry, huckleberry, blackberry, raspberry, currants, cranberry, grape, strawberry
2 tsp. grated lemon rind
2 tsp. honey
1/8 tsp. lavender

Directions

Puree berries in blender. Blend in lemon rind with honey. Use as a topping for desserts. 1 serving is ¾ cup.

4 servings.

Nutritional serving information: carbohydrate–fruit 1

THE APO E GENE DIET KELLY'S FORE STREET DESSERT

I literally made this dessert hundreds, if not thousands, of times as a young waitress growing up. It was a Kelly's Cornish ice cream favorite. People came from all over England to have one of these. I have modified the recipe to be heart-healthy.

Ingredients

6 oz. vanilla soy frozen yogurt

2 tbsp. dark chocolate (70%), melted

1 banana

¼ cup Apo E Scottish Fruit Pottage

2 tbsp. chopped almonds

½ cup berries

Directions

Slice banana in half lengthwise. Place in glass dessert dish, with one half on either side of dish. Place vanilla frozen yogurt in between the banana halves. Add chocolate sauce and fruit pottage, and then berries and nuts.

2 servings.

Nutritional serving information: carbohydrate–fruit 2

protein ½

fat 1

THE APO E GENE DIET ENGLISH VANILLA CUSTARD

This is the modified English custard, perhaps also known as the classic traditional British dessert sauce.

Ingredients

1 tsp. vanilla essence extract

1 cup egg substitute

2 oz. honey

1 cup skim or soy milk

1 tbsp. arrowroot

Directions

Place milk and vanilla in a saucepan. Place over a low heat. Heat to just below boiling point. While the milk is heating, whisk the egg substitute, arrowroot, and honey together in a medium bowl, using a balloon whisk. Then, while whisking the egg mixture with one hand, slowly pour the hot milk into the bowl. When it's all in, immediately return all the ingredients back to the saucepan, then place on a low gentle heat as you continue stirring until the custard is thick and creamy.

4 servings.

Nutritional serving information: protein 1

THE APO E GINGER BISCUITS

Ingredients

1 cup unbleached whole wheat flour

2 tsp. baking soda

1 tsp. cinnamon

¼ tsp. vanilla

¾ cup canola oil

½ cup applesauce unsweetened

1 cup unbleached white flour

Pinch of salt

1 pinch of clove spice

¾ tsp. freshly grated ginger

½ cup brown sugar

2 egg whites

Directions
Preheat oven to 350° F. Sift all dry ingredients together. In another bowl mix canola oil and sugar, add the ginger. Add all the wet ingredients to the canola mixture, and mix well. Slowly add the dry ingredients. Roll into 1-inch balls and place on a nonstick cookie sheet. Bake in the oven for 12–14 minutes, until lightly browned. Allow to cool before removing from cookie sheet.

24 servings.

Nutritional serving information: carbohydrate–grain ½
fat ½

THE APO E GENE DIET LEMON GINGER BISCUITS

Ingredients

1 cup unbleached whole wheat flour	1 cup unbleached white flour
2 tsp. baking soda	Pinch of salt
1 tsp. cinnamon	¾ tsp. grated lemon rind
¼ tsp. vanilla bean extract	¾ tsp. freshly grated ginger
¾ cup canola oil	½ cup brown sugar
½ cup applesauce	2 egg whites

Directions
Preheat oven to 350° F. Sift all dry ingredients together. In another bowl mix canola oil and sugar, add the ginger. Then add all the wet ingredients to the oil and sugar mix, and mix well. Then slowly add the dry ingredients. Make 1-inch balls and place on a nonstick cookie sheet. Bake in the oven for 12–14 minutes or until done. Allow to cool on a cooling sheet.

Nutritional serving information: carbohydrate–grain ½
fat ½

THE APO E GENE DIET RASPBERRY GINGER BISCUITS

Ingredients

1 cup unbleached whole wheat flour	1 cup unbleached white flour
2 tsp. baking soda	Pinch of salt
1 tsp. cinnamon	¼ tsp. vanilla
¾ tsp. freshly grated ginger	¾ cup canola oil
½ cup brown sugar	½ cup applesauce and raspberries
2 egg whites	

Directions

Preheat oven to 350° F. Sift all dry ingredients together. In another bowl, mix canola oil and sugar, add the ginger. Mix all the wet ingredients together. Slowly add the dry ingredients. Mix well. Make one-inch round balls on a nonstick cookie sheet. Bake in the oven for 12–14 minutes, or until done. Allow to cool on a cooling sheet.

24 servings.

Nutritional serving information: carbohydrate–grain ½
fat ½

THE APO E ORANGE GINGER BISCUITS

Ingredients

1 cup unbleached whole wheat flour	1 cup unbleached white flour
2 tsp. baking soda	Pinch of salt
1 tsp. cinnamon	¼ tsp. vanilla extract
¼ tsp. grated orange rind	¾ tsp. freshly grated ginger
¾ cup canola oil	½ cup brown sugar
¼ cup unsweetened applesauce	1/8 cup orange juice
2 egg whites	

Directions

Preheat oven to 350° F. Sift all dry ingredients together. In another bowl mix canola oil and sugar, add the ginger. Then add all the wet ingredients, mix well. Then slowly add the dry ingredients. Make one-inch round balls on a nonstick cookie sheet. Bake in the oven for 12–14 minutes. Or bake until done. Allow to cool on a cooling sheet.

24 servings.

Nutritional serving information: carbohydrate–grain ½
fat ½

Teas and Other Fluids

What to drink? As we have learned, pure water is one the best fluids for the human body, but what we put into our water can be either beneficial or harmful. Drinking only water all the time can be boring for many people—a fact that drives our beverage industry. However, adding flavors in the form of teas and herbal infusions or other beneficial substances such as polyphenols can do a body good. I have added some interesting options here for you to try. I enjoy these flavors and so do my patients.

We have been using plants and foods as medicines for thousands of years, ever since humans learned to draw medicinals from a plant by extracting substances through steeping leaves in hot or cold water. From these ancient practices come some of our foundational beverage traditions, such as the tradition of steeping tea and coffee. However, other plants and beans have been used for beverages for hundreds of years. Today, we are exploring various steeped beverages for their health benefits, such as tea.

A famous evening tea I know well from my childhood is chamomile tea, known for its gentle calming effects. And, of course, I think the best variety of chamomile is English (Chamaemelum nobile). Growing up in England, we were all told the stories of our little furry friend, Peter Rabbit. As the story goes, Peter Rabbit's mother used chamomile tea to help calm him down and send him off to sleep after his adventures in Mr. MacGregor's garden.

My patients ask me all the time: "What do you drink if you don't drink soda or coffee? Water is boring." Here are a few delicious substitutes.

Simple Teas

HOT GREEN TEA

1 bag of green tea

HOT GINGER GREEN TEA

1 Bag of green tea   1 Bag of ginger tea

THE APO E GENE DIET HOT CHAMOMILE HIBISCUS TEA

1 oz. dried chamomile flowers   1 bag of hibiscus tea
                                     or 3 bags of chamomile tea

THE GREEN AND RED TEA

(This is a pretty drink)
1 bag of green tea   1 bag of hibiscus tea
1 slice of lemon

HIBISCUS ELDER TEA

1 bag of hibiscus elder tea   1 serving of natural honey if desired

HOT CHAMOMILE PEACH HERBAL TEA

1 bag of chamomile tea   1 bag of peach tea

HOT DECAF PEACH HERBAL TEA

1 bag of chamomile tea   optional slice of peach

Directions
To a warmed, dry teapot, add any of these tea combinations. Add boiling water. Wait 2–5 minutes for the tea to infuse. Serve in your favorite teacup. Take a moment to rest and sip your delicious drink.

GINGER AND TURMERIC TEA

Ginger and turmeric have been found to be beneficial for reducing inflammation in the body. Adding these delicious herbs as an anti-inflammatory drink to your daily diet may be very helpful in reducing your risk of inflammatory diseases.

Ingredients
1 cup boiling water   ½ tsp. ginger powder
½ tsp. turmeric powder   ¼ tsp. cloves
1 tbsp. honey   Juice of ½ lime or lemon

Directions
In your teapot, place ginger, cloves, and turmeric. Add boiling water, steep for 5 minutes. Add honey and lemon to taste. Best drunk immediately.

BLACK CURRANT, GINGER, AND TURMERIC TEA

Ingredients

1 cup boiling water   2 tsp. black currant
½ tsp. ginger powder   ½ tsp. turmeric powder
¼ tsp. cloves   1 tbsp. honey

Directions
In your teapot, place ginger, cloves, and turmeric. Add boiling water, steep for 5 minutes. Add honey and blackcurrant juice. Best drunk immediately.

HOT LEMON GINGER GREEN TEA

Ingredients

Bag of green tea   squeeze of fresh lemon
slice of fresh ginger

Directions
To a warmed, dry teapot, add your favorite bag of green tea and a squeeze of fresh lemon, and a slice of fresh ginger. Add boiling water. Wait 2–5 minutes for the green tea, ginger, and lemon to infuse. Serve in your favorite teacup. Take a moment to rest and sip your delicious tea.

HOT WHITE TEA WITH CRANBERRIES

Ingredients

1 bag of white tea   1 bag of cranberry tea
A few fresh cranberries

Directions
In a warmed, dry teapot, add your favorite bag of white tea and a bag of cranberry tea. Add a few fresh cranberries to your cup. Add boiling water. Wait 2–5 minutes for the tea to infuse. Serve in your favorite teacup. Take a moment to rest and sip your delicious tea, and reflect on your day.

WHITE MINT TEA

Ingredients

1 oz of your favorite loose leaf   1 sprig of fresh mint
1 bag of mint tea, white tea or 1 white tea bag

Directions
To a warmed, dry teapot, add 1 oz of your favorite loose-leaf white tea or 1 white tea bag and 1 bag of mint tea and a sprig of fresh mint. Add boiling water. Wait a few minutes for the tea to infuse. Serve in your favorite teacup. Take a moment to rest and sip your delicious tea.

HOT GINGER GREEN TEA

Ingredients

1 bag of green tea   1 bag of ginger tea

Directions
To a warmed, dry teapot, add your favorite bag of green tea and 1 bag of ginger tea. Add boiling water. Wait a few minutes for the tea to infuse. Serve in your favorite teacup. Take a moment to rest and sip your delicious tea.

CLASSIC ENGLISH TEA WITH MILK

(A classic afternoon tea break drink)

English people believe in taking a break and a rest in the afternoon—try adding a little British into your day, and take a break. It doesn't have to be long, even five or 10 minutes. You will be surprised how much better you feel after your break.

Ingredients

1 English China teapot—warmed   1 English China teacup
Loose-leaf tea or tea bags   Skim milk or soy milk, if desired

Directions
To your china teapot add 1 serving per person of either loose-leaf tea or traditional tea bags—1 tsp. or bag per person and 1 for the pot. Add freshly boiled water to the pot, then brew for 3–5 minutes. Not longer or shorter—shorter doesn't give you all the flavor, longer can make it bitter. Pour your piping hot tea into an English china teacup. If you prefer milk in your tea, pour a little milk in the bottom of the teacup before you pour the hot tea in (skim or soy milk). Sip your tea and dream of your perfect day.

CORNISH PIXIE GREEN ROSE LEMONADE

Ingredients

1 bag green tea   1 bag hibiscus herbal tea
lemon juice   slices of lemon
baby rose petals

Directions

Add boiling water to tea, allow to cool. Squeeze juice of lemons. Mix tea and juice together and pour over freshly crushed ice. Drop sliced lemons and baby rose petals to the top of your drink and glasses. Listen for the whispers of the fairies and pixies. For the moms of the world, this is a very good drink to sip with little girls while you share a story about fairies.

LEMON LIMEADE WITH WILD MINT

Ingredients

1 bag basic green tea   1 bag wild mint tea (or use fresh mint)
Squeeze of lemon and lime juices   Slices of lemon and lime

Directions

Brew 1 bag of your favorite basic green tea with 1 bag of wild mint herbal tea. You can use fresh mint if you have it. Add boiling water. Brew your tea and allow to cool. Squeeze juice of lemons and lime mix tea and juice together and pour over freshly crushed ice. For the top: Add sliced lemons and limes to the top of your drink and glasses.

Waters

Earlier in the book I encouraged you to drink fresh pure water. Plain water is refreshing if it has no added substances. However, water can be a wonderful beverage if fresh fruit juices, berries and herbs are added. Consider the following combinations for a refreshing change to your water.

SPARKLING LIME JUICE ICED WATER

crushed ice

lime slices

sparkling water

juice of 1 ½ limes

SPARKLING ORANGE ICED WATER

crushed ice

orange slices

sparkling water

juice of 1 ½ oranges

SPARKLING LEMON ICED WATER

crushed ice

lemon slices

sparkling water

juice of 1 ½ lemons

SPARKLING HIBISCUS ICED WATER

crushed ice

lemon slices

sparkling water

hibiscus juice

Herbs for Cooking and Health

TURMERIC (CURCUMA LONGA):

A yellow spice generally used in Asian and Indian food, turmeric is akin to the ginger family and has been shown to reduce inflammation. Some research states this herb can reduce the development of beta amyloids in the brain of patients who are prone to, or have, Alzheimer disease. Turmeric has also been shown to provide some anti-cancer benefits with melanoma, colorectal cancer, and breast cancer.

GINGER (ZINGIBER OFFICINALE):

This spice is a root or underground stem with a highly pungent spiced bite to it. It also has anti-inflammatory properties.

CHAMOMILE (ANTHEMIS NOBILIS):

Chamomile is a plant found throughout Europe. As a child in England, I saw it growing wild as a common weed. This plant is used mainly as an infusion that can help with intestinal colic, fever, and mild acid indigestion. Chamomile is commonly used for restlessness.

PEPPERMINT MENTHA (PIPERITA):

A flavor historically used in candy, gum, toothpaste, tea, and ice cream. Medicinal benefits include reducing gastric upset and helping to the body to relax.

CAYENNE CAPSICUM (BACCATUM):

Cayenne is a spice of the nightshade family. This is a hot spice. It also has some anti-inflammatory properties to it.

GARLIC (ALLIUM SATIVUM):

Garlic is part of the family Alliaceae and genus Allium, and it is connected to leeks, shallot, and the onion families. Garlic has a very strong flavor and odor, and it has some benefits for cardiovascular health and diabetes.

PARSLEY (PETROSELINUM CRISPUM):

Parsley is a pretty leafy green herb, with a mild flavor. Commonly used as a garnish for food, parsley has been known to help with high blood pressure and enhancing the immune system.

CHIVES (ALLIUM SCHOENOPRASUM):

Connected to the onion family Alliaceae, chives grow in clusters and have very pretty purple flowers. Chives have been known to relieve pain.

TARRAGON (ARTEMISIA DRACUNCULUS):

Tarragon is an herb with a smooth, spicy flavor. National Institutes of Health Botanical Research Center is carrying out a research project at this time investigating the actions of Russian tarragon on insulin in the human body.

THYME (THYMUS):

You may be familiar with many varieties of this herb. Garden thyme (T. vulgaris), citrus thyme (T. citriodorus), and wild thyme (Thymus serpyllum) are a few of the most common varieties. Thyme has been said to aid with inflammation in the body.

BASIL (OCIMUM BASILICUM):

Basil is an herb traditionally found in Asia. It has a unique flavor and has been said to have anti-bacterial and anti-fungal benefits.

ROSEMARY (ROSMARINUS OFFICINALIS L.):

Rosemary's translated Latin name is "dew of the sea." It is a multicolored, flowering herb plant and a distant relation of the mint family. Thanks to its a unique flavor, rosemary can be used in many ways from fish and poultry to lemonade. It has a potential to aid with memory.

SAGE (SALVIA OFFICINALIS):

Sage grows as a beautiful light purple flower. It was first cultivated in the southern parts of Europe. Sage is a common herb often used at Christmas and Thanksgiving as a poultry seasoning. Sage can help settle the digestive system and calm the mood.

DILL (ANETHUM GRAVEOLENS):

This herb has a rugged white and yellow flower. Dill was originally found in Asia, but now has a strong British connection, and the word "dill" has a British meaning of soothing or calming. Dill has some pain-relieving properties.

Appendix A

OPTIMAL NUTRITION FOR BABIES AND YOUNG CHILDREN

My first advanced practice education was a women's health care nurse practitioner program. Prior to this advanced practice course, I worked in a labor and delivery unit at a local hospital for eight years. At this hospital I worked with not only uncomplicated births, but also high-risk deliveries, C-sections and highly technological IVF (*in vitro* fertilization) surgeries.

All these medical situations had the same end result—a brand new baby. Once a baby is on the way, the parents need to make a host of decisions. By the time of the birth, some have already been made, but others are still pending. I was most surprised to observe the decision-making process new mothers went through about what to feed their new little person. They were given so little information about feeding their babies, which puzzled me. They seemed ill-prepared, confused, and often did not make the decision until the baby was 30 minutes to an hour old. Some feeding decisions were made with no nutritional health considerations whatsoever. With regard to breast feeding, I have heard mothers say many negative things, ranging from it being too messy or two much work, to the mother wanting to quickly get back into her pre-pregnancy clothes or take a scheduled trip and not have to worry about breast feeding.

Whether to use breast or bottle is certainly up to the new mother. However, part of the vacuum in which the new mother makes such decisions is a medical system that often does not provide adequate guidance. Another factor influencing her decision is cultural, in that some cultures don't even consider bottle feeding as an option. That can change when a mother from a breast feeding culture gives birth in a culture that emphasizes bottle feeding.

If we look at the history of infant feeding we can see that, like other products from the processed food industry, infant formulas make a good profit. In the early 1920s the dairy industry improved its sanitation practices, and milk storage was facilitated by the invention of the home icebox. These two environmental improvements allowed the public to increase their use of milk and milk products—including processed infant formula. As a result, breast feeding rates declined from the late 1920s through the early 1970s. Instead, cow's milk and strained solid foods, called "baby food," were given to babies at increasingly earlier ages, which led to iron-deficiency anemia.[36] In response, "iron fortified" formulas were introduced.

By 1970 the World Health Organization and UNICEF were becoming extremely concerned about the decline in breast feeding. In the United States, thanks to a small but vocal group, La Leche League International, breast feeding rates began to increase.

Historically the medical field has moved at a slow-as-molasses pace, and by the time the information reaches the patient it can be several months, or even years, later. We need to act now with respect to the children. One major factor that can help with our obesity epidemic in very young children is the use of appropriate choices when deciding how to feed our babies. The more we learn about human genomics, our internal genetic instruction, and the role of nutrition and how it can affect the health of physical bodies, the sooner we will be guided in making the decisions nature intended us to make where nutrition is concerned.

This can begin when that little person is born. Which is best? Feeding a baby processed food products or feeding a baby breast milk? My answer is nature's way is best. Give your baby what nature intended—breast milk—if breast feeding is possible for you. How and what to feed your baby is a decision that should be based on optimal nutritional outcome—not on what is most convenient for the mother. Furthermore, the mother's diet during pregnancy and during the breast feeding period is extremely important to a baby's health. There is no longer any question about this; it is a fact.

36 Committee on Nutrition. Iron Fortification of Infant Formulas. *J Am Acad Pediatr.* 1999;104(1):119-123. http://pediatrics.aappublications.org/cgi/content/full/104/1/119. Accessed July 22, 2007.

Breast Milk and the Apo E Gene

The human body has an innate intelligence that has been serving the human race for hundreds of thousands of years. It is odd to think that baby food companies could provide a better food than nature. The American Academy of Pediatrics (AAP) has issued clear guidelines stressing that breast milk is the foundation of good infant nutrition. As parents and health care providers, we need to listen to this recommendation.

In my own practice, I am finding with some patients that breast milk provides a perfect diet for babies based on the mother and baby's Apo E genotype. For example, women who are positive for the Apo E 4 gene have a certain percentage of fat content in their breast milk for their babies—between 50 to 75 percent less total fat in breast milk than an alternative Apo E genotype mother.

We also know that the correct proportions of the fatty acid DHA and the omega-3 and omega-6 ratios for each Apo E genotype is critical for the baby's brain development and eye health. Breast milk is perfect in this respect, too. There is some major research with regards to conditions such as anxiety disorders, mood disorders, hyperactivity disorders, learning disabilities, and even autism as they relate to fat content of an infant's diet and mother's genetics. All these diseases could potentially be greatly reduced by feeding babies breast milk rather than processed formula milk.

Advice of the American Academy of Pediatrics

The AAP recommends that infants be fed *exclusively* breast milk (no water, formula, or other liquids) for approximately the first six months after birth and continue to be breast fed for *at least* the next six months while solid foods are introduced. Infants weaned before 12 months should not receive cow's milk but an iron-fortified infant formula. Science reveals the extreme benefits of breast feeding both to mother and infant to at least one year, and ideally as long as mother and baby desire. While 71 percent of American mothers presently at least attempt to breast feed their children, only 46 percent of these babies are being breast fed *exclusively* at three months. That number drops to 13 percent by six months. Once solid foods are introduced in the second half of the first year, the numbers drop further. By a year, only 16 percent of infants receive *any* breast milk at all, and even fewer get the two or more years of breast feeding recommended by the World Health Organization.

Nutritional Value for Breast Milk

Breast milk contains all the ingredients that a baby needs to thrive. Formulas based on cow's milk provide *only 60* of the 200 nutrients found in breast milk. Formula makers simply cannot duplicate breast milk. Why? Because each human body is as individual as our fingerprints, yet mother's body knows exactly what nutrients to produce for her baby's optimal health. Breast milk includes antibodies and other immune-system enhancing ingredients as well as growth factors, hormones, and other substances that help the baby grow and develop at an appropriate rate. Vitamin D supplementation is recommended for babies who live in northern latitudes because people today spend so much time indoors they often don't get enough sunlight to help their bodies produce adequate Vitamin D.

With no long-term data on what any formulas will do to an infant's health, we do not really know the outcomes of adding artificial vitamin and fat supplements to man-made infant formula. Does this type of supplementation cause inflammation? We just don't know. It is only logical to stay with what nature intended, and choose breast milk over formula.

Not only is breast milk the perfect food, but it is ready to drink at any time, day or night. When it comes to the baby's Apo E genotype, it is likely that any formula we pick will contain serious mismatches and not promote the health of the baby as well as breast milk would have done.

In addition to perfect nutrition, there are a host of other benefits, both physical and psychological, for both mother and baby to consider, including more eye contact, connection via touch and the scent of the mother's body, plus the benefit to the central nervous system from the movement of the mother carrying her child around as she nurses.[37] In addition, mouth and tooth development does not unfold as designed when an infant does not suckle on a normal human breast. A big benefit for mothers later on is that breast cancer rates drop precipitously after several years of using breasts for their intended purpose.

Formulas can't even begin to match the natural balance of breast milk and all the other factors that go along with the process of breast feeding. Research shows that babies' serum cholesterol is elevated as a result of being fed formula and other processed foods.[38] From this we can conclude they are experiencing

37   See Alliance for Transforming the Lives of Children's Blueprint of Principles and Actions www.aTLC.org Brown, A. J. and Roberts, D.C. (1991). The effect of fasting triacylglyceride concentration and apolipoprotein E polymorphism on postprandial lipemia. Arteriosclerosis and Thrombosis, 11:1737-44

38   Kallio, M. J. T., Salmenpera, L., Shes, M. A., Perheentupa, J., Gylling, H., and Miettinen, T. A. Apoprotein E phenotype determines serum cholesterol in infants during both high cholesterol breast feeding and low-cholesterol formula feeding. J. Lipid Res. 1997;38:759–764.

early inflammatory conditions, along with behavioral and immune dysfunction. Here are some common illness trends I have noticed in my primary care practice with babies fed on formula:

- allergies
- behavioral disorders—concentration, attention, anger, sleep disorders
- ear infections
- obesity
- anxiety
- abnormal cholesterol levels
- tooth decay
- blood pressure abnormalities
- stomach or intestinal conditions and infections
- digestive problems such as diarrhea or constipation
- skin diseases such as eczema, psoriasis, atopic dermatitis

I encourage parents to ask lots of questions! Read about baby nutrition from a reputable source that is *not* promoting a particular product. Talk with a medical provider who has been trained in pediatric medicine and nutrition. If breast feeding is truly not possible (a rarity), you can make better choices and feel good about the choice you are making for the life of your baby.

I have cared for hundreds and hundreds of moms and new babies. Most parents want what is best for their baby, no matter whether it is their first or their seventh. With a more evidence-based nutritional education, we will see an entirely new level of health appearing with our children and much less chronic disease in adults. Pediatric medicine has taken care of most infectious illnesses that once plagued children, and we can now begin preventing early chronic illnesses with just a few small changes in the nutrition of our babies and children.

Infant Nutrition and the Apo E Gene

The following table lists the nutritional requirements of infants from birth to 12 months of age. After two years the caloric requirement needs to be adjusted based on the individual child's caloric needs, related to the Apo E Genotype, lean mass and activity level.

AGE	0-6 months	6-10 months	10-12 months
PROTEIN	Breast milk	Breast milk	Breast milk
CARBS (grains and starches)	Begin iron-fortified baby cereal mixed with breast milk	Continue baby cereal. Begin adding other breads and cereals	Baby cereal until 18 months. Total of 4 servings per day; 1 serving =1/4 slice bread
CARBS. (fruits and veg.)	None	Begin 2-4 oz soft fruit and vegetables—mashed; slowly adding soft pieces or cooked fruit and vegetables	4 servings per day 2-8 tbsp. fruit and vegetables
FAT	From breast milk	From breast milk	From breast milk
NUTS and LEGUMES	None	Slowly introduce soft purée plant protein, lentils, beans, legumes, soy, yogurt	2-3 1/2oz servings per day. Nut or nut butters before 1 year

Birth to 2 years old:

Recommendation by Age and Genotype

Age 0-6 months:
Apo E 2/2   Apo E 2/3   Apo E 3/3
Nutritional recommendation–100% breast milk
Apo E 4/2   Apo E 4/3   Apo E 4/4
Nutritional recommendation–100% breast milk

Age 6 months to 1 year
Over the next 6 months to a year the slow introduction of solid plant-based whole foods begins. Give infants a combination of these foods plus breast milk.

- Breast milk
- Whole grain cereal. Consider appropriate preparation for your baby's eating ability. Consider iron-fortified cereal.
- Rice—gluten free to begin.
- Small amounts of non-citrus organic whole fruit—appropriately prepared for your baby's eating ability.
- Yellow vegetables—appropriately prepared for your baby's eating ability.
- Green vegetables—appropriately prepared for your baby's eating ability.
  - Good fats—appropriately prepared for your baby's eating ability.
  - Small amounts of plant proteins—appropriately prepared for your baby's eating ability

Suggested Schedule for Introducing Solid Food Types
Serving size vary

6-12 months old

rice cereal	carrots	yam
sweet potato	squash	apricots
apple	blackberries	blueberries
banana	cherries	grapes
prunes	pears	peaches
cauliflower	broccoli	beets
split pea	millet	oats and oatmeal
apples	basmati rice	green string beans
blueberries	peas	papaya
nectarines	soy beans	lima beans

Apo E 2/2   **Apo E 2/3**   **Apo E 3/3**
Breast milk
With solid foods during the day

Apo E 4/2   **Apo E 4/3**   **Apo E 4/4**
Breast milk
With solid foods during the day

Schedule for Introducing Solid Foods
Age 1- 2 years

pearl barley	other green leafy vegetables	asparagus
acorn squash	avocado	brown rice
honey	eggplant	garlic
shallots	cabbage	turnips & turnip greens
rye	lettuce	fish
buckwheat	egg whites	corn
nuts ground—	citrus fruits—	peanuts
almonds, walnuts,	lemons, limes,	sunflower seeds
cashews	oranges, pineapples	shell fish
wheat foods with yeast	lentils	

Depending on Apo E Genotype meat in small amounts of preferably an organic source can be added to the diet. Source: chicken, cornish game hen, turkey, wild meats. No more than once every 24-48 hours.

Apo E 2/2   **Apo E 2/3**   **Apo E 3/3**
Breast milk
Increased solid foods during the day.

Apo E 4/2   **Apo E 4/3**   **Apo E 4/4**
Breast milk
At this age begin to increased solid foods during the day.
Animal protein to be limited.
Use protein primarily from plant-based sources.
Provide high-quality animal protein not more than every 24-48 hours.
Fat from a monounsaturated and polyunsaturated sources.

After age 2—
Follow carbohydrate, fat, and protein percentages more closely once breast feeding has stopped. Use caloric recommendations based on the American Heart Association—see the included calorie chart by age.

Macronutrient Recommendations for Apo E Genotypes

Apo E 2/2
Carbohydrate: 50% of total calories
Protein 15% of total calories
Fat: 35% of total calories

Apo E 3/3
Carbohydrate: 55% of total calories
Protein: 20% of total calories
Fat: 25% of total calories

Apo E 4/4
Carbohydrate: 55% of total calories
Protein: 25% of total calories
Fat: 20% of total calories

Apo E 4/3
Carbohydrate: 55% of total calories
Protein: 25% of total calories
Fat: 20% of total calories

Apo E 4/2
Carbohydrate: 55% of total calories
Protein: 20% of total calories
Fat: 25% of total calories

Apo E 2/3
Carbohydrate: 50% of total calories
Protein: 20% of total calories
Fat: 30% of total calories

General dietary recommendations for children with daily estimated calories and recommended servings—American Heart Association. For Whole Grains, Fruits, Vegetables, and Milk/Dairy by Age and Gender. When making fat, carbohydrate and protein choices—Apo E Gene Diet guidelines are to be considered.

Caloric Intake Guidelines[ab]

Yrs.	1 Yr.	2-3* Yrs.	4-8 Yrs.	9-13 Yrs.	14-18 Yrs
Calories	900 kcal	1000 kcal			
Female Kcal			1200 kcal	1600 kcal	1800
Male Kcal			1400 kcal	1800 kcal	2200
Fat	30-40% kcal	30-35% kcal	25-35% kcal	25-35% kcal	25-35% kcal
Milk/Dairy[c]	2 cups[c]	2 cups	2 cups	3 cups	3 cups
Lean Meat/ Beans	1.5 oz	2 oz		5 oz	
Female			3 oz		5 oz
Male			4 oz		6 oz
Fruits[d]	1 cup	1 cup	1.5 cups	1.5 cups	
Female					1.5 cups
Male					2 cups
Vegetables[e]	3/4 cup	1 cup			
Female			1 cup	2 cups	2.5 cups
Male			1.5 cup	2.5 cups	3 cups
Grains	2 oz	3 oz			
Female			4 oz	5 oz	6 oz
Male			5 oz	6 oz	7 oz

*for children older than 2 years, consider following Apo E Fat percentage guidelines for genotype.

a. Dietary Guidelines for Americans (2005)14; http://www.healthierus.gov/dietaryguidelines. Calorie estimates are based on a sedentary lifestyle. Increased physical activity will require additional calories: add 0–200 kcal/d if moderately physically active; add 200—400 kcal/day if very physically active.

b. http://www.americanheart.org/presenter.jhtml?identifier=3033999

c. Milk listed is fat-free (except for children under the age of 2 years). If 1%, 2%, or whole-fat milk is substituted, this will utilize, for each cup, 19, 39, or 63 kcal of discretionary calories and add 2.6, 5.1, or 9.0 g. of total fat, of which 1.3, 2.6, or 4.6 g. are saturated fat.

d. For 1-year-old children, calculations are based on 2% fat milk. If 2 cups of whole milk are substituted, 48 kcal of discretionary calories will be utilized. The American Academy of Pediatrics recommends that low-fat/reduced fat milk not be started before 2 years of age. Adapted from the Executive Office of the President of the AAP and the Department of Health and Human Services.

Appendix B

APO E GENE RESEARCH

Arbonés-Mainar JM, et al. (2006). Trans-10, cis-12- and cis-9, trans-11-conjugated linoleic acid isomers selectively modify HDL-apolipoprotein composition in apolipoprotein E knockout mice. *Journal of Nutrition,* 136:353–359.

Bray MS (2000). Genomics, genes, and environmental interaction: the role of exercise. Journal of Applied Physiology, 88:788–792.

Brown AJ and Roberts DC (1991). The effect of fasting triacylglyceride concentration and apolipoprotein E polymorphism on postprandial lipemia. *Arteriosclerosis and Thrombosis,* 11:1737–44.

Berenson GS, et al. Influence of apolipoprotein E polymorphism on the tracking of childhood levels of serum lipids and apolipoproteins over a 6-year period. The Bogalusa Heart Study. *Atherosclerosis.* 1996 Nov 15;127(1):73-9.

Corder EH, Saunders AM, Strittmatter WJ, et al. Gene dose E type 4 allele and the risk of Alzheimer's disease in late, *Science.* 1993; 261:921-923.

de Andrade M, Thandi M, Brown S, Gotto A, Patsch W, and Boerwinkle E, (1995). Relationship of the apolipoprotein E polymorphism with carotid artery atherosclerosis. *American Journal of Human Genetics,* 56:1379–1390.

Djousse L, et al. (2004) Apolipoprotein E polymorphism modifies the alcohol-HDL association observed in the National Heart, Lung, and Blood Institute Family Heart Study. *American Journal of Clinical Nutrition,* 80(6):1639–1644.

Dreon DM, Fernstrom HA, Williams PT and Krauss RM, (2000). Reduced LDL particle size in children consuming a very low-fat diet is related to parental LDL subclass patterns 1,2,3. *American Journal of Clinical Nutrition*, Vol. 71, No. 6, 1611–1616.

Farrer LA, Brin MF, Elsas L, et al. (1995) Statement on use of Apolipoprotein E testing for Alzheimer disease. *JAMA*; 274:1627–1629.

Ghebremedhin E, et al. (2005) Relationship of apolipoprotein E and age at onset to Parkinson disease neuropathology. *American Journal of Medical Genetics: Part B Neuropsychiatric Genetics*, 5:136(1):72-74.

Green RC, (2002) Genetic testing for Alzheimer's disease: has the moment arrived? *Alz Care Quarterly* 208–214.

Heyer EJ, et al. (2005). ApoE-epsilon4 predisposes to cognitive dysfunction following uncomplicated carotid endarterectomy. *Neurology*, 13;65(11):1759–1763.

Huang X, Chen P, Kaufer DI, Troster AI, and Poole CJ, (2006). Apolipoprotein E and dementia in Parkinson's disease: a meta-analysis. *Neuropathology Experimental Neurology*, 65(2):116–23.

Kallio MJ, et al. (1997). Apoprotein E phenotype determines serum cholesterol in infants during both high-cholesterol breast feeding and low-cholesterol formula feeding. *Journal of Lipid Research*, 38:759–764,

Lapinleimu H, et al. (2000). Impact of gender, apolipoprotein E phenotypes, and diet on serum lipids and lipoproteins in infancy. *Atherosclerosis*, 152(1):135–141.

Lehtinen S, et al.(1993). Gene dose of apolipoprotein E type 4 allele and the risk of Alzheimer's disease in late onset families. *Science*, 261:921–923

Lim GP, et al. (2005). A diet enriched with the omega-3 fatty acid docosahexaenoic acid reduces amyloid burden in an aged Alzheimer mouse model. *USA Neurology*, 13;65(11):1759–63.

McConnell LM, Koenig BA, Greely HT, Raffin TA, and the Alzheimer Disease Working Group of the Stanford Program in Genomics, Ethics, & Society. (1998) Genetic testing and Alzheimer disease: has the time come? *Nat Med*: 4:757–759.

Mahley RW, Apolipoprotein E: cholesterol transport protein with in cell biology. *Science*. 1988;240:622-630.

Mahley RW (1995). Apolipoprotein E polymorphism, serum lipids, myocardial infarction and severity of angiographically verified coronary artery disease in men and women. *Atherosclerosis*, 114:83–91.

Martinez M, et al. (2006). Apolipoprotein E 4 is probably responsible for the chromosome 19 linkage peak for Parkinson disease. American Journal of Medical Genetics Part B: *Neuropsychiatric Genetics*, 37(2):364–370.

Maury CP, Liljestrom M, Tiitinen S, Laiho K, Karela K, and Ehnholm C, (2001). Apolipoprotein E phenotypes in rheumatoid arthritis with or without amyloidosis. *Amyloid*, 8(4):270–273.

Miura Y, et al. (2001). Tea catechins prevent the development of atherosclerosis in apoprotein E—Deficient mice. *Journal of Nutrition* 131:27–32.

Minihane, et al. Apo E polymorphism and fish oil supplementation in subjects with anatherogenic lipoprotein phenotype. *Arterioscler Thromb Vasc Biol.* 2000; 20:1990-1997.

Moore RJ, Chamberlain RM, and Khuri FR, (2004). Apolipoprotein E and the risk of breast cancer in African-American and non Hispanic white women: A review. *Oncology*, 66:79–93.

Moreno JA, et al. (2005) The apolipoprotein E Gene Promoter (—219G/T) Polymorphism determines insulin sensitivity in response to dietary fat in healthy young adults, *Journal of Nutrition,* 135:2535–2540.

José López-Miranda, et al.(2004). The effect of dietary fat on LDL: Size is influenced by apolipoprotein E genotype in healthy Subjects. *Journal of Nutrition,* 134:2517–2522.

Pertovaara M, et al. (2004). Presence of apolipoprotein E epsilon4 allele predisposes to early onset of primary Sjogren's syndrome. *American Journal of Clinical Nutrition,* 80(6):1639–1644.

Roberts JS, Green RC, Relkin N, et al. (2003) How do participants rate the impact of genetic susceptibility testing for Alzheimer's disease? *Neurology* 60:A453.

Roses AD (1997). Genetic testing for Alzheimer disease: practical and ethical issues. *Arch Neurol* 54:1226–1229.

Roter DL, Stewart M, Putnam, S, et al. (1997) Communication patterns of primary care physicians. *JAMA* 270:350–355.

Sarkkinen E, Korhonen M. Erkkila A, Ebeling T, and Uusitupa M, (1998). Effect of apolipoprotein E polymorphism on serum lipid response to the separate modification of dietary fat and dietary cholesterol. *American Journal of Clinical Nutrition,* 68, 1215–1222.

Simell O, et al. Impact of gender, apolipoprotein E phenotypes, and diet on serum lipids and lipoproteins in infancy, *J Pediatr.* 1997 Dec;131(6):825-32.

Simell O, et al. Apolipoprotein E4 phenotype increases non-fasting serum triglyceride concentration in infants - the STRIP study. *Atherosclerosis.* 2000 Sep;152(1):135-41.

Sisto T, et al. Apolipoprotein E polymorphism, lipids, myocardial infarction and severity of angiographically artery disease in men and women. *Atherosclerosis.* 1995;114:

Sudlow C, Gonzalez, Martinez, NA, Clark, Kim, JC, (2006). Does apolipoprotein E genotype influence the risk of ischemic stroke, intracerebral hemorrhage, or subarachnoid hemorrhage Systematic review and meta-analyses of 31 studies among 5961 cases and 17,965 controls. *Stroke,* 37(2):364–370.

Superko HR, Haskell WL. The effect of apolipoprotein E genotype on postprandial lipoprotein in patients matched for triglycerides, LDLcholesterol, and HDL-cholesterol. *Artery.* 1991:18:315-325.

Taimela S, et al. (1996). The effect of physical activity on serum total and low density lipoprotein cholesterol concentrations varies with apolipoprotein E phenotype in male children and young adults: The Cardiovascular Risk in Young Finns Study. *Metabolism,* 45:797–803.

Tammi A, et al. (1996). Apolipoprotein E 4 phenotype increases non-fasting serum triglyceride concentration in infants—the STRIP study. *Cardiorespiratory Pediatrics,* 98(4 Pt 1):757–62.

Thompson PD, et al. (2006). Angiotensin-converting enzyme genotype and adherence to aerobic exercise training. *Preventive Cardiology,* 9(1):21–24.

Zick CD, Matthews C, Roberts JS, et al. (2005) Genetic susceptibility testing for Alzheimer's disease and its impact on insurance behavior. *Health Aff.* 24(2):483–490.

Zhongyin Z, Hesheng L, Jun L, and Jihong C. (2006). Association of serum lipids and apolipoprotein E gene polymorphism with the risk of colorectal adenomas. *Saudi Medical Journal,* 27(2):161–164.

Appendix C

ANONYMOUS APO E AND ADVANCED CHOLESTEROL TESTING

For those of you who are concerned about protecting your privacy with regards to these tests and your medical records, we are offering test kits so you can anonymously do Apo E gene and advanced cholesterol testing. You can order a protected Apo E Gene test kit or an advanced cholesterol panel testing kit, with detailed instructions to get your test results.

Select the Testing Kit You Want

Go to the website, www.ApoEGeneDiet.com and find the section called Apo E Gene Testing for more information.

Two different testing kits can be ordered:

- Test Kit One is an anonymous Apo E gene testing kit with detailed instructions on how to get your Apo E gene test and keep your medical record private and confidential.

- Test Kit Two is an advanced cholesterol testing kit. This test sequence checks 13 different types of cholesterol and other important chemistries that will help you identify critical risk factors.

Apo E Gene Seminars

Apo E Seminar 1: This Apo E testing-only seminar provides information about the Apo E gene, as well the Apo E gene test and/or Advanced cholesterol testing.

Apo E Seminar 2: This seminar provides a step-by-step solution for accomplishing behavior change—after a person has received his or her Apo E gene test result.

Index

basal metabolic rate   226

bathroom scale. *See* weight, measuring

Before the Heart Attacks   xiv, 173

belief structure   26

Big Three
    caloric requirements   30
    described   77–82
    percentages in diet   13

bio-impedance test   226, 228

blood sugar   178

BMI. *See* body mass index

BMR. *See* basal metabolic rate

body. *See* mind/emotion/body connection

body composition and arterial health   24

body composition test   228

body mass index   227, *231–232*

brain and aging   180

breakfast recipes   331–341

breast milk
    See also infant nutrition
    Apo E gene and   393, 397
    nutritional information   394
    omega-3 and -6   393

breathing. *See* mindful breathing

C

calcium   92

calming awareness response   198

calorie requirements
    calculating   33–34
    children   400
    daily   225–226
    determining   225–226
    generally   32–33

cancer
    garlic and   166
    inflammation and   13, 105
    mushrooms and   167

candy bars   98

carbohydrates
    Apo E 2 gene and   24
    Apo E 4 gene and   23
    described   77–80

Food Exchange List   237–239
    glucose and   82

cardiovascular disease
    Apo E gene and   15
    garlic and   166
    inflammation and   12, 13
    physiology of   16

changes, making
    See also nutritional change
    expressive arts therapy and   209–210
    meditation and   211–215
    mindful breathing and   210–211

chemical additives
    list of those to avoid   94–95
    preserving and processing   92
    US corporate use of   92

children, dietary recommendations   400

chiropractors   57

chlorine   165

chocolate   171

cholesterol
    Apo E 4 and   25
    coffee and   97
    exercise and   131
    garlic and   166
    inflammation and   13
    mushrooms and   167
    patient story   7
    physiology of   109–110
    sources of   110

cholesterol levels   28
    Apo E gene and   23–24
    high levels, patient stories   37–38, 50–51
    optimum levels   23–24

cholesterol medications and alcohol   177

cholesterol panel   7, 18, 45

cholesterol particles and the Apo E gene   18

chromosome   10

chronic illness   13

chronic inflammation, physiology of   104–106

chronic kidney disease   12

About the Author

Pamela McDonald, RNFA, WHCNP, APCNP, PNP, FNP
Integrative Medicine Fellow

Pamela McDonald, a leading integrative medicine nurse practitioner, is devoted to the prevention of heart disease and chronic illness. A certified nurse practitioner and graduate of Andrew Weil MD's Program in Integrative Medicine, University of Arizona, Pamela has used her advanced specialty training in surgery, women's health care, adult primary care, pediatrics, pediatric obesity, family practice, cardiovascular and heart disease prevention, nutrition, exercise sports medicine, mind-body medicine, energy medicine, and botanical medicine to develop the ground breaking Apo E Gene Diet. Through her private practice and her work in primary care, she uses this program to help patients work with their own genotypes in order to reach optimum health and prevent disease.

Pamela was born in Paisley, Scotland, and grew up in the southernmost part of England. Originally trained as a nurse at the Royal Hospital of St. Bartholomew's in London, England, she now lives in Northern California with her husband, Rick, and three children. In addition to her clinical work, Pamela also lectures to public and private groups.

Healing Magic

You say you are a healer,
binding up wounds and
applying potions and salves
for a broken humanity.

Tell me, kind healer,
have you found on your journey
a wound deeper
than lovelessness?
A person more broken
than the one who's own heart
was long ago abandoned
in search of what we do not know,
if not for Love itself.

And tell me gentle healer,
how do you bind the wound
of lovelessness?
What potions and salves
do you carry
in your black bag
that can mend a broken heart?

"I'm sorry," you say, "I have nothing,
there is nothing I can do."
And that, dear friend,
is where you are wrong

Put down the bag:
Leave go of the rummaging
for magic other than your own;
open your heart,
pick up a hand,
Gaze into an eye,
Share in
one
true
moment,
and watch healing begin.

Many thanks to Janet Quinn PhD RN
Source: Quinn, Janet, (1996). *Alternative Therapies.*

Many thanks to the following people:

Andrea Holwegner BSc, RD

Carole Dobson, MAN, RD

Health Stand Nutrition Consulting Inc. www.healthstandnutrition.com

John MacArthur, Editor

Sherman Keen, Design / Editor

Tom Joyce, CreativeWerks www.creativewerks.com

Ray Rimmer, Ray Rimmer Studios

Jessica Keet, Editor

Deidre Lingenfelter, imagesbydeidre.com

John W Travis, MD, Editor

Meryn Callander, Editor

Barbara Stahara, Editor

Marla Wilson, Printed Page Productions

Doug Parks, Spirit 2000

Dawson Church, Elite Books

Heather Hamilton, Art Design

Alex Hamilton, Art Design www.alexhamilton.net

Gayle T. Vivere, The Vivere Design Team www.viveredesign.com